Readings in Contemporary Sexuality

Second Edition

John P. Elia, Ph.D.

Albert J. Angelo, M.S.Ed.
with Ivy Chen, MPH

San Francisco State University

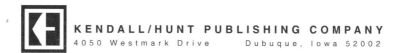
KENDALL/HUNT PUBLISHING COMPANY
4050 Westmark Drive   Dubuque, Iowa 52002

Cover image courtesy of Corel.

Copyright © 2000, 2005 by Kendall/Hunt Publishing Company

ISBN 13 978-0-7575-3198-9
ISBN 10 0-7575-3198-9

Printed in the United States of America
10 9 8 7 6 5 4 3 2

Contents

Preface

The knowledge produced in human sexuality studies has exploded over the past several years. There are an increasing number of textbooks specially written for survey human sexuality courses. The authors of such texts are faced with a Herculean task of trying to do justice to myriad aspects of human sexuality. However, no matter how meticulous and thorough the authors are, much information never finds itself included in these textbooks. Rarely are these books truly comprehensive. Clearly, then, there is a need to supplement such texts with the information that either gets a scant mention or is totally absent in current textbooks in the field. Students in general, survey human sexuality courses need to be exposed to most if not all of the major areas and issues in human sexuality studies to get a well rounded educational experience.

College and university professors constantly bemoan the fact that the textbooks they use are sorely lacking, or that they have this or that slant and ignore this or that issue. We are no exceptions! The genesis of this second edition of *Readings in Contemporary Sexuality* grew out of our continued interest to provide students with a supplemental text, as the majority of textbooks for general, survey courses on human sexuality have fallen short of being truly comprehensive.

After several conversations and going back and forth about the merits of one text over another, we realized that we had similar complaints about human sexuality textbooks. Some themes emerged. Upon a closer and more systematic examination—by doing an informal content analysis of various textbooks—we found that there were readily identifiable areas of human sexuality that were either given brief mention—an academic "hit and run"—or were ignored entirely.

It is our hope that *Readings in Contemporary Sexuality* will be used to supplement the major texts in the field. While the majority of the writings we chose were previously published articles in journals and popular press publications, other chapters were specially solicited for this volume. By no means do we consider this text to be a comprehensive coverage of contemporary sexuality. Rather, it is intended to supplement texts in the field. However, this volume may stand alone and be read as a collection of thought-provoking essays about contemporary sexual matters. We hope it proves to be informative, provocative, interesting, and that it spurs discussion.

Also, there is a *Student Guide* to accompany this volume. It is designed to help students master the content of each chapter in the main text and to encourage them to think more deeply about the issues raised. Each chapter of the *Student Guide* begins with a summary of the corresponding chapter in the main text, and then moves on to exercises. For instance, the summary of each chapter is followed by identification items (important names, concepts, and terms) that students should locate in the chapter and not only familiarize themselves with these items but also place them in proper context in terms of their significance in the chapter. Next, discussion items are listed to spur conversations about significant aspects of the chapter in question. Then, study questions are posed. Finally, sample test questions (e.g., true and false and multiple-choice items) are provided to provide students with feedback about how well they mastered the material in the main text.

We express deep gratitude to our hundreds of students in Health Education 320, "Contemporary Sexuality," over the past several years who have been committed to discussing contemporary sexual issues with unflagging eagerness in an attempt to assess where they stood on such issues to make their sex lives more meaningful and fulfilling.

An acknowledgement from Albert Angelo: This book is dedicated to five very important people in my life: John Elia, Juliet Olson, Al Vernacchio, David Whitaker, and Lance Barshinger. I sincerely thank you for many years of friendship, support, and unconditional love.

An acknowledgement from John Elia: Many thanks are in order to my co-editors, Albert Angelo and Ivy Chen. I respect your commitment to comprehensive sexuality education, and your unflagging dedication to help create more sexual and social justice in the world. I appreciate your friendship, and the academic work we do together. It has certainly helped me to think more deeply about various aspects of human sexuality, and my own work is better as a result.

I (John Elia) am also grateful to many wonderful individuals who have made such a positive impact on my life. I am grateful to: Don Arnstine, Rosa Barragan, Norma and Roger Bautista, John De Cecco, Debbie Elia, Amanda Goldberg, Roma Guy, Kirk Hinman, Richard Hoffman, Mike Kurokawa, Mary Beth Love, Lisa Moore, Michael Quimpo, Daniel (Danny) Silver, Rowena Tack, Bruce Whaley, and Gust Yep. All of you have enriched my life in so many ways, and I am incredibly pleased and comforted to have you in my life.

I (John Elia) dedicate this book to my partner, Gina Bloom and her son, Brian, who have been, and continue to be, great sources of joy and inspiration in my life. Being part of a family with you two has taken my life in a direction that I could have never anticipated. It is a wonderful journey, and I look forward to continuing it for many years to come. The love, care, and commitment you have shown me are truly reciprocal. You are very special to me.

John P. Elia, Ph.D., Albert J. Angelo, M.S.Ed., and Ivy Chen, MPH *San Francisco, California*

Introduction:
The Landscape of Contemporary Sexuality

John P. Elia, Ph.D., Albert J. Angelo, M.S.Ed., and Ivy Chen, MPH

There are many aspects of sexuality that are taken for granted and rarely discussed by scholars and non-scholars alike. As indicated in the preface to this volume, many authors of human sexuality textbooks have been either negligent for providing only a superficial coverage or totally remiss in addressing some of fundamental aspects of human sexuality. This volume is an attempt to address some of these important yet often overlooked aspects of human sexuality. This volume begins with a section on sexuality in history, culture, and the media, including information on the historical and future considerations of human sexuality, epistemological questions, Asian-American sexuality, and media influences on sexuality. Then the volume turns to an exploration of adolescent sexuality, dealing with a range of issues such as sexual maturation of girls, teen pregnancy, oral sex, and contraceptive use. Next, the book turns to an extremely topical and contentious aspect of human sexuality, *viz.,* school-based sexuality education. This section contains chapters on comprehensive sexuality education, and facts, issues, & answers about sexuality education in the United States.

Moving on to an equally important area of human sexuality that also has not enjoyed thorough treatment in human sexuality texts is sexual preference, which is the subject of the next section. Here, bisexual, gay, lesbian, and transgender (bglt) issues are covered. Following the section on bglt aspects, the volume offers a coverage of parenting, relationships, and sexual behavior, which includes works on ending romantic/sexual relationships, sperm donors, subjective experience of the loss of virginity in the U.S., and conceptual models of sexual activity. The next section deals with the broad area of sexual health, including reproductive health, HIV/AIDS, aging, sexual offenders, sexual victimization, and disabilities. Next, the volume turns to the issue of sexuality and spirituality. This small section contains a chapter on Eastern spiritual traditions and sexuality, which offers alternative ways of viewing sexuality spiritually-speaking. Finally, the volume turns to a treatment of the sex industry and technology. This section, while relatively small, deals with a plethora of issues, such as an interdisciplinary treatment of sex work, including the history of the sex trade, different jobs within the sex industry, legal aspects, international issues, sexual abuse within the industry, feminism, and sex workers' organizations. Additionally, this section contains information about the commercialization of sex on the Internet.

The Mission of This Book

As indicated in the preface, this book is intended either to supplement general human sexuality textbooks or to be read on its own and viewed as a volume that provides readers with a number of thought-provoking chapters on various aspects of contemporary sexuality. It is not meant to be a comprehensive coverage of the field. However, this volume is intended to get readers to think more deeply about many contemporary sexual issues to foster a better understanding of the human sexual experience. Many of the chapters in this book challenge traditional notions of sexuality and gender, and expand upon areas of sexuality that have been at least somewhat neglected by sexologists. If this book, in part, gets readers to think more deeply, thoughtfully, and critically about sexual matters, spurs lively discussions or debates, fosters an appreciation for the complexity of human sexuality, or helps individuals with their own sexual lives in one way or another, then this book has fulfilled its mission.

Section I

Sexuality in History, Culture, and the Media

The History and Future of Sex

Marty Klien, Ph.D.

C H A P T E R

Researching this paper, I realized how much I don't know about many things important to sexology. I realized how little I know about Prohibition, the Civil War, the Depression, segregation, and the history of technology, to name just a few. And I realized anew how important topics like those are for our field.

I also realized that the field of sexology knows a lot more about the phenomenology of sex than it does about social science. We know more about what individual people say they do and how they feel than about the role sexuality plays in the pageant of world events. While this is legitimate knowledge, it means that sexology has a limited perspective. History, economics, law, technology, religion, and other large-scale social forces dramatically shape people's sexual consciousness and behavior—which is what we sexologists purport to study. And so examining the past and looking toward the future are essential for sexological sophistication. Doing so demonstrates, as we are always saying, just how critical an interdisciplinary perspective is for our work. As we seek to understand sexuality, there is very little that is irrelevant.

Let's start with some examples of how technology in general drives history in unexpected ways.

1. In the 13th century, the flying buttress and the gothic vault were invented. These architectural structures took much of the weight off the external walls of churches. Within five years, a whole new kind of cathedral was being built, such as Westminster Abbey. The reduced weight on the walls made large windows possible, which allowed a brand new art form to develop: stained glass.
2. During the mid-19th century, train speeds increased every few years. Eventually, travellers who started in place A with their watches set correctly would arrive in place B with watches that were now incorrect, because they had traveled so far so quickly. To eliminate this problem, time zones were invented in 1883.

3. At the beginning of the 20th century, zippers were considered a novelty. Then World War I required American soldiers to go abroad for the first time. Because they were going to exotic foreign countries, they wanted to hide their money when they traveled. The holder of the zipper's patent sold money belts with zippers to the American government for its soldiers—and zippers became popular overnight.

4. Until the early 1960s, college administrations were expected to act "in loco parentis"—as substitute parents, making lifestyle decisions for students. For hundreds of years, students had to conform to college rules about dress, religion, sexual activity, and recreation. This arrangement ended in American colleges in the mid- and late-1960s because of the Vietnam War draft. Millions of young people reasoned that if they were old enough to get drafted and killed, they were old enough to run their own lives.

Throughout history, technological advances and social changes have had very different outcomes than were originally planned or predicted. This is the rule, not the exception. And it's true regarding sexuality.

Societal developments affect sexuality in two ways: directly and indirectly. Examples of direct influences include the invention of the birth control pill, the discovery of ovulation, and the invention of vasectomy.

But events can also affect sex indirectly. For example, during World War II, the few young men who were left in America's cities were suddenly a scarce commodity, and women started to compete for them. One way they did this was with sex—and quickly, initiating dates and being sexually aggressive became more culturally acceptable.

Interestingly, the indirect effects on sexuality are far more numerous and much more powerful than the direct sexual effects. Now, nobody is going to argue that the invention of the birth control pill or the discovery of ovulation are trivial. Nevertheless, as we look back over history, the indirect forces shaping sexual expression have been enormously important. Here is a small sample of historical events that shaped the course of human sexuality—indirectly:

The story of Adam and Eve
The story of 12 male apostles
The invention of paper
The destruction of the Roman Empire
The development and spread of Islam
The invention of the clock
The founding of the Protestant church
The Salem witchcraft trials
Allowing women to act on stage
The vulcanization of rubber

The invention of photography
The relocation of Mormans to Utah
The transcontinental railroad
The belief that conception required female orgasm
The installation of gas lights for theaters
No-fault divorce

Let's examine just one of these: the installation of gaslights in theaters. Up until then, theater productions did not take place at night, only in the daytime. Once theaters could install gas lighting, however, they could present shows at night. People could now go there on dates at night; they could go to the dark places in the theater, hold hands and cuddle—which totally changed courting forever.

In every era, new technologies are always adapted to sexual uses. Here are some examples:

pottery > pornography
car > drive-in
VCR > porn films
telephone > phone sex
printing > penny dreadfuls
photography > pornography
vulcanization > condoms
hormone research > contraception
Internet > cybersex

Let's look at a few examples.

Originally developed as a form of transportation, the car was quickly adapted for so-cial uses, such as privacy. The "backseat of a car" even became a synonym for not-quite-legitimate privacy. Once the car became popular, motels outside of town were invented. Before then, there were hotels in town, for people who were travelling. Remember, trav-elling long distances in those days was a huge hassle. But once people had mobility and could use a car to get out of town for, say, half a day or just overnight, there was a reason for motels—outside of town.

The VCR was not invented for sexual purposes, but the VCR only took off as a con-sumer item when low-cost porn videotapes became available. The resulting demand for machines then lowered their price, making them affordable for everyone. In fact, the com-mercial battle over which tape format would become standard ended when Sony decided not to participate in pornography—which doomed Betamax to extinction. Over 500 mil-lion X-rated videotapes are now rented every year.

Soon after the telephone became a standard item in the American home, teenagers started using it. Domestic battling about phone use was one of the common themes of stand-up comedy in the mid-1950s and '60s. What the telephone actually made possible was that people could lay in their beds and talk to their sweetheart privately, could talk about sex, romance, and intimacy. Until that time, such conversations had been highly regulated by the physical separation of lovers required by the rules of courtship. Before the invention of the telephone, only married people had the opportunity to regularly lay in bed and cuddle with or whisper to their sweetheart.

Now let's look at some developments in the 20th century that had important—and unintended—sexual impacts.

- **Municipal electricity**

At the start of the century, the widespread installation of municipal electricity allowed people to go out at night, and lighted places attracted people who wanted to see other people. Downtowns were transformed from places to go shopping during the day, to places where people congregated at night, places of evening entertainment—and suddenly there was nightlife all over the United States. Remember that when electricity became common in American cities, more than half of the country still lived in towns of less than 20,000 people. At that time, the idea of a downtown where people could congregate and go to a movie or have a soda together at night was quite risque.

- **Bicycles**

Before the bicycle was invented, the average American woman had to wear an average of 37 pounds of clothes just to go out of the house. Once women started to ride bicycles, this wasn't practical anymore, and within two years, women were wearing less than half that amount to go out. Imagine the change that must have been in people's lives. The bicycle also led to the development of female athletics because it proved that women could exercise without physical harm.

- **High-density housing**

Around the turn of the century, immigration and industrialization led people in cities to live in apartments. This meant that there was no more front porch, and courting could no longer take place within the bounds of the family's home. This led to unchaperoned dating for the first time.

- **Psychoanalysis**

Psychoanalysis was the first intellectual movement in this country to suggest that sexual repression actually had an effect on people. It became quite a parlor game for people to sit around and speculate about criminals or others who were socially inappropriate—what sort of sexual repression was this or that person acting out? Psychoanalysis gave people a vocabulary with which to talk about sexual norms and libido, something they hadn't had before.

- **Prohibition**

During Prohibition, drinking became sexy. It was an outlaw activity, something that sophisticated and wealthy people did. There were clubs where people gathered to drink—speakeasies—and a new genre of popular music. Like cigarette smoking in the 1960s, drinking became a symbol of eroticism during Prohibition. The glorification of alcohol, of course, heavily affected people's sexual decision-making and functioning.

• The Depression

During the Depression there weren't enough jobs, so instead of going to work, teenagers went to high school. Suddenly, high school kids were surrounded not by adults but by other high school kids. Hanging out with so many of their peers, high school kids developed their own jargon, their own culture, and courtship patterns. "Dating" became an adolescent institution.

• Gay Civil Rights

The last 25 years have seen a swell of rights for gay and bisexual people. This battle isn't finished yet, but one of the unexpected outcomes of the increased visibility of gay sexuality is that a certain amount of non-normative sexual activity has gone mainstream. I don't think it's a coincidence that the popular culture now talks so much more about S&M, anal sex, and non-monogamy.

During the 20th century there have been, of course, many developments specifically aimed at shaping sexuality. At the turn of the century there was a massive anti-masturbation campaign. The government, medical profession, Boy Scouts, army, and other institutions went out of their way to spread frightening lies about masturbation, whose legacy people are still dealing with.

Another thing that has shaped sexuality in this century is the invention and acceptance of sanitary pads and tampons, which are still not used in every country. In rural Russia, for example, a lot of women use pieces of cloth, and it's their mother-in-law's job to wash these out once a month. There is all this ritual and social meaning around it. You can imagine how the invention of menstrual supplies put individual women more in control of their periods, including the information about whether or not they were pregnant. Of course it also changed their relationship with the local grocer.

Other things in this century that have had a direct sexual impact include, the Kinsey Report, AIDS, pantyhose, birth control pills, Playboy magazine, the discovery of the clitoris and G-spot, penicillin, and the most important sex-related court case of the 20th century, Baird v. Eisenstadt. Named after the courageous Bill Baird, this decision gave people the right to use birth control even if they were single—less than fifty years ago. That established the constitutional right to privacy, cited several times a few years later in Roe v. Wade.

So now we are in the present, which only a few years ago was the past. And that past, and its past, could have helped us predict the future—which is now. Here are a few ways in which our current sexual challenges were predictable, if only we'd had a better grasp of history and the other social sciences:

Present:	Medicalization of sexuality & depression
Past:	Medicalization of "hysteria" and "self-abuse"

Present:	Mixed gender workplaces
Past:	Impact of the Industrial Revolution & factories

Present:	AIDS
Past:	Impact of the plague, TB, other epidemics

Present:	Anti-gay & anti-porn campaigns
Past:	The purity movements of 1910, 1930, & 1950

Present:	Internet & cybersex
Past:	Impact of the cinema, radio, & telephone

For example, the last 25 years has seen the increasing medicalization of sexuality and depression. This is no surprise when we look at history, because a hundred years ago we saw the medicalization of hysteria—a "woman's disease"—and of "self-abuse"—masturbation. A century ago, the medical profession became completely involved in these "problems'" diagnosis, treatment, and language. Most of what "modern" lay people knew about hysteria and self-abuse came from the medical profession. If sexology had studied that more we would be better able to understand the current medicalization of depression and sexuality.

The mixed-gender workplace is, according to the Institute for the Future's Wendy Everett, a turning point in human history. I think we could understand it better if we would examine the impact of the Industrial Revolution and factories on people's sexual and erotic relationships. What happened to families in England, France, and Germany in the 1700s or 1800s when, for the first time, women actually left the house early in the morning and went to a factory and were surrounded by other women and other men? That must have been an enormous change. In fact, some historians say that a key trigger of the French Revolution was all the masses of people now walking to work every morning, with all that time to discuss how unhappy they were. This couldn't happen when people worked isolated among their families, but with industrialization they were walking ten abreast to the factories—complaining.

AIDS continues to have an enormous impact on sexuality. One of the ways we could better understand it is to look at the impact of other plagues, from the Bubonic in the thirteenth century to influenza, less than a hundred years ago. Pandemics are not just medical phenomena, they are social and cultural phenomena. Bioethicist Ina Roy says that one of the reasons society is having so much trouble dealing with AIDS today is because it's been conceptualized as a sexually transmitted disease rather than a communicable disease. She says if we talked about it more like tuberculosis than syphilis, we'd have more medical and social options. Looking at the impact other pandemics had on their respective cultures could give us clues about how to handle AIDS.

The dreadful anti-gay and anti-porn campaigns that we've been suffering through in the last 20 years are not unique in America. Back around 1910, again around 1930, and again around 1950, both of these campaigns of fear and hate were in vogue. Their structure looked similar to what we see now. It seems everyone is now talking about the Internet. This includes anti-pornography crusaders talking about how awful it is. Well, virtually every invention has been used for pornography when possible. People have always complained about other people—including "the children"—getting sexual information the newest form of telecommunications instead of from their families (or not at all).

When the cinema first became popular around 1915, self-appointed public guardians went crazy because they were afraid that the moving images would seep into people's brains, control their thinking and undermine their values. The same was said about radio, comic books, television, and now the Internet.

Another predictable thing is how the Right and certain elements of feminism are in bed together around issues of pornography and non-normative sexuality. This is not new; we have seen this coalition before, with the Women's Christian Temperance Union and other groups. In the 1900s and 1910s a group of right-wing religiously-oriented people wanted to "reform" Americans' behavior around issues such as sex, alcohol, tobacco, and language. A group of feminist women aligned with them, even though those people were against women working outside the home and women's suffrage. These regressive feminists aligned with these men because they recognized a joint goal—supporting the "purity of the home." So today's coalition is not new.

Now that we've looked at history, let's explore the future. I believe the future of sex will be determined along three dimensions—demographic, technologic, and cultural.

• Demographic Trends

The fact that kids have so much private time after school is a huge change. When I came home from school as a kid, my mom was there with milk and cookies. This was true for most American kids for the first two-thirds of the century—a mother or grandmother providing after-school supervision. We now have an enormous number of young people coming home from school with no supervision. Some of them are watching soap operas, some of them are talking on the phone, some of them are smoking dope, some of them are having sex with each other, and, I suppose, some of them are doing their homework.

Another demographic trend is the enormous push for abstinence education and anti-abuse programs. Some 20 years ago sex education was mandated in schools throughout the United States, a wonderful, progressive accomplish of SIECUS. The problem is that a lot of schools have twisted this mandate and now provide abstinence education instead of sex education. This is harming these children, and it will undermine their sexuality as adults.

Schools are also getting government money to provide anti-abuse programs, teaching seven-year-olds how to protect themselves from so-called bad touch. While we all want kids to be safe, I think it's a big mistake for kids to learn about all the ways they can be sexually exploited without learning about all the wonderful ways they can be involved in sexuality.

Unfortunately, this fits in with what a lot of younger parents: they're anxious that their kids are going to be kidnapped, terrified that their kids are going to be molested, they're overwhelmed by this social narrative of sexual danger, as if we were living in an erotic war zone—which, in reality, we're not. But there's a whole cohort of parents right now being trained by the media about how vulnerable their kids are. Even worse, this generation of kids now getting anti-abuse training is going to be parents one day, perpetuating this ugly mythology.

Another demographic change is that the population is aging. Many adults alive right now will live to be 100. Even more amazing, one out of three babies born in the year 2000 will live to be a hundred, so those of you who are looking for a marketing niche should consider eroto-gerontology. Issues that involve aging are going to be sexual issues as well, whether it's chronic pain, second, third, and fourth marriages, or how to be sexual when your medication steals your sexual desire. All of the lifestyle issues associated with aging are going to become sexual issues. Analgesics will soon be considered aphrodisiacs.

College cohorts are becoming much more heterogeneous. When I was in college all the students were the same age. Now in four-year colleges the ages of the students are much more mixed, even more so in two-year schools. So college students now spend several years in close proximity to people of widely varying ages. That means they're going to be exposed to various sexual cultures. It also means that the issue of student dating across generations will eventually be a cultural issue. As it is, colleges are already restricting the rights of students to have sex with the faculty. Not just faculty's rights to be sexual with students, but students' rights. People will soon be debating whether or not younger and older students should be allowed to have sex together, because the same power issues could be alleged.

There's also an increase in American society's cultural diversity. The amount of cross-ethnic and cross-racial cohabiting and marriage is skyrocketing, which obviously involves a mixing of sexual cultures. My therapy practice has lots of couples consisting of, say, an Indian engineer married to an American woman, or a Chinese engineer married to a Jewish man. Or it's two people from Thailand in an arranged marriage.

Western psychotherapy depends on concepts of individuation, decision-making, and personal responsibility. But what do we do when a guy comes in with erection problems and says he's in an arranged marriage? He's a responsible professional, an adult; but he says "this is who my mother told me to marry, so of course I did." We can't argue with that. But we are going to see more and more cultural diversity issues affecting people's sexual expression—and I frankly don't think we're prepared for it.

• Technologic Trends

We've already discussed that technology is always adapted to sexual uses, frequently in unanticipated ways. Take cell phones—invented for business situations in which telephones were unreliable, they are now in the hands of every junior high school kid. This completes the circle of privacy started by old-fashioned telephones, which established a person's private little world. Cell phones facilitate that private little world anyplace, anytime, and that's going to have an enormous sexual impact.

Everybody all over the country is getting access to the Web and getting hip to the Internet. For better or worse, the Net will be an increasing source of sexual information, as well as a means for people to meet. Virtual sex is an increasingly important part of many people's lives, and truly virtual sex is only a few years away. It will be interesting to see how this capability affects the use patterns of traditional pornography.

Pornography is everywhere now, more so than ever before. I don't think we have a clue as to what the impact of this is going to be.

All sexologists have their ideas about pornography, positive or negative. Regardless of our judgements, we're now looking at a whole new phenomenon. Porn started out restricted, and history has gradually democratized it via the printing press, nickelodeon, telephone, etc. With the Internet, everybody now can have as much of it as they want, whenever they want it, in as narrow a niche as they want. For example, there's actually a website called "Wet and Messy Shoes." You can see pictures of women who are fully clothed, wearing high heels—some of their shoes are caked with mud, some of them are dripping with milk, some of them are dangling in swimming pools. I don't think we have a clue about what the effect of all this pornography is going to be. We shouldn't be frightened, just very, very curious.

The medicalization of sexual dysfunction and its treatment is an increasing trend. Viagra is hot right now, but before Viagra there were Caverject, urethral suppositories, crude papaverine injections, and penile implants. So in the last 25 years we've watched the gradual medicalization of certain kinds of sexual difficulties—and we're going to see more and more of this.

A sublingual pill and even a topical cream to facilitate erection are in the works. Viagra is now being studied for its effects on women. Other scientists are investigating drugs that will help women have orgasms more easily.

While there's an exciting side to all this, I'm concerned about the relationships in which these pharmaceuticals are used. How often will these treatments imbalance or damage relationships in which people are accustomed to the erectile problem or the anorgasmia? Some women will think, "now that you can get it up, how do I know you won't be unfaithful?" And some men will think, "well, now that you come so easily, you're a slut."

We would like those people to get couples counseling along with their meds, but most are not interested in counseling. They just want to have decent sex. So we're going to see an increasing medicalization of sexual complaints. That means that insurance companies will be key players. You may remember that when Viagra first became available, people wondered how many pills their insurance company was going to cover—two a year? An unlimited supply? For many insurance companies, it's now five pills a month. It would be interesting to look at their company decision-makers. You can imagine six people sitting around a conference table and the first guy says, "Oh, three or four pills a month," and the second guy says, "Oh, three or four pills a month," and the third guy says, "Oh, I don't know, 20 a month . . ."

So we're going to see the pharmaceutical and insurance industries increasingly involved with sexuality. How much of our input are they getting? And how much of their process do we understand? We shouldn't be turning our backs on the drug companies. We should be pestering them and saying, "Hey, what about me? I know something that maybe you people haven't considered." We need to educate them, not reject or pooh-pooh them.

The disappearing line between contraception and abortion is an exciting development. I am really looking forward to the day when we're done with all of this fighting about abortion. I am against unwanted pregnancies. Sooner or later we're going to see the line between contraception and abortion completely wiped out. We already have the morning-after pill. There's a website where you can go and learn about the morning-after pill, even take the first steps toward ordering it. Sooner or later we're going to have RU486 (or its equivalent) legally and easily available in this country; it's a technologic and economic steamroller that just can't be stopped. The sense of desperation in the anti-choice people is not just that they want to stop abortion, it's that they realize that this is coming. Sooner or later a woman will be able to take a pill in the privacy of her own home that eliminates conception after the fact, and the fight over abortion will be over.

• Cultural Trends

The first thing is ideas. Ideas have an enormous impact on sexuality. For example, in 19th century England people were quite certain that a woman had to have an orgasm in order to conceive. This was a medical fact, all the smart people knew this, and doctors taught their patients that if you're having trouble conceiving, it's because she's not climaxing, so do something about that. Ideas about what's normal, of course, have a big impact on sexuality.

The question of what is infidelity is now very interesting. Not whether infidelity is a good thing or bad thing, but the definition of it. Because with all of the technological ways that people now experience sex, it isn't so clear. For example, if somebody is having phone sex with a third party, is that infidelity? If somebody is masturbating while they're typing an e-mail, is that infidelity? I get people coming into my office and one of them wants to end the marriage because of the other's infidelity, and the partner says, "What are you so upset about? It was just a lap-dance, I don't even know the woman's name!" Or, "We typed some messages back and forth and I jacked off. What's wrong?" Conflicts like this will continue to escalate as technology creates more and more ways for people to be sexual together.

Most American religions are now facing internal power struggles. Who gets ordained—women? Gays? Divorced people? Will same-gender unions be blessed? Some clergy are saying they are obligated by their vows to God to perform same-gender marriages. And will traditional liturgies be rewritten—will it be God the Father or God the Incredible Cosmic Mother?

Since the 1970s, people have increasingly turned to the courts for guidance on their sexual rights. Do you have the right to be protected from unwanted sexual imagery at your job? Do you have the right to be protected from somebody making a pass at you? Do college students have the right to be sexual with professors? In Menlo Park, California, for example, one of the most liberal cities in the known world, a woman actually sued the city because there was a classic Greek nude statue in the lobby of the civic building where she worked. She said that this was sexual harassment and went to court.

One of the things we sexologists should be asking, is, which features of modern life are shaping the future of sexuality this very moment? What is it that we need to pay attention to in order to understand sexuality in the coming decade—or century? Examples might include:

Amazon.com & e-commerce
the mainstreaming of s/m
the disappearance of downtowns
life expectancy beyond age 100
tampons
artificial fertility technologies
female clergy
unsupervised free time for kids
virtual sex
low-fat diets
public jack-off clubs
talk radio
John Gray's Mars/Venus paradigm
Internet blocking software
chlamydia
the rise in cohabiting
female athletics
new pain medications
young adults moving back home
expanding definitions of date rape
the normalization of female masturbation
e-mail instead of written love letters
the end of the Cold War
the coming stock market crash
bisexual chic
people entering college in their 20s & 30s

increasing interracial dating & marriage
Internet penetration of daily life
RU486
the ubiquity of pornography
the decreasing stigma of extramarital sex
the increase in religiosity
the disappearing availability of abortion
female police & emergency personnel
repetitive stress injuries
cybersex
increasing acceptance of psychotherapy
pharmaceuticals that facilitate desire, arousal, & orgasm
expanding definitions of "child molestation"
tattoos and piercings
whites becoming a minority
managed health care & HMOs
abstinence education
bans on student-faculty dating
steroids

How are these things shaping our sexual future? And what else is currently shaping our sexual future in ways we don't realize?

Why Do We Know So Little about Human Sex?

Anne Fausto-Sterling, Ph.D.

CHAPTER

Because I am a biologist, my friends have assigned me the role of resident expert on any news, rumor, or fad having even the slightest connection to the life sciences. Questions about human sexuality—that topic of eternal interest to us all—certainly top the list of queries my buddies shoot hopefully in my direction. What causes homosexuality? Do farm boys really experiment with animals? Are kids reaching puberty at ever younger ages? I'm as eager as anyone to talk about these questions, even at some length, but deep down I realize that we know far too little to answer them accurately.

Last summer, for example, the newspapers and weekly magazines buzzed with reports of a finding by Simon LeVay that the brains of male homosexuals and male heterosexuals differed. LeVay had found a structural variation located in the hypothalamus, a part of the brain involved with the regulation of hormones and some sexual activities. Many people think he has obtained evidence of a biological cause of homosexuality. But when, inevitably, my friends asked me what I thought, I came back again and again to what I see as a central flaw: LeVay had no specific information about the sexual behavior of the men in his study.

In LeVay's study either you're gay or you're straight. He thinks that the men from his heterosexual group, whose brains he obtained at autopsy, were straight. But he doesn't really know for sure. They might have been gay but in the closet, or they might have lived straight, married lives yet had an occasional liaison with a man. He also thinks that his homosexual group represented men who engaged in sex with high frequency. But here too he doesn't know what kinds of sex acts they did nor how often they did them.

The presumption that most people are heterosexual and the idea that heterosexuality and homosexuality represent sharply distinct behaviors seem reasonable to most of us. But human behavior is far more complex than that. One survey of gay men and women in San Francisco, for example, used the plural word *homosexualities* to emphasize the diversity of behaviors subsumed under the term *homosexual.* Self-defined homosexuals turned out to live very varied lives. Some were monogamous and in long-term relationships; others engaged in frequent sex with total strangers. Male and female homosexuality were different in practice. They may eventually be shown to differ in origin as well. LeVay surmised that his sample of homosexual men had frequent sex; could the brain differences he found, if confirmed, correlate with frequency of sexual activity rather than with orientation?

We can't understand the origins of human sexual expression without knowing more about how we actually behave. But sexology, the study of human sexual behavior, began only in the twentieth century. The first, and the most famous, modern scientific survey appeared a mere 44 years ago under the title *Sexual Behavior in the Human Male,* coauthored by Alfred Kinsey, Wardell Pomeroy, and Clyde Martin. It underwent nine reprintings in the first year and a half of publication.

Kinsey and his co-workers discovered a continuum of sexuality. They developed a heterosexual-homosexual rating scale, which they divided into seven categories, from exclusively or predominantly heterosexual to exclusively or predominantly homosexual. Where sex is concerned, it turned out, you find all sorts of shades of gray. They found that 37 percent of the male population surveyed had some overt homosexual experience, that most of these experiences occurred during adolescence, and that at least 25 percent of adult males had more than incidental homosexual experiences for at least three years of their lives.

Not surprisingly, howls of protest met the Kinsey study's conclusions. When it comes to the scientific investigation of sexuality, European-American culture does not have a good track record. Pioneer sexologists included the German Richard von Krafft-Ebing and the Englishman Havelock Ellis, and many found their work dangerous. In 1897 Ellis published a book that treated homosexuality in neutral, scientific tones. His British publisher quickly faced criminal prosecution for issuing a "lewd, wicked, bawdy, scandalous, and obscene" book. In *The Well of Loneliness,* written a couple of decades later, novelist Radclyffe Hall describes the lesbian protagonist as she comes across one of Krafft-Ebing's books, which her father has forgotten to return to its locked cabinet. Trembling, she reads for the first time a description of her "condition." Hall's fictional revelation of these secrets led to a 1928 court declaration banning the novel as obscene. The judge ordered all copies seized.

In 1919 in Germany, Magnus Hirschfeld founded the Institute for the Study of Sexual Behavior, which housed more than 20,000 volumes, numerous photographs, and archival material. Interest in the topic grew, and by the 1930s about 80 sex-reform organizations opened clinics in which professionals and laypeople offered medical and sexual information. The flourishing of such knowledge didn't last long. In 1933, months after their rise to power, the Nazis attacked Hirschfeld's institute and burned its books and papers in the street.

Nor did Kinsey escape unscathed. In 1954 the American Medical Association attacked him for contributing to "a wave of sex hysteria." Conservative congressman Louis

Heller called for an investigation, urging that Kinsey's work be barred from the U.S. mails. He accused him of contributing to "the depravity of a whole generation" and "the spread of juvenile delinquency." Under political pressure from the House Committee to Investigate Tax-Exempt Foundations, the Rockefeller Foundation, which had funded Kinsey's work, withdrew its support. Kinsey died of a heart attack two years later, a death some say was hastened by the vilification of his work.

Regrettably, this story turns out to have a contemporary echo. Over the past three years conservative House members and senators have again intervened to halt studies and a new national sex survey that would have provided us with the first truly comprehensive accounting of sexual behavior in this country since the Kinsey report. Current epidemiological estimates of the spreading patterns of sexually transmitted diseases still rely on Kinsey's data even though they are badly out of date. Behavior has certainly changed in the interim, and Kinsey's sample, large as it was, did not represent a cross section of the American population.

Indeed, such is our state of ignorance that in 1989 scientists from the National Research Council warned in a report that we don't know enough to win the war against sexually transmitted diseases, including AIDS. To devise a sensible strategy, they reported, we need to know the prevalence of sexually risky behaviors associated with AIDS transmission in low-risk as well as in high-risk groups. We also have to understand the social contexts promoting risky behavior, and the relationships among sex, drug use, and alcohol consumption.

The report called for longitudinal studies—following the behavior of groups of teens for several years, for example—and for research on how to accurately gather information about behavior that many feel squeamish discussing. There are still many puzzles about AIDS transmission. Among them is that in developing countries the virus is spread mostly by heterosexual sex. But in the United States heterosexual sex seems a minor means of transmission, at least so far, compared with homosexual sex or intravenous drug use. What makes our country so different? At the time of the National Research Council report, studies to answer some of these questions were just getting under way, but since then projects have ground to a sudden and discouraging halt.

Here's what happened. About four years ago the National Institute of Child Health and Development (NICHD) awarded a contract to Edward Laumann, dean of the division of social sciences at the University of Chicago. He was to plan an update of the outmoded Kinsey report and amass the kind of information that would guide public health decisions. Laumann assembled a national team to design a survey that would throw light on practices relating to contraception, fertility, and disease prevention. The researchers wanted the science in the study to be beyond reproach, so they worked hard to solve difficult methodological problems. They asked very basic questions: How would they get the answers they needed from people without violating their privacy? Could they control for interviewer bias—would a male respond differently to a female interviewer than to a male interviewer? How would they check the validity of the answers?

But Laumann and his co-workers wanted to do more than simply gather raw statistics. They wanted to know how social networks influence behavior. Most epidemiological models of the spread of sexually transmitted diseases use estimates of the average number of sexual partners a person has in a given population. For example, statistics might show that on average, women born after 1950 have ten partners in their lifetime. Traditional models would presume that their mating is more or less random. Laumann thinks this is a poor way to model the spread of sexually transmitted diseases. People engage in different patterns of sexual activity at different times of their lives. For instance, after a burst of experimentation in her teens and twenties, a woman might remain monogamous for 20 years, divorce, and have several sexual partners before returning to monogamy. Hence you might expect a different pattern of disease spread in a population where most women are under age 30 than in one where most women are older. Social and economic status also play a role. Sex between partners of the same age, ethnic group, and economic standing may be more openly negotiated, thereby lessening the risk of unprotected sex.

So Laumann proposed a model of sexual behavior as something done by couples living in social networks, rather than by randomly acting individuals, as most epidemiological models presume. His proposal was of such high quality that the NICHD was set to launch the national study when, in 1989, Senator Jesse Helms (Republican of North Carolina) and Congressman William Dannemeyer (Republican of California) caught wind of it. When they were done, the Office of Management and Budget and the House Appropriations Committee had withdrawn funding for the project.

Meanwhile, researchers at the Carolina Population Center (part of the University of North Carolina) had designed a longitudinal study of teenage sexuality of the sort called for by the National Research Council. They planned to study teens' sexual behavior, ranging from contraceptive use to homosexual activities, taking into account education, religion, and family and peer-group interactions. Their proposal was submitted to the NICHD (the appropriate branch of the National Institutes of Health), was peer-reviewed, and received a high-priority score; in 1991 the researchers received their first year of funding for a five-year survey of 24,000 teenagers and their parents. In July 1991, however, Helms and Dannemeyer reentered the scene and successfully pressured Secretary of Health and Human Services Louis Sullivan into canceling the project.

The story doesn't end there. In October 1990 Laumann applied for a grant from the NICHD to do a more limited adult sex study, using the approaches developed for his ill-fated national survey. His application received rave reviews and a funding priority placing him in the top 2 percent of grants reviewed at the time. Funding seemed all but assured. The following year NICHD director Wendy Baldwin told him it would be "political suicide" to award him the money.

It so happened that on September 12, 1991, Senator Helms had introduced an amendment to the NIH appropriations bill, which determines the money allotted to projects and individual institutes within the NIH. Helms proposed that the money earmarked for sex surveys be removed from the NIH budget. Instead, he wanted the same dollar amount transferred to that portion of the Adolescent Family Life Act devoted to encouraging premarital celibacy (that is, just say no). Voting on the amendment, he argued, would "provide senators with a clear choice between right and wrong." In a one-two punch Congressman Dannemeyer introduced the same amendment in the House. The amendment passed in the Senate, failed in the House, and the House-Senate Conference Committee later dropped it from the final bill. Nevertheless, the debate on both the House and Senate floors had the desired effect. Funding for Laumann's research is on indefinite hold.

Why were the surveys canceled? A broad cross section of the scientific and medical community felt they represented cutting-edge research. The quality of the science had never been in question. Instead, it seems that Senator Helms and Congressman Dannemeyer's deep-seated hatred and fear of homosexuality are at issue. Last August Dannemeyer told a *Los Angeles Times* columnist that he believes the sex surveys are the idea of a conspiratorial cell of homosexuals who operate inside the Department of Health and Human Services. The following month Helms took the Senate floor to say: "The NIH funds these sex surveys . . . to 'cook the books,' so to speak, in terms of presenting 'scientific facts'—in order to do what? To legitimize homosexual life-styles, of course."

"Mr. President," he went on, "let me just say that I am sick and tired of pandering to the homosexuals in this country."

The surveys, Helms argued, are not really intended "to stop the spread of AIDS. The real purpose is to compile supposedly scientific facts to support the leftwing liberal argument that homosexuality is a normal, acceptable life-style. . . . As long as I am able to stand on the floor of the U.S. Senate," he added, "I am never going to yield to that sort of thing, because it is not just another life-style; it is sodomy."

Helms concluded by gay-baiting both of Laumann's coinvestigators—distinguished social scientists and acknowledged homosexuals—repeating that "the surveys are part and parcel of the homosexual movement's agenda to legitimize their sexual behavior."

And so the battle rages on. On one side stands the social science and medical community, which wants to know what people do behind closed doors. These researchers don't want to gain prurient pleasure from it, or judge it, or encourage it. They wish merely to devise sound public health policies aimed at stopping the spread of a deadly disease. On the other stand two powerful legislators and their conservative constituencies. Their approach to stopping the spread of sexually transmitted diseases is simple: just say no to any kind of sexual activity other than heterosexual relations within the confines of marriage. During the past three rounds of the fight, the top managers at Health and Human Services have put their money on the conservatives. Who will be left standing at the end of the fight remains to be seen.

Influences of Culture on Asian Americans' Sexuality

3

CHAPTER

Sumie Okazaki

Asian Americans comprise a population group that is characterized by an enormous demographic, historical, and cultural heterogeneity, yet Asian Americans also share many Asian cultural characteristics such as the primacy of the family and the collective's goals over individual wishes, emphasis on propriety and social codes, the appropriation of sexuality only within the context of marriage, and sexual restraint and modesty. Although there are significant gaps in the scientific literature concerning Asian Americans' sexuality, the existing data point to notable differences between Asian Americans and other ethnic groups on major aspects of sexual behavior. For example, relative to other U.S. ethnic group cohorts, Asian American adolescents and young adults tend to show more sexually conservative attitudes and behavior and initiate sexual intercourse at a later age. There are indications that as Asian Americans become more acculturated to the mainstream American culture, their attitudes and behavior become more consistent with the White American norm. Consistent with their more sexually conservative tendencies in normative sexual behavior, Asian American women also appear more reluctant to obtain sexual and reproductive care, which in turn places them at a greater risk for delay in treatment for breast and cervical cancer as well as other gynecological problems. Available data suggest that the prevalence rate of sexual abuse in Asian American communities appear lower than those of other groups, although it is not clear to what extent the low rates are due to cultural reluctance to report shameful experiences.

Preparation of this manuscript was supported in part by a grant from the National Insitute of Mental Health (MH-01506). I thank Gordon C. Nagayama Hall for comments on an earlier version of this article.

Address correspondence to Sumie Okazaki. Department of Psychology, University of Illionois at Urbana-Champaign, 603 E. Daniel St., Champaign, IL 61820; e-mail: okazaki@uiuc.edu.

From *Journal of Sex Research,* Vol. 39, No. 1, February 2002. Permission conveyed through Copyright Clearance Center.

While sharing their Asian ancestry and vestiges of Asian cultural heritage to varying degrees, Asian Americans comprise an ethnic minority group that defies simple characterizations. Consisting of approximately 4% of the total U.S. population, Asian Americans trace their roots to one or more of 28 Asian countries of origin or ethnic groups. The largest proportions of Asian Americans in 1990 were Chinese (24%) and Filipino (20%), followed by Japanese, Korean, and Asian Indian at approximately 11% to 12% each and Vietnamese at 9% (U.S. Bureau of the Census, 1993). However, the continuing influx of new immigrants from Southeast Asia and South Asia as well as from China and Korea provide a backdrop for diversity among Americans of Asian ancestry on important dimensions such as national origin, language, nativity, generational status, religion, acculturation to the mainstream American values and customs, and so on. The majority (66%) of Asian Americans in 1990 were born in foreign countries (U.S. Bureau of the Census, 1993).

The present review concerning the impact of Asian and Asian American cultures on sexuality will first examine aspects of various Asian cultural traditions and values that influence sexual attitudes and behavior among Asian Americans, then examine the available scientific literature in several major areas (but excluding materials related to HIV, other STDs, and safe sex practices). Some topics, namely sexual dysfunction and treatment, are not covered because no data exist. Most studies that are reviewed here do not specifically test the link between aspects of Asian or Asian American culture and sexual variables but instead use Asian American ethnicity as a proxy for culture.

Cultural Roots

Sexuality is linked to procreation in most Asian cultures. Gupta (1994) argues that sexuality was not a taboo subject in ancient Hindu culture granted that it was discussed within the context of marriage. Rather, sexuality was openly discussed in religious and fictional texts (e.g., the Kama Sutra) and depicted in paintings and sculptures, some with explicit erotic details. Japanese and Chinese erotica also date back to ancient times. On the other hand, sex is a taboo subject in contemporary Chinese culture, where sex education in schools is minimal and parents as well as health professionals are reluctant to discuss sexuality and sexual information (Chan, 1986). Traditional Cambodian society believed that a lack of knowledge regarding sexuality would prevent premarital sexual activity that would tarnish the family honor; consequently, discussions of information regarding sexual intercourse and sexuality were kept to a minimum (Kulig, 1994). Filipino culture, with the strong influence of Catholicism, tends to have a strong moral undercurrent that scorns premarital sex, use of contraceptives, and abortion (Tiongson, 1997).

Regardless of each Asian culture's degree of openness surrounding sexual discourse, expressions of sexuality outside of marriage are considered highly inappropriate in most Asian cultures. Most Asian cultures are highly collectivistic and patriarchical; thus, sexuality that is allowed open expression (particularly among women) would represent a threat to the highly interdependent social order as well as to the integrity of the family. Many Asian cultural traditions place emphasis on propriety and the observance of strict moral and social conduct, thus modesty and restrained sexuality are valued (Abraham, 1999). The sexually conservative beliefs and behavior that many Americans of Asian ancestry may exhibit may, in turn, be misinterpreted by the larger American society as asexual (Tsui, 1985).

Sexual Knowledge, Attitudes, and Norms

Available data regarding the sexual knowledge, attitudes, and norms among Asian Americans reflect relative conservatism. In a 1993 study in British Columbia comparing 346 Asian Canadian and 356 non-Asian Canadian[1] university students enrolled in introductory psychology courses, Meston, Trapnell, and Gorzalka (1998) found that Asian Canadians held more conservative sexual attitudes and demonstrated less sexual knowledge than non-Asian Canadians. Among Asian Canadians, the more acculturated they were to the Canadian culture the more permissive their sexual attitudes. In a survey of 574 girls in sixth through eighth grades at public junior high schools in southern California, East (1998) compared the girls' sexual, marital, and birth expectations across four ethnic groups (White, Black, Hispanic, and Southeast Asians). Southeast Asian American (Vietnamese, Cambodian, Laotian; $n = 70$) girls reported the oldest "best" age for first intercourse ($M = 21.7$) and first birth ($M = 24.4$) and the oldest "desired" age for first birth ($M = 26.4$) of the four ethnic group girls. Southeast Asian American girls indicated the least desire to have children, the last likelihood of having children out of wedlock, and the least intention of having sexual intercourse in the near future. In a survey of 452 unmarried young adults (ages 18 to 25) attending 2-year community colleges, Feldman, Turner, and Araujo (1999) also found that Asian Americans ($n = 104$) held significantly later normative and personal sexual timetables for initiating all types of sexual behavior relative to other ethnic groups. In another survey with 474 college students in the Southwest (17 of whom were Asian American) regarding sex education, Asian Americans' reported age at which they understood what sexual intercourse was ($M = 15.1$) and the age at which they plan to begin their future children's sex education ($M = 14.1$) were older than those of any other ethnic group (Harman & Johnson, 1995).

There are some data suggesting that Asian Americans' sexually conservative attitude may erode with higher degrees of exposure to the American culture. Abramson and

---

[1]In this and all other studies conducted by Meston et al. (1996, 1997, 1999), individuals born in South Asia (India and Pakistan) were classified as non-Asians rather than Asians. (South Asians are considered in this review as Asians, following the convention in Asian American scholarship and the U.S. Census classification.) However, because South Asian Canadians typically constituted less than 3% of Meston et al.'s (1996, 1997, 1999) non-Asian samples, the results of their ethnic comparisons are likely to be reliable. The Asian Canadian group in their studies consisted primarily (70%) of ethnic Chinese.

Imai-Marquez (1982) administered a measure of sex guilt to three different generations of Japanese American men and women and matched groups of White Americans in the metropolitan Los Angeles area. The researchers found that each subsequent younger generation of Japanese Americans and White Americans reported less guilty thoughts and feelings concerning sexual matters, although Japanese Americans still reported more sex guilt than White Americans within each age cohort group. However, in a different study of 18 Japanese American, 22 Mexican American, 20 African American, and 27 White American parents in Los Angeles regarding their attitudes toward sex education, the attitudes of Japanese American parents were found not to differ from those of other ethnic group parents once father's education and mother's religiosity were controlled for (Abramson, Moriuchi, Waite, & Perry, 1983). Notably, all of the Japanese American parents were born in the U.S.

Sexual Behavior

Most studies of sexual activity among Asian Americans have been conducted with adolescents and college students. The most comprehensive survey of American adults' sexual behavior, the National Health and Social Life Survey conducted in 1992, did not oversample Asian American individuals (Laumann, Gagnon, Michael, & Michaels, 1994). Consequently, only 2% of the total sample was Asian American, making it difficult to sufficiently characterize the sexual behavior of Asian American (particularly female) adults in the general population.

ADOLESCENTS

In a survey of 2,026 high school students in Los Angeles County, Asian American adolescents ($n = 186$) were more likely to be virgins (73%) than African American (28%), Latino (43%), and White Americans (50%) (Schuster, Bell, & Kanouse, 1996). Further analyses of the same data revealed that Asian American adolescents were less likely to have initiated a vaginal intercourse at an early age and were less likely to report having participated in other heterosexual genital sexual activities during the prior year than their non-Asian counterparts as well (Schuster, Bell, Nakajima, & Kanouse, 1998). The researchers found that Asian American nonvirgins also reported the lowest number of lifetime partners for vaginal intercourse, even though the reported frequency of sexual activity did not differ from those of other ethnic group adolescents. Asian American adolescents in homes where English is the primary language spoken were more likely than other Asian Americans to be nonvirgins and to have engaged in heterosexual genital sexual activities. Asian American adolescents were also more likely than non-Asian Americans to think that their parents and friends would disapprove if they had vaginal intercourse and that people their own age should not have vaginal intercourse.

Another study of an ethnically diverse sample of 877 Los Angeles County youths (Upchurch, Levy-Storms, Sucoff, & Aneshensel, 1998) found that Asian American males had the highest median age of first sex (18.1) and that Asian American females (as well as Hispanic females) had rates of first sex that was about half that of White females. Finally, an analysis of the national Youth Risk Behavior Survey data (total $N = 52,985$) collected by the Centers for Disease Control and Prevention (Grunbaum, Lowry, Kann, & Pateman, 2000) also found that Asian American high school students were significantly less likely than Black, Hispanic, or White students to have had sexual intercourse or to have had four or more sex partners. Only 28% of Asian American students reported lifetime experience of sexual intercourse compared to 77% of Black, 55% of Hispanic, and 48% of White students. However, among those who were currently sexually active, Asian American students were found to be as likely as other groups to have used alcohol or drugs during last sexual intercourse or to have used a condom at last intercourse. It should be noted that there is variability among Asian ethnic groups with respect to sexual behavior. Horan and DiClemente (1993) reported that among 11th and 12th grade students in San Francisco, only 13% of Chinese American students were sexually active but 32% of Filipino students were sexually active.

COLLEGE STUDENTS

The patterns found with Asian American adolescents also extend to college students. In a 1982 survey of 114 Chinese American college students in northern California (60% of whom were U.S.-born), Huang and Uba (1992) found that the majority (over 60%) approved of premarital sexual intercourse when partners are in love or engaged to be married; however, only 37% of the men and 46% of the women surveyed had ever engaged in coitus. In this sample, Chinese American women were generally more sexually experienced than men, with more women having engaged in kissing, necking, and petting, although men ($M = 18.5$) and women ($M = 18.8$) did not differ in age of first vaginal intercourse experience. There was a positive correlation between the level of acculturation to the U.S. and engagement in premarital sexual intercourse, and those Chinese Americans dating only White Americans consistently had more sexual experience than those dating only Chinese Americans. Huang and Uba concluded that Chinese American college students were not avoiding premarital sex because they do not find it permissible. Rather, the authors speculated that Chinese Americans' sexual behavior and gender differences may reflect internalized racism (e.g., less positive body images), more conservative standards for engaging in premarital sexual relations, and racialized stereotypes of Asian American men as asexual and undesirable sexual partners.

In a 1987–1988 survey of 153 Asian American college students in Souther California (half of whom were born in the U.S.), Cochran, Mays, and Leung (1991) found that 44% of the men and 50% of the women had engaged in heterosexual sexual intercourse at least once. The rate of Asian Americans who were sexually active (47%) was significantly lower than their age cohorts in other ethnic groups. Among those who were sexually active, the rates of engagement in oral sex was high (86% for women, 75% for men). In an analyses of their 1993 data on 346 Asian and 356 non-Asian Canadian college students, Meston, Trapnell, and Gorzalka (1996) found significant and substantive ethnic differences in all measures of interpersonal sexual behavior (i.e., light and heavy petting, oral sex, intercourse) and intrapersonal sexual behavior (i.e., frequency of fantasies, masturbation incidence and frequency, and ideal frequency of intercourse), and all sociosexual restrictiveness measures (e.g., lifetime number of partners, number of partners in the past year, predicted number of partners, lifetime number of one-night stands). Overall, 35% of Asian Canadian college students in this survey reported having experienced intercourse. This study did not find any differences among Asian Canadians in their sexual behavior according to their length of residency in Canada.

A survey of 148 White American and 202 Asian American college students in Southern California (McLaughlin, Chen, Greenberger, & Biermeir, 1997) also found that Asian American men (over 55%) and women (60%) were significantly more likely than White American men (25%) and women ($<$ 30%) to be virgins. Among those who were sexually experienced, Asian American men ($M = 2.3$) and women ($M = 2.2$) reported fewer lifetime sexual partners than White American men ($M = 5.5$) and women ($M = 3.5$). Within the Asian American sample, women from least acculturated families were more likely to be virgins (77%) than those from moderately or highly acculturated families (52% and 53%, respectively). This pattern did not hold for Asian American men. Of note, Asian Americans and White Americans endorsed casual sex to a similar degree even though the groups differed significantly in the number of partners. McLaughlin et al. interpreted this attitude-behavior inconsistency among Asian American college students as possibly reflecting the larger and more effective role that their parents play in controlling the adolescents' behavior.

In sum, the available data indicate that Asian Americans tend to be more sexually conservative than non-Asian Americans of the same age group, particularly with regard to the older age of initiation of sexual activity. One exception is a study by Sue (1982), who reported in a survey of 36 Asian American college students enrolled in a human sexuality course that rates of premarital sexual behavior did not differ from those of non-Asian students. However, Sue's anomalous data are likely the result of the selective nature of Asian American students who voluntarily enrolled in a human sexuality course.

Sexual and Reproductive Health

Almost all studies examining sexual and reproductive health among Asian Americans have been conducted with women. The studies of participation in breast and cervical cancer screening among the Asian American population paint a fragmented picture.

Some studies have shown moderate rates of cancer screening among Asian American women. For example, 57% of 189 Chinese American women in Michigan, aged 50 or older, had had mammograms in the past 2 years (Yu, Seetoo, Tsai, & Sun, 1998), and over 70% of the Chinese American women sampled in San Francisco had had a mammogram, Pap test, clinical breast examination (CBE), and breast self examination (BSE) (Lee, 1998).

However, the majority of the studies have found extremely low rates of screening in Asian Americans compared to the non-Asian American population. In a study conducted in the Puget Sound area, Asian American women were found to be less likely than other ethnic group women to enroll in breast cancer screening programs even when out-of-pocket expenses for the screening tests were paid by managed care (Tu, Taplin, Barlow, & Boyko, 1999). In a study of women 18 to 74 years old in the San Francisco Bay Area, Chinese American and Vietnamese American women had the lowest rates of first time utilization and recent utilization of breast and cervical cancer screening among all the ethnic groups (Hiatt et al., 1996). Specifically, 33% of Chinese American women had never obtained a pap test and 30% had never performed BSE, whereas 58% of Vietnamese American women had never had a Pap test and 66% had never performed BSE. An interview study of 332 Chinese American women (ages 40–69) recruited through a two-stage probability sampling method in the Chinatown area of Chicago (Yu, Kim, Chen, & Brintnall, 2001) also found a low level of knowledge of cancer screening tests and low use rates. Only 52% and 54% of the Chinese American women surveyed had ever heard of the CBE and Pap smear test, respectively, for cancer screening purposes, and much lower percentages had actually undergone screenings (35% for CBE, 12% for mammogram, 26% for BSE, and 36% for Pap test). Levels of education, English fluency, and source of health care (Eastern vs. Western medicine) were significant predictors of reproductive health behavior in this population.

The pattern of low use of screening also extends to younger age groups. Only 14.9% of 174 Chinese American students at a midwestern university practiced BSE (Lu, 1995). In a 1996 reproductive and sexual health survey of 674 Asian American women (age 18–35; the majority foreign-born) in California, 67% of the women reported having had at least one sexual partner in their lifetime, yet half of the women (50%) had not received any reproductive or sexual health services within the past year and 25% had never received such services in their lifetime (National Asian Women's Health Organization, 1997). More than one third of the respondents reported that they had never discussed pregnancy, sexually transmitted diseases, birth control, or sexuality in their households. A survey of high school students in Los Angeles County also found that Asian American adolescents reported lower levels of communication with physicians about sexual activity and risk prevention than other ethnic groups (Schuster, Bell, Peterson, & Kanouse, 1996).

In a rare study that specifically examined the role of Asian cultural variables, Tang, Solomon, Yeh, and Worden (1999) studied BSE and cervical cancer screening behavior in

156 Asian American and 50 White American female college students. In this sample, 48% of Asian American and 68% of White American women reported having had sexual intercourse with a male partner. The ethnic differences extended to screening behavior, as only 27% of Asian American women reported performing BSE at least once in their lifetime in contrast to 47% of White American women. Similarly, only 32% of Asian American but 70% of White American women reported having had at least one Pap test in their lifetime. Asian American women were found to have more cultural barriers to screening (more communication barrier with mother surrounding sexual and gynecological issues, less openness around sexuality and more modesty, less prevention orientation in health care, and less utilization of Western medicine). Even after controlling for differences between the two ethnic groups (e.g., mother's education, year in college, family history of breast or cervical cancer, knowing someone with breast cancer, being sexually active, etc.), Asian Americans were still less likely than White Americans to have had BSE and pap test. However, Asian American women who were more acculturated were more likely to participate in these screening behaviors.

Consistent with Tang et al.'s (1999) results, similar cultural reasons for the low utilization of reproductive health services were elucidated through a qualitative analysis of interview data with 9 Asian American health care practitioners and educators who worked with Asian American women and focus group data with 6 second-generation Asian American women (National Asian Women's Health Organization, 1995). This study found that Asian American women's sense of risk regarding reproductive and sexual health appeared to be downplayed, as the women tended to view gynecological services as important and legitimate only when they concerned reproductive functions or when the pain or symptoms of infection became unbearable or interfered with daily functioning. In the interviews, health advocates and practitioners agreed that recent immigrants in particular may perceive gynecological exams such as Pap tests as invasive and inappropriate prior to marriage, and that the perception that gynecological care is only acceptable after marriage likely prevents many Asian American women from accessing appropriate care. Additionally, Mo (1992) argued that the idea of a visit to a medical doctor for a checkup without receiving some form of intervention (namely medication) does not fit immigrant Chinese patients' expectations. Mo explained that a Cantonese term, *ham suup,* which is a colloquial term for sexuality that is most often used in a derogatory manner, is used to describe anyone who is sexually inappropriate. Talking about or touching one's body and being knowledgeable about the body are considered as *ham suup,* thus discouraging traditional and immigrant Chinese women from gaining knowledge regarding sexuality and sexual health. In sum, there appears to be a pervasive tendency for Asian American girls and women to be more reluctant than White American girls and women to seek care for their sexual and reproductive health.

As a possible consequence of their relatively low use of screening, Asian American women tend to be diagnosed with more advanced stages of cervical cancer (Frisch & Goodman, 2000) and breast cancer (Jenkins & Kagawa-Singer, 1994) than White

American women, thereby increasing the disease burden at diagnosis (Hedeen, White, & Taylor, 1999). Cervical cancer rates among Vietnamese American women was the highest of all ethnic groups in the U.S., with the incidence of 43 per 100,000, a rate that is almost five times that of White American women (Miller et al., 1996). These statistics indicate that there are high health costs associated with Asian American women's reluctance to become knowledgeable about, and to engage in, sexual and reproductive health practices.

One study regarding the sexual and reproductive health issues of Asian American men does exist. A telephone survey of 802 English speaking Asian American men between the ages of 18 and 65 was conducted in Los Angeles, San Francisco, and New York (National Asian Women's Health Organization, 1999). Over half of the respondents (54%) were single and the majority (75%) was foreign-born. Although 87% of the surveyed Asian American men had at least one sexual partner in the past year, the vast majority of the respondents (89%) had never received sexual or reproductive health care services.

Sexual Abuse and Aggression

The scope of sexual abuse in the Asian American community is unknown, as most state and national agencies that collect such data fail to segregate the data for Asian American victims. Where data are available, the reported incidence among Asian Americans appears relatively low compared to other ethnic groups, possibly due to their lack of access or reluctance to use mental health services and public agencies (Kenny & McEachern, 2000). However, many service providers assert that the actual incidence is much higher than reported (Okamura, Heras, & Wong-Kerberg, 1995). High rates of history of sexual victimization among Cambodian American refugees women and children, which they suffered during the Khmer Rouge reign of terror or at refugee camps, have been extensively documented (e.g., Mollica, Wyshak, & Lavelle, 1987; Rozée & Van Boemel, 1989; Scully, Kuoch, & Miller, 1995). In a study of abuse history among 102 Vietnamese Amerasian refugee young adults in the Philippine Refugee Processing Center who were awaiting placement in the United States, 12% of men and 9% of women reported having been sexually abused (McKelvey & Webb, 1995).

Those who work with Asian American communities speak of the Asian American victims' extreme reluctance to disclose or report sexual abuse or assault (Okamura et al., 1995; Tsuneyoshi, 1996). For example, most Southeast Asian refugees surveyed by Wong (1987) stated that they would respond to sexual abuse in their own family by keeping it a family secret. Further, sexual abuse within the context of marriage may be fatalistically tolerated among some Asian American communities. As a result, immigrant Asian American women may be at a higher risk of marital sexual abuse than U.S.-born Asian American women because they may have been socialized to believe that they had fewer sexual rights than their husbands (Lum, 1998). An analysis of interviews with 25 South Asian immigrant women who were abused by their spouses found that 60% of the women reported being forced to have sex with their husbands against their will, and sexual abuse took many forms such as marital rape and violence and the husbands' control of women's reproductive choices (e.g., forcing the wife to get an abortion, refusal to allow the use of contraceptives, etc.) (Abraham, 1999). Similarly, an interview study with 150 immigrant Korean American women in Chicago revealed that 60% of the women reported being battered, and 37% of those who were physically abused also reported being forced to have sex by their partners (Song, 1996).

Given the cultural tendency to hide sexual abuse from others, it is difficult to ascertain the accuracy of sexual abuse reports.[2] A review of 158 Asian American cases referred for child maltreatment to a San Diego social service agency serving Asian American immigrants and refugees found that sexual abuse constituted only 5% of the total cases, with most sexual abuse victims being Filipino and female (Ima & Hohm, 1991). Another retrospective chart review study of a child abuse clinic in San Francisco generated 69 substantiated cases of sexual abuse between 1986 and 1988 in which the victims were Asian Americans (Rao, DiClemente, & Ponton, 1992). A comparison of this sample of Asian American child sexual abuse victims with randomly selected samples of other ethnic group counterparts found that Asian American victims tended to be older ($M = 11.5$ years) and more likely to be living with both parents than other ethnic group victims. Notably, Asian American victims were much less likely to display inappropriate sexual behaviors or express anger and hostility but most likely to express suicidal ideation or attempt suicide. Although Asian American mothers were as likely as White Americans and Hispanic Americans to be the primary caretakers to the child victims, they were much less likely than the other groups to have brought the abuse to the attention of authorities and most likely to disbelieve the report of the abuse. Asian American victims were also the least likely to disclose sexual abuse to their mothers; 61% either never spontaneously disclosed the abuse or disclosed the abuse to someone other than their mothers. Asian American victims were also the most likely group to be abused by a male relative (including the father).

Meston and her colleagues (Meston, Heiman, & Trapnell, 1999; Meston, Heiman, Trapnell, & Carlin, 1999) conducted a survey of 466 Asian Canadian and 566 non-Asian Canadian undergraduates regarding abuse experience before age 18 and their current sexuality. The researchers found that 25% of Asian Canadian women and 11% of Asian Canadian men had at least one experience with sexual abuse (defined here as being involved in some sexual activity against their wishes). In contrast, 40% of non-Asian Canadian women and 11% of non-Asian Canadian men reported at least one experience with sexual abuse. However, associations between early abuse and adult sexual behavior did not differ significantly between Asian and non-Asian Canadians, and reports of sexual abuse were not significantly correlated with socially desirable responding in either group. In another survey of 243 college women (38 of whom were Asian American), rates of reported childhood sexual

---

[2]For a more in-depth discussion of cultural factors that may influence in the reporting and treatment of child sexual abuse in Asian American communities, see Futa, Hsu, and Hansen (2001).

abuse and being a victim of rape among Asian American college women (21% and 11%, respectively) were lower than those of their White American and African American counterparts (Urquiza & Goodlin-Jones, 1994). The researchers also found that for White and African Americans, women with a history of childhood sexual abuse were three times as likely to be raped as an adult than women without a history of childhood sexual abuse. However, this pattern did not hold for Asian American women.

Hall and Barongan (1997) noted that there appeared to be a lower prevalence of sexual aggression in Asian American communities. A national survey of sexual aggression found that fewer Asian American men perpetrate rape and fewer Asian American women are victims of rape than other ethnic groups (Koss, Gidycz, & Wisniewski, 1987). In their review of risk and protective factors for sexual aggression among Asian Americans, Hall, Windover, and Maramba (1998) argued that the patriarchical aspects of Asian culture, in which women hold subordinate status to men, may create a risk for, and a tolerance of, sexual aggression by Asian American men. On the other hand, Asian cultural emphases on self-control and interpersonal harmony may serve as protective factors for sexual aggressive behavior among Asian Americans. To test culture-specific models of sexual aggression, Hall, Sue, Narang, and Lilly (2000) examined intra- and interpersonal determinants of Asian American and White American men's sexual aggression. In this sample of college students, 33% of Asian American and 38% of White American men reported that they had perpetrated some form of sexual aggression. Whereas a path model for White American men suggested that only an intrapersonal variable (misogynous beliefs) predicted sexual aggression, both interpersonal (concern about social standing) and intrapersonal (misogynous beliefs, alcohol use) variables were predictive of Asian American sexual aggression.

Other studies point to a possible role of Asian cultural factors in the attitudes toward sexual violence. For example, a study of 302 Asian American and White American college students (Mori, Bernat, Glenn, Selle, & Zarate, 1995) found that Asian Americans were more likely to endorse negative attitudes toward rape victims and greater belief in rape myths than their White counterparts. Moreover, less acculturated Asian Americans held more negative attitudes toward rape victims than more acculturated Asian Americans. A telephone survey about domestic violence attitudes with 262 Chinese Americans in Los Angeles County (Yick, 2000) found that although 89% of the respondents agreed that sexual aggression constituted domestic violence, the respondents' gender role beliefs (traditional or egalitarian) emerged as a significant factor that shapes their definitions of abuse. In summary, certain facets of traditional Asian cultures (e.g., traditional gender roles, concerns about loss of face) appear to be implicated in Asian Americans' attitudes toward, reporting of, and perpetration of sexual abuse and aggression.

Sexual Orientation

Little empirical research exists concerning sexual orientation and sexual identity among Asian Americans apart from the HIV-risk studies, although a body of scholarly work (largely in the humanities) regarding Asian American gay, lesbian, and bisexual identities and sexual orientation exists (e.g., Leong, 1994, 1996). One study of 13 Japanese American gay men revealed that only half of their respondents were open with their families regarding their gay identity (Wooden, Kawasaki, & Mayeda, 1983). In a survey of 19 women and 16 men (ages 21–36) who identified as both Asian American and lesbian or gay, Chan (1989) found that they tended to be more involved in social and political activities in the lesbian-gay community than in the Asian American community. More than half of the respondents (57%) reported being more comfortable in the lesbian/gay community than in the Asian American community and identified more strongly with the gay or lesbian aspects of their identity, although a minority of the respondents reported a synthesized ethnic and sexual identities. Although the majority (77%) had come out to a family member (e.g., sibling), only 26% had disclosed their gay identity to their parents because of fear of rejection.

Finally, in a study investigating whether cultural backgrounds moderate the relationship between sexual orientation and gender-related personality traits, Lippa and Tan (2001) found that participants from more gender-polarized cultural backgrounds (Hispanics and Asian Americans) showed larger homosexual-heterosexual differences in gender-related traits than White Americans for both men and women. That is, Hispanic and Asian American gay men assumed more feminine roles and Hispanic and Asian American lesbians assumed more masculine roles with respect to occupational and hobby preferences as well as self-ascribed masculinity and femininity. Hispanic and Asian American gays and lesbians were also found to fear social disapproval of their homosexuality more than their White counterparts. Taken together, the findings from the few existing studies on sexual orientation among Asian Americans suggest possible influences of cultural and community factors in their sexual identity, disclosure of homosexuality, and gender-related traits.

Conclusion

Although there are significant gaps in the social science literature concerning Asian Americans' sexuality and sexual behavior, the existing data converge on notable differences between Asian Americans and other ethnic groups on major aspects such as sexual timetables and behaviors and attitudes surrounding sexuality, reproductive health, and sexual abuse. Many characteristics of the Asian Americans' sexual attitudes and behavior have significant implications for public health and clinical work. The next generation of empirical work must begin to test specific hypotheses regarding the Asian cultural characteristics as well as the impact of minority status on sexuality of Asian Americans.

References

Abraham, M. (1999). Sexual abuse in South Asian immigrant marriages. *Violence Against Women, 5,* 591–618.

Abramson, P. R., & Imai-Marquez, J. (1982). The Japanese-American: A cross-cultural, cross-sectional study of sex guilt. *Journal of Research in Personality,* 16, 227–237.

Abramson, P. R., Moriuchi, K. D., Waite, M. S., & Perry, L. B. (1983). Parental attitudes about sexual education: Cross-cultural differences and covariate controls. *Archives of Sexual Behavior, 12,* 381–397.

Chan, C. S. (1989). Issues of identity development among Asian-American lesbians and gay men. *Source Journal of Counseling & Development, 68,* 16–20.

Chan, D. W. (1986). Sex misinformation and misconceptions among Chinese medical students in Hong Kong. *Archives of Sexual Behavior, 19,* 73–93.

Cochran, S. D., Mays, V. M., & Leung, L. (1991). Sexual practices of heterosexual Asian-American young adults: Implications for risk of HIV infection. *Archives of Sexual Behavior, 20,* 381–391.

East, P. L. (1998). Racial and ethnic differences in girls' sexual, marital, and birth expectations. *Journal of Marriage & the Family, 60,* 150–162.

Feldman, S. S., Turner, R. A., & Araujo, K. (1999). Interpersonal context as an influence on sexual timetables of youths: Gender and ethnic effects. *Journal of Research on Adolescence, 9,* 25–52.

Frisch, M., & Goodman, M. T. (2000). Human papillomavirus-associated carcinomas in Hawaii and the mainland U.S. *Cancer, 88,* 1464–1469.

Futa, K. T., Hsu, E., & Hansen, D. J. (2001). Child sexual abuse in Asian American families: An examination of cultural factors that influence prevalence, identification, and treatment. *Clinical Psychology: Science & Practice, 8,* 189–209.

Grunbaum, J. A., Lowry, R., Kann, L., & Pateman, B. (2000). Prevalence of health risk behaviors among Asian American/Pacific Islander high school students. *Journal of Adolescent Health, 27,* 322–330.

Gupta, M. (1994). Sexuality in the Indian subcontinent. *Sexual & Marital Therapy, 9,* 57–69.

Hall, G. C. N., & Barongan, C. (1997). Prevention of sexual aggression: Sociocultural risk and protective factors. *American Psychologist, 52,* 5–14.

Hall, G. C. N., Sue, S., Narang, D. S., & Lilly, R. S. (2000). Culture-specific models of men's sexual aggression: Intra- and interpersonal determinants. *Cultural Diversity & Ethnic Minority Psychology, 6,* 252–267.

Hall, G. C. N., Windover, A. K., & Maramba, G. G. (1998). Sexual aggression among Asian Americans: Risk and protective factors. *Cultural Diversity & Ethnic Minority Psychology, 4,* 305–318.

Harman, M. J., & Johnson, J. A. (1995). Cross-cultural sex education: aspects of age, source, and sex equity. *TCA Journal, 23*(2), 1–11.

Hedeen, A. N., White, E., & Taylor, V. (1999). Ethnicity and birthplace in relation to tumor size and stage in Asian American women with breast cancer. *American Journal of Public Health, 89,* 1248–1252.

Hiatt, R. A., Pasick, R. J., Perez-Stable, E. J., McPhee, S. J., Engelsatd, L., Lee, M., Sabogal, F., D'Onofrio, C. N., & Stewart, S. (1996). Pathways to early cancer detection in the multiethnic population of the San Francisco Bay Area. *Health Education Quarterly, 23 (Suppl.),* S10–S27.

Horan, P. F., & DiClemente, R. J. (1993). HIV knowledge, communication, and risk behavior among White, Chinese-, and Filipino-American adolescents in a high-prevalence AIDS epicenter: A comparative analysis. *Ethnicity & Disease, 3,* 97–105.

Huang, K., & Uba, L. (1992). Premarital sexual behavior among Chinese college students in the United States. *Archives of Sexual Behavior, 21,* 227–240.

Ima, K., & Hohm, C. F. (1991). Child maltreatment among Asian and Pacific Islander refugees and immigrants: The San Diego case. *Journal of Interpersonal Violence, 6,* 267–285.

Jenkins, C. N. H., & Kagawa-Singer, M. (1994). Cancer. In N. W. S. Zane, D. T. Takeuchi, & K. N. J. Young (Eds.), *Confronting critical health issues of Asian and Pacific Islander Americans,* (pp. 105–147). Thousand Oaks, CA: Sage.

Kenny, M. C., & McEachern, A. G. (2000). Racial, ethnic, and cultural factors of childhood sexual abuse: A selected review of the literature. *Clinical Psychology Review, 20,* 905–922.

Koss, M. P., Gidycz, C. A., & Wisniewski, N. (1987). The scope of rape: Incidence and prevalence of sexual aggression and victimization in a national sample of higher education students. *Journal of Consulting & Clinical Psychology, 55,* 162–170.

Kulig, J. C. (1994). Sexuality beliefs among Cambodians: Implications for health care professionals. *Health Care for Women International, 15,* 69–76.

Laumann, E. O., Gagnon, J. H., Michael, R. T., & Michaels, S. (1994). *The social organization of sexuality: Sexual practices in the United States.* Chicago: The University of Chicago Press.

Lee, M. (1998). Breast and cervical cancer early detection in Chinese American women. *Asian American & Pacific Islander Journal of Health, 6,* 351–357.

Leong, R. (Ed.) (1994). Dimensions of desire [Special issue]. *Amerasia Journal, 20*(1).

Leong, R. (Ed.) (1996). *Asian American sexualities: Dimensions of the gay and lesbian experience.* New York: Routledge.

Lippa, R. A., & Tan, F. D. (2001). Does culture moderate the relationship between sexual orientation and gender-related personality traits? *Cross-Cultural Research, 35,* 65–87.

Lu, Z. J. (1995). Variables associated with breast self-examination among Chinese women. *Cancer Nursing, 18,* 29–34.

Lum, J. L. (1998). Family violence. In L. C. Lee & N. W. S. Zane (Eds.), *Handbook of Asian American psychology,* (pp. 505–525). Thousand Oaks, CA: Sage.

McKelvey, R. S., & Webb, J. A. (1995). A pilot study of abuse among Vietnamese Amerasians. *Child Abuse & Neglect, 19,* 545–553.

McLaughlin, C. S., Chen, C., Greenberger, E., & Biermeier, C. (1997). Family, peer, and individual correlates of sexual experience among Caucasian and Asian American late adolescents. *Journal of Research on Adolescence, 7,* 33–53.

Meston, C. M., Heiman, J. R., & Trapnell, P. D. (1999). The relation between early abuse and adult sexuality. *The Journal of Sex Research, 36,* 385–395.

Meston, C. M., Heiman, J. R., Trapnell, P. D., & Carlin, A. S. (1999). Ethnicity, desirable responding, and self-reports of abuse: A comparison of European- and Asian-ancestry undergraduates. *Journal of Consulting & Clinical Psychology, 67,* 139–144.

Meston, C. M., Trapnell, P. D., & Gorzalka, B. B. (1996). Ethnic and gender differences in sexuality: Variations in sexual behavior between Asian and non-Asian university students. *Archives of Sexual Behavior, 25,* 33–72.

Meston, C. M., Trapnell, P. D., & Gorzalka, B. B. (1998). Ethnic, gender, and length-of-residency influences on sexual knowledge and attitudes. *The Journal of Sex Research, 35,* 176–188.

Miller, B. A., Kolonel, L. N., Bernstein, L., Young, J. L., Swanson, G. M., West, D., Key, C. R., Liffy, J. M., Glover, C. S., Alexander, G. A., et al. (Eds). (1996). *Racial/ethnic patterns of cancer in the United States, 1988–1992, NIH Publication No. 96 4104.* Bethesda, MD: National Cancer Institute.

Mo, B. (1992). Modesty, sexuality, and breast health in Chinese-American women. *Western Journal of Medicine, 157,* 260–264.

Mollica, R., Wyshak, G., & Lavelle, J. (1987). The psychological impact of war trauma and torture on Southeast Asian refugees. *American Journal of Psychiatry, 144,* 1567–1571.

Mori, L., Bernat, J. A., Glenn, P. A., Selle, L. L., & Zarate, M. G. (1995). Attitudes toward rape: Gender and ethnic differences across Asian and Caucasian college students. *Sex Roles, 32,* 457–467.

National Asian Women's Health Organization. (1995). *Perceptions of risk: An assessment of the factors influencing use of reproductive and sexual health services by Asian American women.* San Francisco: Author.

National Asian Women's Health Organization. (1997). *Expanding options: A reproductive and sexual health survey of Asian American women.* San Francisco: Author.

National Asian Women's Health Organization. (1999). *The Asian American men's health survey: Sharing responsibility.* San Francisco: Author.

Okamura, A., Heras., P., & Wong-Kerberg, L. (1995). Asian, Pacific Island, and Filipino Americans and sexual child abuse. In L. A. Fontes (Ed.), *Sexual abuse in nine North American cultures: Treatment and prevention* (pp. 67–93). Thousand Oaks, CA: Sage.

Rao, K., DiClemente, R. J., & Ponton, L. E. (1992). Child sexual abuse of Asians compared with other populations. *Journal of the American Academy of Child & Adolescent Psychiatry, 31,* 880–886.

Rozée, P. D., & Van Boemel, G. (1989). The psychological effects of war trauma and abuse on older Cambodian refugee women. *Women & Therapy, 8*(4), 23–50.

Schuster, M. A., Bell, R. M., & Kanouse, D. E. (1996). The sexual practices of adolescent virgins: Genital sexual activities of high school students who have never had vaginal intercourse. *American Journal of Public Health, 86,* 1570–1576.

Schuster, M. A., Bell, R. M., Nakajima, G. A., & Kanouse, D. E. (1998). The sexual practices of Asian and Pacific Islander high school students *Journal of Adolescent Health, 23,* 221_231.

Schuster, M. A., Bell, R. M., Petersen, L. P., & Kanouse, D. E. (1996). Communication between adolescents and physicians about sexual behavior and risk prevention. *Archives of Pediatric and Adolescent Medicine, 150,* 906–913.

Scully, M., Kuoch, T., & Miller, R. A. (1995). Cambodians and sexual child abuse. In L. A. Fontes (Ed.), *Sexual abuse in nine North American cultures: Treatment and prevention* (pp. 97–127). Thousand Oaks, CA: Sage.

Song, Y. I. (1996). *Battered women in Korean immigrant families.* New York: Garland.

Sue, D. (1982). Sexual experience and attitudes of Asian American students. *Psychological Report, 51,* 401–402.

Tang, T. S., Solomon, L. J., Yeh, C. J., & Worden, J. K. (1999). The role of cultural variables in breast self-examination and cervical cancer screening behavior in young Asian women living in the United States. *Journal of Behavioral Medicine, 22,* 419–436.

Tiongson, A. T., Jr. (1997). Throwing the baby out with the bathwater. Situating young Filipino mothers and fathers beyond the dominant discourse on adolescent pregnancy. In M. P. P. Root

(Ed.), *Filipino Americans: Transformation and identity* (pp. 257–271). Thousand Oaks, CA: Sage Publications.

Tsui, A. M. (1985). Psychotherapeutic considerations in sexual counseling of Asian immigrants. *Psychotherapy, 22,* 357–362.

Tsuneyoshi, S. (1996). Rape trauma syndrome: Case illustration of Elizabeth, an 18–year-old Asian American. In F. H. McClure & E. Teyber (Eds.), *Child and adolescent therapy: A multi-cultural relational approach* (pp. 287–320). New York: Harcourt Brace College Publishers.

Tu, S., Taplin, S. H., Barlow, W. E., & Boyko, E. J. (1999). Breast cancer screening by Asian-American women in a managed care environment. *American Journal of Preventive Medicine, 17,* 55–61.

Upchurch, D. M., Levy-Storms, L., Sucoff, C. A., & Aneshensel, C. S. (1998). Gender and ethnic differences in the timing of first sexual intercourse. *Family Planning Perspectives, 30,* 121–127.

Urquiza, A. J., & Goodlin-Jones, B. L. (1994). Child sexual abuse and adult revictimization with women of color. *Violence & Victims, 9,* 223–232.

U.S. Bureau of the Census. (1993). *We the Americans: Asians.* Washington, DC: U.S. Government Printing Office.

Wong, D. (1987). Preventing child sexual assault among Southeast Asian refugee families. *Child Today, 16,* 18–22.

Wooden, W. S., Kawasaki, H., & Mayeda, R. (1983). Lifestyles and identity maintenance among gay Japanese-American males. *Alternative Lifestyles, 5,* 236–243.

Yick, A. G. (2000). Domestic violence beliefs and attitudes in the Chinese American community. *Journal of Social Service Research, 27,* 29–51.

Yu, E. S. H., Kim, K. K., Chen, E. H., & Brintnall, R. A. (2001). Breast and cervical cancer screening among Chinese American women. *Cancer Practice, 9,* 81–91.

Yu, M. Y., Seetoo, A. D., Tsai, C. K., & Sun, C. (1998). Sociodemographic predictors of Papanicolaou smear test and mammography use among women of Chinese descent in Southeastern Michigan. *Womens Health Issues, 8,* 372–381.

Mass Media Influences on Sexuality

Jane D. Brown

4

CHAPTER

The mainstream mass media (television, magazines, movies, music, and the Internet) provide increasingly frequent portrayals of sexuality. We still know relatively little about how this content is used and how it affects sexual beliefs and behaviors. The few available studies suggest that the media do have an impact because the media keep sexual behavior on public and personal agendas, media portrayals reinforce a relatively consistent set of sexual and relationship norms, and the media rarely depict sexually responsible models. More longitudinal research, especially with early adolescents is needed to learn more about how media content is attended to, interpreted, and incorporated into developing sexual lives.

The mass media are an increasingly accessible way for people to learn about and see sexual behavior. The media may be especially important for young people as they are developing their own sexual beliefs and patterns of behavior, and as parents and schools remain reluctant to discuss sexual topics.

In the United States, young people spend 6 to 7 hours each day on average with some form of media. A national survey in 1999 found that one third of young children (2 to 7 years old) and two thirds of older children and adolescents (8 to 18 years old) have a television in their own bedroom. Many of those televisions also are hooked up to cable and a Videocassette Recorder (VCR) (Roberts, 2000).

Sexual talk and displays are increasingly frequent and explicit in this mediated world. One content analysis found that sexual content that ranged from flirting to sexual intercourse had increased from slightly more than half of television programs in 1997–1998 to more than two-thirds of the programs in the 1999–2000 season. Depiction of intercourse (suggestive or explicit) occurred in one of every 10 programs (Kunkel, Cope-Farrar, Biely, Farinola, & Donnerstein, 2001).

From *Journal of Sex Research,* Vol. 39, No. 1, February 2002. Permission conveyed through Copyright Clearance Center.

One fifth to one half of music videos, depending on the music genre (e.g., country, rock, rap) portray sexuality or eroticism (DuRant et al., 1997). Two thirds of Hollywood movies made each year are R-rated; most young people have seen these movies long before they are the required 16 years old (Greenberg et al., 1993). Although teen girls' and women's magazines, such as *Seventeen* and *Glamour* have increased their coverage of sexual health issues over the past decade, the majority of advertising and editorial content in these magazines remains focused on what girls and women should do to get and keep their man (Walsh-Childers, Gotthoffer, & Lepre, 2002).

Gay, lesbian, bisexual, and transgender youth rarely find themselves represented in the mainstream media. Although a few of the youth-targeted programs such as "Dawson's Creek" and "Will and Grace" have included gay characters, what some have called *compulsory heterosexuality* prevails (Rich, 1986; Wolf & Kielwasser, 1991).

The Internet has increased dramatically the availability of sexually explicit content. Computer and Internet use is diffusing more rapidly than any previous technology; as of the end of 1999, more than half (56%) of all adults in the United States were online. It is expected that by 2010 most U.S. homes with children will have access to the Internet (Taylor, 1999).

The word *sex* is the most popular search term used on the Internet today (CyberAtlas, 2001). The Internet may have both positive and negative effects on sexual health. According to one national survey of young people (10–17 years old) who regularly used the Internet, one out of four said he or she had encountered unwanted pornography in the past year, and one out of five had been exposed to unwanted sexual solicitations or approaches (Finkelhor, Mitchell, & Wolak, 2000). At the same time, a number of sites, such as the American Social Health Association's iwannaknow.org, promote healthy sexual behavior and provide young people with advice on communication in relationships as well as methods for protecting against sexually transmitted diseases.

Despite increasing public concern about the potential health risks of early, unprotected sexual activity, most of the mass media rarely depict three C's of responsible sexual behavior: Commitment, Contraceptives, and consideration of Consequences. Although more than half of the couples who engage in sexual intercourse on television are in an established relationship, 1 in 10 are couples who have met only recently; one quarter do not maintain a relationship after having sex (Kunkel et al., 2001).

Only about 1 in 10 of the programs on television that include sexual content mentions the possible consequences or the need to use contraceptives or protection against STDs. Unintended pregnancies rarely are shown as the outcome of unprotected sex, and STDs other than HIV/AIDS are almost never discussed (Kunkel et al., 2001). Abortion is a taboo topic, too controversial for commercial television and magazines (Walsh-Childers et al., 2002).

Do audiences learn about sex from this array of sexual information and portrayals? The perceived sensitivity of sex as a research topic and a focus on television to the exclusion of other media unfortunately has restricted the kind of research that has been done. Much of the empirical work has been analyses of content that allow only speculation about what effects the content might have on audiences. But an emerging set of studies that go beyond content to address how audiences select, interpret, and apply sexual content suggests that the media may plan an important role, especially for young people (Steele, 1999).

Selection of Sexual Media Content

When asked where they have learned the most about sex, younger adolescents (13–15 years old) rank the mass media fourth behind parents, friends, and schools. Older adolescents (16–17 years old) put friends first, then parents, and then the media (Yankelovich Partners, 1993). More than half of the high school boys and girls in a national survey in 1997 said they had learned about birth control, contraception, or preventing pregnancy from television; almost two thirds (63%) of the girls (and 40% of the boys) said they had learned about these topics from magazines (Sutton, Brown, Wilson, & Klein, 2002).

The media are used as sources of information about sexuality at some times more than others. One qualitative study found three patterns of sexual media use among early adolescent girls (11–15 years old) that suggested that sexual portrayals in the media were attended to more when girls were interested personally in learning about relationship norms, strategies for establishing relationships, and tips on how to get sexually attractive. Some girls still found depictions of sex in the media (e.g., nudity in advertisements) "gross" and "disgusting," while other girls had papered their walls with images of media models they lusted after or aspired to be. Still other girls, typically those who had been involved in sexual relationships, were less enamored with the mainstream media's sexual fantasy and had turned to "oppositional" media (e.g., fringe music groups, teen-produced magazines, aka 'zines) that spoke more to the kinds of relationships they wanted (Brown, White, & Nikopoulou, 1993).

We know that patterns of media use differ dramatically by age, gender, race/ethnicity, and socioeconomic level. Girls and women typically choose softer music, and more relationship-oriented television programs, movies, and magazines, while boys and men prefer more action and activity-oriented media and sports programming, heavier rock and rap music, action and adventure movies, music, and sports magazines. African Americans typically view more television than Whites, prefer television programming and movies that feature Black characters, and listen to different genres of music (Roberts, 2000; Roe, 1998). Thus, it is important to consider the media's effects on sexuality within subgroups: All people will not be seeing the same set of sexual messages—some will see much more than others, some will be seeking out the sexual content, some will try not to be exposed to it.

Interpretation

All members of an audience also will not see or interpret the same messages in the same way (Zillmann & Bryant, 1985). One striking example of differences in interpretation was found in an analysis of one of rock star Madonna's early music videos, "Papa Don't Preach." When first released, newspaper columnist Ellen Goodman called it "a commercial for teenage pregnancy," while the religious right said it was a stand against abortion. College students who saw the video differed in their "reading" of the video, too. Although most White females thought the video was about a teen girl deciding to keep her unborn child ("baby"), Black males were more likely to think the girl (Madonna) in the video was singing about wanting to keep her boyfriend "baby." Since the young men were identifying primarily with the dilemma of the boyfriend in the video, they were less likely than the female viewers to see or hear the cues that suggested pregnancy (Brown & Schulze, 1990).

Other studies also conclude that young males and females interpret media content differently. Ward and her colleagues (Ward, Gorvine, & Cytron, 2001) have shown college students portions of situation comedies such as "Roseanne" and "Martin." They find that young women are more likely than young men to think the sexual scenes they see are realistic, and the women are more approving than the men of behaviors that are relationship-maintaining (e.g., jealous husband protecting wife) and less approving of relationship threats (E.g., man contemplating cheating).

Application

As people attend to and interpret sexual media content, they also evaluate and may or may not incorporate what they are seeing in their own developing sense of sexuality. This is the step that we traditionally have thought of as media effects. Does the sexual content in the media influence how people behave sexually? Are people having sex earlier, with more partners, without protection or affection because of what they see in the media?

The answer to these questions is a qualified "yes." Qualified, because even though we know a fair amount about the ubiquity of sexual content in the media, we still have only sparse research on the effects of sexual media content. According to classic social scientific methods, an ideal test of the effects of sexual media content would involve either randomized assignment to different sexual media diets, or longitudinal surveys. Such studies would establish whether media exposure or behavior came first, and would allow for generalizations about what kinds of media content cause what kinds of behaviors.

The relatively few correlational and still fewer experimental studies of the relationship between exposure to sexual media content and effects suggest that the media do have an impact in at least three ways: (a) by keeping sexual behavior on public and personal agendas, (b) by reinforcing a relatively consistent set of sexual and relationship norms, and (c) by rarely including sexually responsible models. Three theoretical perspectives often used by communication researchers: (a) Agenda Setting/Framing, (b) Cultivation, and (c) Cognitive Social Learning Theory, help to explain why we expect these outcomes.

Agenda Setting/Framing

Agenda Setting and Framing Theories propose that the media tell people both what is important in the world around them, and how to think about the events and people who inhabit that world (Kosicki, 1993). Although rarely thought of as sex educators, even the news media help keep sexual behavior salient. The American public and policy makers frequently are faced with news stories about abandoned babies, sex-enhancing drugs, and even presidential sexual affairs. Topics and images that are frequent and prominent in the media become topics that audiences think are important.

Early coverage of the AIDS epidemic provides a good example of how agenda setting and framing work in relation to a sexual health issue. When AIDS was first discovered, the media were slow to cover the story because it was considered a problem only for gay men, intravenous drug users, and a few Hemophiliacs. It took a number of years and the deaths of celebrities such as Rock Hudson for the media to put the problem higher on the news agenda, and even longer for the frame to shift from one of a problem of morality to one of a threat to the public's health (Rogers, Dearing, & Chang, 1991).

The media are in a unique position to get people thinking and talking about specific issues, while keeping other issues from the public eye. The people who are cited or figure prominently in the stories become known as the heroes or the villains, while some solutions and not others are offered. People use the stories they see both in the news and in entertainment media as reference points about what's important and to compare what they already know, or think they know about what's good and bad, and what should be done about problems. The result often reinforces stereotypes and helps define what is considered appropriate and inappropriate behavior in the culture (Iyengar, 1991).

Cultivation Theory

According to Cultivation Theory, television is the most powerful storyteller in the culture, one that continually repeats the myths and ideologies, the facts and patterns of relationships that define and legitimize the social order. According to the cultivation hypothesis, a steady dose of television, over time, acts like the pull of gravity toward an imagined center. This pull results in a shared set of conceptions and expectations about reality among otherwise ??erse viewers (Gerbner, Gross, Morgan, & Signorelli, 1994).

Tests of the hypothesis have found, for example, that junior and senior high school students who frequently viewed daytime soap operas were more likely than those who watched less often to believe that single mothers have relatively easy lives, have good jobs, and do not live in poverty (Larson, 1996). Exposure to stereotypical images of gender and sexuality in music videos had been found to increase older adolescents' acceptance of nonmarital sexual behavior and interpersonal violence (Greeson & Williams, 1986; Kalof, 1999). Heavier television viewers also have been found to have more negative attitudes toward remaining a virgin (Courtright & Baran, 1980).

Others have shown that prolonged exposure to erotica leads to exaggerated estimates of the prevalence of more unusual kinds of sexual activity (e.g., group sex, sadomasochistic practices, bestiality), less expectation of sexual exclusivity with partners, and apprehension that sexual inactivity constitutes a health risk (Zillmann, 2000). In one experimental study, college student who were exposed to about 5 hours of sexually explicit films over 6 weeks were more likely than a control group to express increased callousness toward women and trivialize rape as a criminal offense (Zillmann & Bryant, 1982).

Two correlational studies have found relationships between the frequency of television viewing and initiation of intercourse in samples of high school students. However, because these were only cross-sectional analyses, it was not possible to say with certainty which came first—the TV viewing or the sexual behavior (Brown & Newcomer, 1991; Peterson, Moore, & Furstenberg, 1991). It is possible that teens who were becoming interested in sex had turned to sexual content in the media because it was now salient in their lives. It also is possible that the teens saw the ubiquitous and typically risk-free sexual media content as encouragement for them to engage in sexual behavior sooner than they might have otherwise. It is most likely that both causal sequences are operating, but longitudinal studies of young adolescents are needed to conclude that with more certainty.

Cognitive Social Learning Theory

Cognitive Social Learning Theory and its earlier variant, Social Learning Theory, predict that people will imitate behaviors of others when those models are rewarded or not punished for their behavior. Modeling will occur more readily when the model is perceived as attractive and similar and the modeled behavior is possible, salient, simple, prevalent, and has functional value (Bandura, 1994). Thus, the theory predicts that people who attend to media content that includes depictions of attractive characters who enjoy having sexual intercourse and rarely suffer any negative consequences will be likely to imitate the behavior.

A related idea is that the media provide cognitive scripts for sexual behavior that people may not be able to see anywhere else (Gagnon & Simon, 1973). Sexually inexperienced people especially may use the media to fill in the gaps in their understanding about how a particular sexual scenario might work (e.g., kissing goodnight at the end of a date, having sex with a new or multiple partners). Walsh-Childers (1990) found that viewers' own expectations for using condoms were affected by depiction of condom use in a soap opera, for example.

What's typically missing from the media's current sexual script, however, is anything having to do with the possible negative consequences of sexual activity or ways to prevent negative outcomes, so it is unlikely that protective behavior could be imitated. Content analyses suggest that media audiences are most likely to learn that sex is consequence-free, rarely planned, and more a matter of lust than love (Kunkel et al., 1999; Ward, 1995). From the most sexually explicit media content, now more readily available than ever before on the Internet, cable TV, and videocassettes, they are likely to learn patterns of aggressive sexual behavior, as well (Zillmann, 2000).

Conclusion

In sum, the relatively few existing studies of the selection, interpretation, and application of sexual content in the media suggest that the mass media can affect awareness of, beliefs about, and possibly actual sexual behavior. More research is needed to say more precisely with which audiences, under what circumstances, and with which content effects occur. Such research is especially relevant as access to increasingly explicit sexual material increases and other potential perspectives on sexually responsible behavior, such as parents, schools, and faith communities, remain relatively reticent.

References

Bandura, A. (1994). Social cognitive theory of mass communication. In J. Bryant & D. Zillman (Eds.), *Media effects: Advances in theory and research* (pp. 61–90). Hillsdale, NJ: Lawrence Erlbaum.

Brown, J. D., & Newcomer, S. (1991). Television viewing and adolescents' sexual behavior. *Journal of Homosexuality, 21,* 77–91.

Brown, J. D., & Schulze, L. (1990). The effects of race, gender, and fandom on audience interpretation of Madonna's music videos. In B. S. Greenberg, J. D. Brown, & N. Buerkel-Rothfuss (Eds.), *Media, sex and the adolescent* (pp. 263–276). Cresskill, NJ: Hampton Press, Inc.

Brown, J. D., White A. B., & Nikopoulou, L. (1993). Disinterest, intrigue, resistance: Early adolescents girls' use of sexual media content. In B. S. Greenberg, J. D. Brown, & N. Buerkel-Rothfuss (Eds.), *Media, sex and the adolescent* (pp. 177–195). Cresskill, NJ: Hampton Press, Inc.

Courtwright, J., & Baran, S. (1980). The acquisition of sexual information by young people. *Journalism Quarterly, 57,* 107–114.

CyberAtlas (2001). Search engines, browsers still confusing many web users. Retrieved August 25, 2001 from the World Wide Web: http://cyberatlas.internet.com/big_picture/traffic_patterns/article/0,,5931_588851,00.html.

DuRant, R., Rome, E. S., Rich, M. Allred, E., Emans, S. J., & Woods, E. R. (1997). Tobacco and alcohol use behaviors portrayed in music videos: A content analysis. *American Journal of Public Health, 87,* 1131–1135.

Finkelhor, D., Mitchell, K., & Wolak, J. (2000). *Online victimization: A report on the nation's youth.* Washington, DC: National Center for Missing and Exploited Children.

Gagnon, J., & Simon, W. (1973). *Sexual conduct: The social sources of human sexuality.* Chicago: Aldine.

Gerbner, G., Gross, L., Morgan, M., & Signorelli, N. (1994). Growing up with television: The cultivation perspective. In J. Bryant & D. Zillman (Eds.), *Media effects: Advances in theory and research* (pp. 17–41). Hillsdale, NJ: Lawrence Erlbaum Assoc.

Greenberg, B. S., Siemicki, M., Dorfman, S., Heeter, C., Lin, C., Stanley, C., & Soderman, A. (1993). Sex content in R-rated films viewed by adolescents. In B. S. Greenberg, J. D. Brown, & N. Buerkel-Rothfuss (Eds.), *Media, sex and the adolescent* (pp. 45–58). Cresskill, NJ: Hampton Press, Inc.

Greeson, L. E., & Williams, R. A. (1986). Social implications of music videos for youth: An analysis of the content and effects of MTV. *Youth & Society, 18,* 177–189.

Iyengar, S. (1991). *Is anyone responsible? How television frames political issues.* Chicago: University of Chicago Press.

Kalof, L. (1999). The effects of gender and music video imagery on sexual attitudes. *The Journal of Social Psychology, 139,* 378–386.

Kosicki, G. (1993). Problems and opportunities in agenda-setting research. *Journal of Communication, 43,* 100–127.

Kunkel, D., Cope, K., Farinola, W., Biely, E., Rollin, E., & Donnerstein, E. (1999). *Sex on TV: A biennial report to the Kaiser Family Foundation, 2001.* Menlo Park, CA: The Henry J. Kaiser Family Foundation.

Larson, M. (1996). Sex roles and soap operas: What adolescents learn about single motherhood. *Sex Roles: A Journal of Research, 35,* 97–121.

Peterson, J., Moore, K., & Furstenberg, F. (1991). Television viewing and early initiation of sexual intercourse. Is there a link? *Journal of Homosexuality, 21,* 93–118.

Rich, A. (1986). *Blood, bread, and poetry: Selected prose 1979–85.* New York: Norton.

Roberts, D. (2000). Media and youth: Access, exposure, and privatization. *Journal of Adolescent Health, 27*(2), 8–14.

Roe, K. (1998). Boys will be boys and girls will be girls: Changes in children's media use. *European Journal of Communication Research, 23,* 5–25.

Rogers, E., Dearing, J., & Chang, S. (1991). AIDS in the 1980's: The agenda-setting process for a public issue. *Journalism Monographs, 126.*

Steele, J. R. (1999). Teenage sexuality and media practice: Factoring in the influences of family, friends and school. *The Journal of Sex Research, 36,* 331–341.

Sutton, M. J., Brown, J. D., Wilson, K. M., & Klein, J. D. (2002). Shaking the tree of knowledge for forbidden fruit: Where adolescents learn about sexuality and contraception. In J. D. Brown, J. R. Steele, & K. Walsh-Childers (Eds.), *Sexual teens, sexual media* (pp. 25–55). Mahwah, NJ: Lawrence Erlbaum Associates, Inc.

Taylor, H. (1999, Dec. 22). Online population growth surges to 56% of all adults. Retrieved June 29, 2000 from the World Wide Web: http://www.harrisinteractive.com.

Walsh-Childers, K. (1990). *Adolescents' sexual schemas and interpretations of male-female relationships in a soap opera.* Unpublished doctoral dissertation, University of North Carolina-Chapel Hill.

Walsh-Childers, K., Gotthoffer, A., & Lepre, C. R. (2002). From "Just the Facts" to "Downright Salacious": Teen's and women's magazines' coverage of sex and sexual health. In J. D. Brown, J. R. Steele, & K. Walsh-Childers (Eds.), *Sexual teens, sexual media* (pp. 153–172). Mahwah, NJ: Lawrence Erlbaum Associates, Inc.

Ward, L. M. (1995). Talking about sex: Common themes about sexuality in the prime-time television programs children and adolescents view most. *Journal of Youth and Adolescence, 24,* 595–615.

Ward, L. M., Gorvine, B., & Cytron, A. (2002). Would that really happen? Adolescents' perceptions of sexuality according to prime-time television. In J. D. Brown, J. R. Steele, & K. Walsh-Childers (Eds.), *Sexual teens, sexual media* (pp. 95–124). Mahwah, NJ: Lawrence Erlbaum Associates, Inc.

Wolf, M. A., & Kielwasser, A. P. (1991). *Gay people, sex, and the media.* New York: Harrington Park Press.

Yankelovich Partners, Inc. (1993, May 24). How should we teach our children about sex? *Time,* 60–66.

Zillmann, D. (2000). Influence of unrestrained access to erotica on adolescents' and young adults' dispositions toward sexuality. *Journal of Adolescent Health, 27*(2), 41–45.

Zillmann, D., & Bryant, J. (1982). Pornography, sexual callousness, and the trivialization of rape. *Journal of Communication, 32*(4), 10–21.

Zillmann, D., & Bryant, J. (Eds.). (1985). *Selective exposure to communication.* Hillsdale, NJ: Lawrence Erlbaum Assoc., Inc.

Section II

Adolescence and Sexuality

Early Sexual Maturation Increasingly Common among Girls

5

C H A P T E R

Henry J. Kaiser Family Foundation

More girls today appear to be reaching puberty at younger ages than their mothers, sparking various theories that try to find a reason for precocious **sexual** development, the AP/Seattle Times reports. At the age of 8, nearly 50% of black girls and 15% of white girls begin to develop breasts or pubic hair, and at 9, these percentages go up to 77% and 33%, respectively. What is "more striking" is that 27% of black girls and 7% of white girls develop these "early puberty signs" at age 7, three years younger than most parents and doctors expect to see them. There is no explanation for the racial differences and no reported figures for Hispanic or **Asian**-American girls. Studies on a possible early pubertal shift for boys have just begun (Neergaard, AP/Seattle Times, 2/13). In a 1997 "landmark study" of 17,000 girls, Dr. Marcia Herman-Giddens of the University of North Carolina "sparked concern" with her findings that "outward signs of puberty that precede menstruation," such as breast buds and pubic hair, were occurring in younger girls. Dr. Gilbert August, a pediatric endocrinologist, said parents worry about the effects of early puberty. "From a psychosocial standpoint, you have a child who looks sexually mature at an age where they can't make judgments associated with their physical appearance" (AP/Detroit Free Press, 2/13). Doctors can administer the drug Lupron to stall puberty, but unless the girls are extremely young or have other medical problems, they more often recommend counseling or support groups instead. The "good news" is that the age of menstruation has held steady since 1960, after it dropped to the ages of 12 and 13 from age 17 in the 19th century (AP/Newark Star-Ledger, 2/13).

Although no one is certain what is causing the shift to earlier physical development, fat is the "leading theory," because childhood obesity has doubled since 1980 and fatter

Reprinted with permission from kaisernetwork.org. You can view the entire Kaiser Daily HIV/AIDS Report, search the archives, and sign up for email delivery at www.kaisernetwork.org/dailyreports/hiv. The Kaiser Daily HIV/AIDS Report is published for kaisernetwork.cor, a free service of The Henry J. Kaiser Family Foundation. (c) 2001 Advisory Board Company and Kaiser Foundation. All rights reserved.

bodies convert more adrenal hormones into the female sex hormone estrogen. Furthermore, overweight children have more insulin in their blood, which also affects maturation, and researchers are studying whether the fat cell-produced protein leptin influences glands that produce sex-related hormones. In addition, overweight children may not be getting enough exercise, an activity that can delay puberty. A more "controversial" explanation for early **sexual** maturation is exposure to chemicals like plastics and cosmetics called phthalates that may "disrupt" girls' normal hormone function (AP/Houston Chronicle, 2/13). A Puerto Rico study of girls with "bafflingly high rates of early breast development" found higher phthalate levels in the blood of girls who matured earlier than others, but researchers agree that more study on this is needed (*AP/Detroit Free Press*, 2/13). In rare cases, a cyst or tumor may cause "extremely early" puberty (*AP/Houston Chronicle*, 2/13).

Decline in Teen Pregnancy Due to Both Less Sexual Activity and More Contraceptive Use: More Evidence That Young People Benefit from a Comprehensive Approach to Sexuality Education

CHAPTER

SIECUS

A report released in the *Journal of Adolescent Health* concluded that less sexual activity and increased contraceptive use among teens are nearly equally responsible for the recent decline in teen pregnancy rates. The pregnancy rate among teens ages 15 to 17 declined by 33% between 1991 and 2000. For this study, researchers analyzed data to estimate how much of this decline could be attributed to changes in sexual behavior and how much could be attributed to contraceptive use.

"We have known for a number of years that more young people are choosing to delay sexual intercourse and that more sexually active young people are using condoms and other contraceptive methods," explained William Smith, director of public policy for the Sexuality Information and Education Council of the United States (SIECUS). "This study affirms that these responsible decisions on the part of young people are having an important impact," Smith continued.

The study found that sexual experience among high school students decreased 16% between 1991 and 2001. At the same time fewer sexually active high school students relied on ineffective methods like withdrawal, or engaged in intercourse without using any method of contraception. Instead, more high school students relied on condoms with use of this important method rising among sexually active students from 37% in 1991 to 46% in 2001.

"This study clearly demonstrates that young people are making a variety of responsible choices and that it is critical for us to provide them with all of the information they need to prevent unintended pregnancy," said Smith. "Unfortunately, too many programs today focus exclusively on abstinence-until-marriage and people may inaccurately use this new research to bolster that unproven approach."

Since 1998, federal and state lawmakers have spent nearly $900 million dollars on abstinence-only-until-marriage programs that discourage the use of condoms and other contraceptive methods to prevent pregnancy. President Bush is seeking to spend an additional $270 million this fiscal year.

"Helping teens delay sexual intercourse is an important goal but we know that over 60% of young people are sexually active before they graduate from high school and it is unconscionable that any program would deprive them of important, medically accurate information about contraception," Smith continued.

"We know what works. Comprehensive education about sexuality that fully informs youth about their sexual health, including messages about abstinence and contraception, has been proven to delay sexual activity and increase contraceptive use," explained Smith. "This study is a testament to all of the progress that young people have made. If abstinence-only-until-marriage programs are allowed to continue unchallenged, however, much this of progress may be reversed," he concluded.

Relationship Type, Goals Predict the Consistency of Teenagers' Condom Use

CHAPTER

Alan Guttmacher Institute

Adolescents who consistently use condoms during sex differ from those who do not in terms of the types of relationships in which they are involved, their goals in relationships and their motivations for having sex, according to a 2001 study of Dutch vocational high school students. Among young people who had had sex with a steady partner but had never had casual intercourse, those who used condoms consistently had a more positive attitude about condom use and perceived more social pressure to use condoms, but needed less intimacy in a relationship and less often had sex to express love than those who engaged in unsafe sex. For those who had had casual sex, consistent condom use was positively correlated with perceived ability to use condoms in difficult situations, attitude regarding condoms and perceived social pressure to use condoms.

To examine whether certain behaviors, attitudes and motives regarding sex and condom use are associated with consistent condom use within casual and steady adolescent relationships, researchers recruited students from five Dutch vocational high schools to complete a questionnaire. Participants answered questions about their sexual history, condom use, attitude toward condom use, perceived social pressure to use condoms, perceived ability to use condoms in difficult situations (i.e., while drunk or highly aroused, when their partner does not want to and during unexpected sex), need for intimacy within relationships and motivations for having sex. The researchers analyzed the data using Pearson correlations, Student's t-tests and discriminant analyses.

Of the 701 students interviewed, 60% were male and 40% were female; their ages ranged between 15 and 23, and averaged 18. The vast majority (89–91%) were born in the Netherlands and still lived at home. Eighty-six percent had ever had a relationship, and 43% were involved in a relationship at the time of the study. Two-thirds of respondents had ever had sex; of these, one-third had had one partner, nearly a third had had

Rosenberg J, Relationship type, goals predict the consistency of teenagers' condom use, Digest, *Perspectives on Sexual and Reproductive Health,* 36(1) January/February 2004, 37.

two partners and slightly more than a third had had three or more partners. Almost all sexually experienced students (93%) had ever had a steady partner, whereas fewer than half (46%) had ever had a casual partner (defined as "someone with whom you do not have a relationship, 'one night stands' "). Respondents who were not sexually experienced were excluded from the analyses.

Among those who had had a steady partner, 23% reported using condoms always, 16% most of the time, 14% sometimes and 47% rarely or never; use of the pill and having known a partner for a long time were the most often cited reasons for inconsistent use or nonuse of condoms with steady partners. Among those who had had sex with a casual partner, 48% reported using condoms always, 28% most of the time, 10% sometimes and 14% rarely or never; use of the pill, unavailability of a condom, substance use and "it did not cross our minds" were the most often cited reasons for inconsistent use or nonuse of condoms. A greater proportion of men than of women had ever had casual sex (56% vs. 39%), and a greater proportion of women than of men had had unprotected sex (85% vs. 68%).

Lifetime number of sexual partners was negatively correlated with students' perceived ability to use condoms in difficult situations and need for intimacy within relationships ($r = -.13$ for both), and was positively correlated with the frequency with which they had sex to please others (.10), to enhance their mood (.15) and to experience pleasure (.14). Lifetime number of casual partners was positively associated with having sex to please others (.20) and to enhance their mood (.23).

Compared with respondents who had ever had casual sex, those who had never had casual sex considered themselves better able to use condoms in difficult situations and were more inclined to seek intimacy in relationships. Respondents who had had a casual partner, however, more frequently had sex to please others, to enhance their mood or to experience pleasure.

Among respondents who had had sex only with a steady partner, those who used condoms consistently had a more positive attitude about condom use and perceived greater social pressure to use condoms, but needed less intimacy in a relationship and less often had sex to express love than those who did not use the method consistently. Having a more positive attitude about condoms, perceiving greater social pressure to use condoms and having sex to express love were correlated with consistent condom use among both males and females. In addition, women who used condoms consistently, compared with those who did not, were more confident that they could use condoms in difficult situations and less often had sex to experience pleasure.

Among respondents who had had casual sex, consistent condom users were more certain that they could use condoms in difficult situations, had a more positive attitude regarding condoms and perceived greater social pressure to use condoms than those who used condoms inconsistently or not at all. Men who consistently used condoms within their casual relationships tended to have a more positive attitude about condoms, a greater perceived ability to use condoms in difficult situations and a stronger perception of social pressure to use condoms than those who had unsafe casual sex. Women who consistently used condoms within their casual relationships had a greater perceived ability to use condoms in difficult situations, expressed a greater need for intimacy within a relationship and were more motivated to have sex to please others or to express love than women who had unsafe casual sex.

The authors comment that according to their findings, the type of relationships in which adolescents are involved and the motivations adolescents have for engaging in sex are associated with consistent condom use. They suggest that interventions that "target specific subgroups and as such take into account the type of relationships (e.g., steady or casual) and the meaning of the relationship and sex itself would be even more effective in promoting safe sex."—*J. Rosenberg*

Reference

Gebhardt WA, Kuyper L and Greunsven G, Need for intimacy in relationships and motives for sex as determinants of adolescent condom use, *Journal of Adolescent Health,* 2003, 33(3):154–164.

Oral Sex among Adolescents: Is It Sex or Is It Abstinence?

Lisa Remez

Over the past few decades, nationally representative surveys have accumulated a wealth of data on levels of adolescent sexual activity. Thanks to such surveys, we know how the proportion of 15–19-year-olds who have ever had intercourse has changed over the years. Similar data exist on age at first intercourse, most recent sexual intercourse and current contraceptive use.

Yet all of these measures focus on—or relate to the possible results of—vaginal intercourse. This is natural, given that attention to adolescent sexual activity arose initially out of concerns over the far-reaching problems associated with teenage pregnancy and childbearing. More recently, infection with sexually transmitted diseases (STDs), particularly with HIV, has fueled further public and scientific interest in teenage sexual behavior.

But to what extent does adolescent sexual activity consist of noncoital behaviors—that is, mutual masturbation, oral sex and anal intercourse—that are not linked to pregnancy but involve the risk of STDs? Some of these activities may also be precursors to vaginal intercourse. Yet, health professionals and policymakers know very little about their prevalence among teenagers.

There are several explanations for this dearth of information. One is the perceived difficulty of getting parents to consent to surveys on the sexual activity of their minor children (generally aged 17 and younger). Another is a generalized fear that asking young people about sex will somehow lead them to choose to have sex. The conflicts and passions usually surrounding the appropriateness of asking young people about sex, especially in public settings such as schools as compared with private households, become even more inflamed when the questions go into behaviors "beyond" intercourse.

Remez, L. Oral sex among adolescents: Is it sex or abstinence? *Family Planning Perspectives* 32(6): 298–304. Used with permission.

Another reason is the federal government's reluctance to sponsor such controversial research into the full range of noncoital behaviors among adolescents.* For example, the highly charged political debate in 1992 over federal financing of comprehensive sexuality studies had a chilling effect on adolescent sexuality research.[1] The Senate's decision, prompted by pressure from a small group of conservative senators, to deny funding for the American Teenage Study of adolescent sexual behavior still reverberates in the scope of research on teenagers. (An amendment sponsored by Sen. Jesse Helms [R.-NC] prohibited the funding of that survey, along with one of adults, "in fiscal year 1992 or any subsequent fiscal year."[2] Despite warnings that ideology was dictating science, the conservative leadership succeeded in casting these endeavors as "reprehensible sex surveys" only undertaken "to legitimize homosexuality and other sexually promiscuous lifestyles."[3])

It has become increasingly clear, however, that the narrow focus on sexual intercourse in research that does get funded is missing a major component of early sexual activity. There is growing evidence, although still anecdotal and amassed largely by journalists, not researchers, that adolescents might be tuning to behaviors that avoid pregnancy risk but leave them vulnerable to acquisition of many STDs, including HIV.

The reports in the popular press that oral sex has become widespread among adolescents cannot be confirmed or refuted because the data to do so have never been collected. Moreover, adults do not really know what behaviors teenagers consider to be "sex" and, by the same token, what they consider to be its opposite, abstinence. All of this leaves health professionals and policymakers without the means to effectively address these issues.

The tendency to equate "sex" with intercourse alone represents long-standing cultural norms of acceptable sexual behavior and certainly applies to adults as well as to adolescents. It also reflects a deeply rooted ambivalence about talking about sex. Recent press reports, however, are forcing a reappraisal of the implications of this exclusive focus on coitus for research and data collection efforts, for STD prevention and treatment, and for the framing and interpretation of abstinence and risk-reduction messages.

This special report draws on interviews and correspondence with roughly two dozen adolescent and health professionals, including researchers, psychologists, abstinence program coordinators and evaluators, sexuality educators and epidemiologists, to explore some of these consequences. The report concentrates on oral sex, as opposed to other noncoital behaviors, because it is currently the subject of public debate in the media and in many schools. It reviews the limited information on adolescents' experience with oral sex, and looks at the even smaller body of evidence on what young people consider to be sex or abstinence.

---

*The exceptions are the National Survey of Adolescent Males, which asked 15–19-year-old males about their experience with oral and anal sex, and other studies that were not national in scope.

Anecdotal Reports in the Media

The first hint in the popular press of a new "trend" in sexual activity among young people appeared in an April 1997 article in *The New York Times*.[4] That article asserted that high school students who had come of age with AIDS education considered oral sex to be a far less dangerous alternative, in both physical and emotional terms, than vaginal intercourse. By 1999, the press reports started attributing this behavior to even younger students. A July *Washington Post* article described an "unsettling new fad" in which suburban middle-school students were regularly engaging in oral sex at one another's homes, in parks and even on school grounds; this piece reported an oral sex prevalence estimate, attributed to unnamed counselors and sexual behavior researchers of "about half by the time students are in high school."[5]*

Other stories followed, such as a piece in *Talk* magazine in February 2000 that reported on interviews with 12–16-year-olds. These students set seventh grade as the starting point for oral sex, which they claimed begins considerably earlier than intercourse. By 10th grade, according to the reporter, "well over half of their classmates were involved."[6] This article laid part of the blame on dual-career, overworked "parents who were afraid to parent," and also mentioned that young adolescents were caught between messages about AIDS and abstinence on the one hand and the saturation of the culture with sexual imagery on the other. In April 2000, another *New York Times* article on precocious sexuality quoted a Manhattan psychologist as saying "it's like a good-night kiss to them" in a description of how seventh- and eighth-grade virgins who were saving themselves for marriage were having oral sex in the meantime because they perceived it to be safe and risk-free.[7]

In a July 2000 *Washington Post Magazine* cover story, eighth graders described being regularly propositioned for oral sex in school. The reporter echoed the assertion made in earlier articles that although overall sexual activity among older, high school-aged adolescents—as measured by the proportion who have ever had penile-vaginal intercourse—seemed to have recently leveled off or slightly declined, middle-school-aged students (aged 12–14) appeared to be experimenting with a wider range of behaviors at progressively younger ages.[8]

What Teenagers Might Be Doing

How valid are these anecdotal reports? Unless and until data to verify them become available, we have only impressions to go on, and there is by no means a consensus among adolescent health professionals. Some believe the level of participation in oral sex and

---

*Around the same time, an *Iris Times* article reported on 14- and 15-year-old Dubliners who, after getting drunk on hard cider, gathered in local parks and paired off for oral sex. (See: Sheridan K, Our children and their sex games, *Irish Times,* July 17, 1999, p. 12.)

other noncoital behaviors is probably higher now than it was in the past, while others have a "hunch" that oral sex is no more common, just much more talked about.

For example, according to Kathleen Toomey, director of the Division of Public Health in Georgia's Department of Human Resources, "anecdotal evidence and some recent data suggest that teenagers are engaging in oral sex to a greater degree than we had previously thought, but whether this represents a true increase is difficult to say, since we have no baseline data for comparison."[9] Susan Rosenthal, a professor of pediatrics and a pediatric psychologist at Cincinnati Children's Hospital Medical Center, notes that in her clinical practice, "girls are clearly talking about oral sex and masturbation (of their partners or by their partners) more frequently than I used to hear about, but whether this is because they talk more openly about it or are doing it more is unclear."[10] Deborah Haffner, a sexuality educator and former president of the Sexuality Information and Education Council of the United States (SIECUS), dismisses the press reports of oral sex among middle-school-aged adolescents as largely media hype, saying that only a very small number of young people are probably involved.[11]

Experts believe that the type of oral sex practiced by young teenagers is overwhelmingly fellatio, not cunnilingus. According to Deborah Tolman, senior research scientist at the Wellesley Center for Research on Women, that distinction is paramount: "We are not fainting in the street because boys are giving girls cunnilingus. Which is not to say that girls and boys never have that experience. They probably do, and just rarely do it again for a really long time, because of how girls feel about themselves and their bodies, how boys feel about girls' bodies, and the misinformation they have about each other's bodies."[12]

Many STDs can be transmitted by either fellatio or cunnilingus, although some are more easily passed than others. According to Penelope Hitchcock, chief of the Sexually Transmitted Diseases Branch of the National Institute of Allergy and Infectious Diseases, saliva tends to inactivate the HIV virus, so while transmission through oral intercourse is not impossible, it is relatively rare.[13] Other viral STDs that can be transmitted orally include human papillomavirus, herpes simplex virus and hepatitis B,[14] while gonorrhea, syphilis, chlamydia and chancroid are among the bacterial infections that can be passed through oral sex.[15]

In the absence of survey data on the frequency of oral sex, the question arises as to whether clinicians are seeing evidence of a rise in STDs that have been acquired orally. The answer depends upon the person asked. Some say they have seen no change in STDs acquired noncoitally, while others report that they are seeing both new types of infections and new types of patients—i.e., teenagers who have not yet initiated coitus but who come in with fears and anxiety over having acquired an infection orally.

Linda Dominguez, assistant medical director of Planned Parenthood of New Mexico and a nurse practitioner with a private practice, reports that at patients' requests, she is performing more oral swabs and throat inspections now than in the past.[16] She affirms that "I have more patients who are virgins who report to me that they are worried about

STDs they may have gotten by having oral sex. There are a lot of questions and concerns about herpes, since they seem to know that there is some risk of 'top and bottom' herpes, as one of my patients put it."

Sharon Schnare, a family planning clinician and consultant in Seattle, remarks that she now sees many teenagers with oral herpes. She adds that "I have also found, though rarely, oral *Condylomata acuminata* [a sexually transmitted condition caused by the human papillomavirus] in teenagers."[17] Moreover, Hitchcock states that "several studies have shown that one-third of the isolates from genital herpes cases in kids right now are HSV1 [herpes simplex virus 1, the oral strain], which suggests a significant amount of oral intercourse is going on."[18] This suggestion is impossible to verify, however, because of the extensive crossover between the two strains. Moreover, trends are especially hard to detect because of past and current problems in the reliability of type-specific testing.

Pharyngeal gonorrhea is one STD that is definitely acquired through oral sex. A few cases of pharyngeal gonorrhea have been diagnosed in adolescent girls in Dominguez's family planning clinic in New Mexico[19] and in one region of Georgia through a community screening project among middle-school students to detect certain strains of meningitis bacteria carried in the throat.[20] In Georgia, the cases caught everyone off guard, according to Kathleen Toomey.[21] The infections were found only because throat swabs were being done for meningitis in a population that would not be considered "sexually active" in the traditional sense of the word.

Many researchers and clinicians believe that young adolescents who are having oral sex before they start coitus might be especially reluctant to seek clinical care. Moreover, adolescents virtually never use condoms or dental dams to protect against STD infection during oral sex, even those who know about the risk and worry that they might become infected.

However little is known about teenagers' experiences with oral sex, even less information is available on their involvement with anal sex, which also carries risks of STD infection, particularly of HIV. While teenage patients now seem much more comfortable talking about oral sex than they were in the past, the taboo against bringing up anal sex is still very much in place.

Attitudes and Motivations

Experts say there are multiple, interrelated reasons for why adolescents might be turning to oral sex. Deborah Roffman, a sexuality educator at The Park School in Baltimore, asserts that "middle-school girls sometimes look at oral sex as an absolute bargain—you don't get pregnant, they think you don't get diseases, you're still a virgin and you're in control since it's something that they can do to boys (whereas sex is almost always described as something boys do to girls)."[22]

This sense of control is illusory, according to Roffman, because engaging in fellatio out of peer pressure or to gain popularity is clearly exploitative of girls who lack the maturity to realize it. The issue of just how voluntary oral sex is for many girls came up repeatedly, especially when the act is performed "to make boys happy" or when alcohol is involved. Roffman relates the experience of a guidance counselor who, after bringing up the topic of rape in this context of coerced oral sex, was told by female students that the term did not apply to their situation, because fellatio "is not really sex."

Teenagers seem to be especially misinformed about the STD risks of oral sex. Experts repeatedly mentioned their concerns over adolescents' perceptions of oral sex as less risky than intercourse,* especially in the context of teenagers' tendency to have very short-term relationships. Several observers mentioned the trap of AIDS education, which often teaches that HIV is transmitted through sexual intercourse, so adolescents think they are avoiding risk by avoiding sexual intercourse. Sarah Brown, director of the National Campaign to Prevent Teen Pregnancy, suggests what some adolescents might be thinking: "Okay, we get it. You adults really don't want us to have sexual intercourse, and you're probably right because of AIDS and pregnancy. But we're still sexual and we're going to do other things."[23]

Haffner's interviews with 11th and 12th graders reveal that they view oral sex as "something you can do with someone you're not as intimate with, while intercourse is, by and large, reserved for that special person."[24] This emotional differential between oral sex and vaginal sex—the assertion that oral sex carries few or no emotional ties—is acknowledged by many professionals who work with adolescents. Linda Dominguez quotes her adolescent patients as thinking "if you're going to avoid intercourse, you're going to resort to oral sex. You're going to do something that is sexual, but in some ways emotionally safer, before you give the big one away."[25]

Adolescent health professionals reinforced the view reported in the popular press that today's adolescents consider oral sex to be less consequential and less intimate than intercourse. "Oral sex is clearly seen as something very different than intercourse, as something other than sex," according to Susan Rosenthal. She also mentions a generational shift in thinking, noting that "if you were to query older women, oral sex might be perceived as something more intimate or equally intimate to vaginal sex (and which frequently happened later on in a relationship); for the teens, oral sex appears to be much less intimate or serious than vaginal intercourse."[26]

---

*For example, in a fall 1999 mall-intercept survey conducted by *Seventeen* magazine and the Henry J. Kaiser Family Foundation, 16% of 15–19-year-old males and females asserted that oral sex was "safe" because it protected against infection with an STD, while 48% labeled the practice as "safe" because it protected against pregnancy. Incidentally, 55% thought that oral sex was "gross," the same proportion who said they had ever done it. (See reference 45.) Moreover, in the *Seventeen*/Kaiser collaborative special section "Sex Smarts," the number-one sex myth listed in the "10 Sex Myths Exposed" was "oral sex is no big thing." (Forman G, 10 sex myths exposed, Sex Smarts Special Section, tearout in *Seventeen,* June 2000.)

Insights from Formal Research

How does the limited published research conducted on oral sex inform the current situation? Because of the difficulties in obtaining funding and consent for conducting this type of research among minors, many of these studies have necessarily relied on small, nonrepresentative samples of college-age students enrolled in human sexuality or psychology classes, which are hardly generalizable to the overall population. Perhaps the best, though still limited, dataset that includes adolescents dates from the early 1980s: In 1982, a marketing research firm collected data from a national panel of households in 49 states.[27] Douglas Kirby, currently of ETR Associates, directed this early research project; he recalls that "we were surprised that there was much more oral sex than we had anticipated."[28]

Roughly one-fifth of the 1,067 13-18-year-olds surveyed in the early 1980s said they had ever had oral sex, and 16% of young women who had performed fellatio had never had vaginal intercourse.[29] To many adolescents, safer-sex in the pre-AIDS era presumably meant avoiding pregnancy. The practice of "outercourse," in fact, was suggested by at least one physician as early as 1972† as an alternative contraceptive method for young teenagers.[30] That physician, John Cobb, asserted that loosening the taboos around noncoital activity might "help significantly in the prevention of unwanted teenage pregnancy and of venereal disease."

Other nonrepresentative research done in the early 1980s focused on adolescents' sexual experimentation as a precursor or predictor of coitus. One longitudinal prospective study conducted in a southern city in 1980 and 1982 found that among a sample of black and white 12–17-year-olds, blacks proceeded more quickly to intercourse, while whites followed a predictable scenario of noncoital activities as substitutes or delay mechanisms.[31] Another study using the 1982 follow-up data set only (545 10th-12th graders) concluded that 24% of the virgins in the sample had had oral sex.[32] The corresponding proportion among those who had initiated coitus was 82%. In 1994-1995, a survey of 291 college undergraduates indicated that among those who were in a serious relationship, virgins were as likely as nonvirgins to have ever had oral sex (although nonvirgins were more likely to have had mutual oral sex).[33]

Few studies focus exclusively on individuals before they are "sexually active." One such effort assessed the range of precoital sexual activities among a volunteer sample of 311 nonvirgin college undergraduates who were surveyed retrospectively, in the 1995–1996

---

†Twenty-five years later, this physician, in a letter to the editor, again advocated encouraging adolescents to practice outercourse (or heavy petting to orgasm without penetration) as a "cost-free, natural and effective way to prevent unwanted pregnancy and STDs while making love." This time, the message was updated with the warning that the advent of HIV meant that "of course, anal or oral intercourse is to be avoided." (See: Cobb JC, Outercourse as a safe and sensible alternative to contraceptives, letter to the editor, *American Journal of Public Health,* 1997, 87(8):1380-1381). Critics of this strategy, however, point to the fact that it has never been adequately evaluated and that since it involves promoting behaviors that are considered themselves predisposing factors for coitus, it may lead to intermittent, unprotected intercourse. (See: Genius SJ and Genius SK, Orgasm without organisms: science or propaganda? *Clinical Pediatrics,* 1996, 35(1):10–17.)

academic year, about their experiences before their first coitus. Seventy percent of the males and 57% of the females reported having performed oral sex at least once before their first intercourse; the proportion ever receiving oral sex was the same for both genders (57–58%).[34]

Two early-1990s surveys based on total high school enrollment, instead of single-subject college classes, came out of efforts to evaluate condom availability programs for HIV prevention.[35] In 1992, baseline data collected for such a program in Los Angeles among 2,026 ninth-12th graders indicated that 29–31% of the virgins in this sample had engaged in masturbation with a partner, and 9–10% of those who had not yet had coitus had nonetheless had oral sex. Very few (1% of noncoitally experienced students) revealed that they had ever engaged in anal intercourse.[36] Another study from 1992, also designed to collect baseline data for a condom program evaluation, was conducted in suburban high schools in the New York City metropolitan area. The director of that study said it unexpectedly uncovered considerably higher rates of oral intercourse than of vaginal intercourse.[37]

Finally, one nationally representative survey—the National Survey of Adolescent Males—asked about a full range of heterosexual genital activities in both 1988 and 1995. Although the overall proportion of 15–19-year-old males who had ever received oral sex did not change significantly from 1988 to 1995 (44% vs. 50%), this proportion more than doubled among blacks (from 25% to 57%).[38] Moreover, among virgin young men, the proportion ever having received oral sex increased from 10% to 17%, although this difference was not statistically significant. [Editors' note: For further details on these data, see pp. 295–297 & 304.]

Data collected in small-scale evaluations of abstinence education programs are an unexpected source of information on adolescents' current experience with oral sex. A few evaluation sites recently used questionnaires that asked about a variety of sexual activities in assessing how middle-school students interpret messages about behaviors to be abstained from. Thus, those who had had oral sex but not coitus could be distinguished from other groups. According to Stan Weed, director of the Institute for Research and Evaluation in Salt Lake City, the responses to these items indicate that "there is a percentage of kids for whom oral sex seems to be a substitute for intercourse; I'm guessing that, although it varies with the sample, for around 25% of the kids who have had any kind of intimate sexual activity, that activity is oral sex, not intercourse."[39]

What Is Sex?

The many, even competing, agendas in the culturally loaded definitions of the term "sex" make sexuality research exceptionally challenging to conduct.* In early fall of 1998, the

---

*For gay men and women, for example, the arrow penile-vaginal intercourse definition is clearly irrelevant. In data recently collected from an Internet sample, adult homosexuals and bisexuals tended to label a greater number of activities as "sex" than did a comparable sample of heterosexuals. The researcher concluded that the implications of such semantic diversity "cannot be underestimated in conducting sexuality survey research, clinical sexual history taking or sex education." (See: Mustanski B, Semantic heterogeneity in the definition of "having sex" for homosexuals, unpublished manuscript, Department of Psychology, Indiana University, Bloomington, IN, 2000).

American public was riveted by President Bill Clinton's claim that he had not perjured himself because he "did not have sexual relations with that woman [White House intern Monica Lewinsky]"; he had, in fact, had something else—oral sex. At the time, according to a Gallup Poll, roughly 20% of adults also believed that oral sex did not constitute "sexual relations."[40] No one knows how many adolescents feel the same way. As Robert Blum, director of the Adolescent Health Program at the University of Minnesota puts it, "we know that there are many sexual practices other than intercourse that predispose young people to negative health outcomes. What we really don't know is, in an age of a focus on abstinence, how young people have come to understand what is meant by being sexually active."[41]

Limited data are available on college undergraduates' perceptions of what is meant by sexual activity. Among roughly 600 students enrolled at a Midwestern university surveyed in 1991, 59% did not believe that oral sex would qualify as sex and only 19% thought the same about anal sex.[42] Females (62%) were more likely than males (56%) to assert that cunnilingus and fellatio were not "sex."

What young adults consider to be "sex" also varies by contextual and situational factors, such as who is doing what to whom and whether it leads to orgasm. In data collected in early 1998 among a sample of college undergraduates who were read hypothetical scenarios and were asked to comment on them, 54% considered that a man would say fellatio did not qualify as sex and 59% that a woman would not consider cunnilingus to be sex;[43] these proportions were even higher once it was specified that oral sex had not resulted in orgasm. Correspondingly, in another study in which these students were asked which acts would define a sexual partner, they were less likely to say that a couple would consider one another as "sexual partners" if they had had oral sex than if they had had vaginal or anal intercourse.[44]

In the face of limited rigorous research in this area, magazines for teenagers serve as an important source of information on what adolescents think about oral sex. Impressions of oral sex are necessarily bound up with views on sexual intercourse, since one is usually cited as either a precursor or substitute for the other. According to a fall 1999 survey conducted by *Seventeen* magazine in which 723 15–19-year-old males and females were approached in malls, 49% considered oral sex to be "not as big a deal as sexual intercourse," and 40% said it did not count as "sex."[45] A summer 2000 Internet survey conducted by *Twist* magazine received 10,000 on-line responses from 13-19-year-old girls, 18% of whom said that oral sex was something that you did with your boyfriend before you are ready to have sex; the same proportion stated that oral sex was a substitute for intercourse.[46]

Adults and adolescents do not necessarily agree on what activities are now inferred by the word "sex." Individuals from across the ideological spectrum who were interviewed for this report acknowledged that the assumption of what "sex" encompasses has changed. As Tom Klaus, president of Legacy Resource Group in Iowa, which produces comprehensive pregnancy prevention and abstinence resources for educators, observes, "we thought we were on the same page as our kids when we talked about 'it.' The new emerging paradigm is that we can't be so certain that we are really talking about the same thing."[47]

What Is Abstinence?

If adolescents perceive oral sex as something different from sex, do they view it as abstinence? Research conducted in 1999 with 282 12-17-year-olds in rural areas in the Midwest probed how adolescents who received abstinence education interpreted the term. students struggled to come up with a coherent definition, although older adolescents had less difficulty than younger ones. The wide-ranging responses covered ground from "kissing is probably okay" to "just no intercourse."[48]

Some of the students brought marriage into their definition of abstinence, and others asserted that it means going only as far sexually as one wanted to or felt comfortable with. The list of behaviors encompassed within virginity was long, and typically ended in statements such as "To me, the only thing that would take away my virginity is having sex. Everything else is permitted." (The very few recent abstinence program evaluations that assessed whether adolescents had engaged in sexual activities other than intercourse did not ask whether they did so under the assumption that they were being abstinent.[49])

In 1994–1995 data from 1,101 college freshman and sophomores in the South, 61% considered mutual masturbation (to orgasm) to be abstinent behavior, 37% described oral intercourse as abstinence and 24% thought the same about anal intercourse.[50] The authors surmised that pregnancy prevention came first in these students' perceptions, so behaviors unlinked to pregnancy then counted as abstinence. On the other hand, nearly one-quarter labeled kissing and bathing or showering together as "not abstinent."

Health educators themselves might be unclear about precisely what the term "abstinence" means. In a 1999 e-mail survey of 72 health educators, for example, nearly one-third (30%) responded that oral sex was abstinent behavior. A similar proportion (29%), however, asserted that mutual masturbation would not qualify as abstinence.[51]

Experts interviewed for this report acknowledged that defining what is meant by abstinence—and accurately communicating that definition to students—has become a crucial issue. While everyone agrees that the implicit meaning of the term is abstaining from vaginal-penile intercourse, especially since the concept is often taught as a "method" of avoiding pregnancy, the consensus stops there. What is the specific behavior that signals the end of abstinence and the beginning of sex?

Given the amount of federal and state money going into abstinence education, the lack of a consensus on whether and how to specify the behaviors to be abstained from warrants close examination. In 1996, Congress established a new abstinence-education program as part of its overhaul of welfare. Title V of the Maternal and Child Health Services Block Grant guarantees $50 million annually in federal support for five years (1998–2004) for abstinence-only education; since state and local governments are obligated to supply $3 for every $4 in federal funds, the total annual expenditure for government-supported abstinence education—which must promote abstinence until marriage—could reach almost $90 million each year.[52]*

Although Title V does not specify an age-range for these activities, the majority of the states that have received funding have targeted teenagers aged 17 and younger. The eight-point official definition in Title V specifies that programs teach "abstinence from sexual activity outside marriage as the expected standard for all school-age children,"[53] but the law does not delineate "sexual activity."

Several experts noted that the different purpose or intent of the teaching of abstinence—i.e., for public health reasons or for moral or religious reasons—will naturally produce a different set of activities to be abstained from. The lack of a consensus definition of abstinence is also a relatively new issue that current events are forcing to the forefront. As Barbara Devaney of Mathematica, a research agency conducting a national evaluation of Title V programs, points out, "at the time that the legislation was written, there was not much public controversy over what abstinence was; this was not yet on the radar screen."[54]

This issue is especially thorny because some abstinence-only programs are committed to being as specific as possible so adolescents do not take away the wrong message about what abstinence is, while others insist that specifying those behaviors violates a child's innocence and amounts to providing a "how-to" manual. Tom Klaus affirms that the inability to specify what activities youth should abstain from is forcing a Catch 22—adolescents cannot practice abstinence until they know what abstinence is, but in order to teach them what abstinence is, they have to be taught what sex is.[55] According to Stan Weed, "there's no settled consensus in the abstinence movement. Some programs are willing to take it head on and say [oral sex] is not an appropriate activity, if you think this is a substitute, you're wrong; others are not even dealing with it."[56]

Amy Stephens of Focus on the Family, a Colorado Springs-based conservative religious organization, asserts that in its curriculum, *Sex, Lies and . . . the Truth,* "our definition is refraining from all sexual activity, which includes intercourse, oral sex, anal sex and mutual masturbation—the only 100% effective means of preventing pregnancy and the spread of STDs."[57] Stephens notes that the different faith communities will use language specific to their congregations (i.e., "chastity" in Catholic circles and "purity" in Christian Evangelical communities). In the official definition of abstinence used by the Chicago-based Project Reality, the "sexual activity" to be avoided until marriage "refers to any type of genital contact or sexual stimulation including, but not limited to, sexual intercourse."[58]

---

*The original Title V legislation had no provision for evaluation at the state level, but nearly every state has committed some funds—an average of 5% of their abstinence education monies. At the federal level, Congress allotted $6 million for a national-level evaluation in the Balanced Budget Act of 1997. (See: reference 52.)

Consequences and Implications

SEXUALITY AND ABSTINENCE EDUCATION

Some adolescent health professionals believe that although the revelation of early oral sex has been shocking, it has had the positive effect of forcing a dialogue with adolescents about the full meaning of sexuality and of the importance of defining sex not as a single act, but as a whole range of behaviors. There is widespread agreement among educators from all along the ideological spectrum that the continuing lack of adult guidance about what sex really means contributes to the desensitized, "body-part" sex talked about in the press, whatever the real prevalence might be. They stress that teachers and parents need to do a better job at helping children interpret the context-free messages of sexuality they are bombarded with in the media, which now includes the still-evolving Internet. Some experts believe that programs are moving in the right direction by teaching adolescents how to identify bad or abusive relationships, but that there is still much work to be done to help them with intimacy and how to recognize good relationships.

The lack of guidelines on what activity is appropriate when is a common concern among professionals who work with adolescents. Educators who endorse comprehensive sexuality education support giving adolescents the criteria they need to decide when to abstain or when to participate across the full continuum of sexual behaviors. Abstinence proponents are wrestling with how to handle an evolving dilemma that pits those who stress the need to be as precise as possible in specifying the range of behaviors to be abstained from against others who insist that such specificity violates the core of abstinence-only education.

RESEARCH AND EVALUATION

What is to be gained by broadening the range of behaviors asked about in surveys of sexual behavior? The simplest public health argument is that doing so would enable researchers to identify individuals whose behaviors place them at risk, so that more appropriate programs and policies can be developed. Many of these youth are now being missed by current survey instruments. By considering only adolescents who have ever had coitus, or only dividing them by whether they had that experience, "we don't get a full understanding of the range of adolescent activity and of the developmental and emotional processes involved," according to Mark Schuster, director, UCLA/RAND Center for Adolescent Health Promotion.[59]

It is also impossible to adequately assess how changes in sexual activity or in contraceptive behavior contributed to recent declines in adolescent pregnancy rates as long as information on sexual activity unlinked to pregnancy remains unavailable. For example, while different groups have attributed a greater or lesser share of the declines in pregnancy rates to increased abstinence,[60] how much of that "abstinence" corresponds to sexual activity other than intercourse is still unknown.

Another advantage to using a broader measure of sexual activity is being able to more fully measure the impact of various programs and curricula that address adolescent sexuality. As Sarah Brown stresses, "if, for example, we found that there was a curriculum that delayed the age of first vaginal intercourse, but increased the preponderance of oral sex, we should know that."[61]

Currently, the principal outcome measures used in evaluations of both comprehensive sexuality and abstinence-based programs are the standard ones of vaginal intercourse, pregnancy and contraceptive use. That holds true for the Mathematica national evaluation of Title V abstinence education programs. The project director, Rebecca Maynard, explains that after much debate, the group that devised the questionnaire settled on the stable outcome measure of intercourse for the first wave of follow-up, to assure that the evaluation was not measuring different definitions of sex, as opposed to different behaviors.[62]

Even if there is agreement on the need to expand the definition of sexual activity to create more accurate research and evaluation tools, getting those items onto survey instruments remains a concern. Some researchers assert that surveys need to be allowed to capture self-reports of these especially sensitive behaviors in the most private setting and mode of administration possible (i.e., using audio computer-assisted self-interviews rather than personal interviews). Others say that should national-level studies prove impossible because of the constraints of funding agencies, then small-area studies would be of value, especially in higher prevalence areas where there might be greater receptivity to gathering such data.

Other professionals are clearly worried about the prospect of gaining parental consent—what Brown terms "the 800 pound gorilla in the room"[63]—especially since many of the adolescents purported to be engaging in sexual activities other than intercourse are younger than 15, the minimum age usually included in traditional surveys. Stan Weed, who has experience drafting questionnaires in the new climate of ostensibly greater participation in oral sex, suggests that advance focus-group research can be helpful in countering objections to questions from parents and school administrators. If findings illustrate that the behavior is prevalent, for example, then the evaluation team can use that information to explain why those questions need to be asked.[64]

Although the well-known technique of asking 18-year-olds to report on their earlier experiences was also mentioned, some experts point out that parents' willingness to grant consent might have recently changed. Joyce Abma, a demographer at the National Center for Health Statistics, for example, is hopeful that "maybe we're in an era where people understand the dire nature of STD transmission and HIV. So if the message is that this could possibly contribute to both a better understanding of and eventual lessening of these serious health conditions, then there might be a greater possibility of cooperation."[65] This belief is echoed by others, who talk of the need to engage parents directly and to not necessarily assume that they would deny permission.

CLINICAL CARE

What are some of the health consequences of continuing to define sex so narrowly and to lack data on a wider range of behaviors? "As public health people, we need to think about how we can address prevention and education, when we don't even know which are the behaviors we are trying to 'prevent,' " Kathleen Toomey says.[66] She notes that the cases of pharyngeal gonorrhea were only uncovered among middle schoolers, who had not sought care otherwise, through a screening project for meningitis, adding "we're probably missing this because we are not routinely doing throat swabs and because we are not asking the right questions."

There is widespread agreement that oral STD risk in adolescent populations has yet to be adequately measured and screened for. This situation is exacerbated by the fact that many of the adolescent patients involved have not yet initiated coitus and thus are unlikely to visit a family planning or STD clinic. When they do, several practitioners assert, more detailed sexual histories, despite the extra time involved, are essential to prevent misdiagnosis and to understand what the patient, rather than the provider, means by "sexual activity." In the absence of an adequate screening protocol, unknowing clinicians might automatically assume that the patient has strep and prescribe antibiotics. The fact that many infections are asymptomatic further complicates the diagnosis when the mode of infection is not easily talked about.

The deeply rooted tendency to define sex as intercourse might not necessarily be working any more in reaching many adolescent patients at risk. How to counsel adolescents about lowering that risk is especially problematic, since many young people consider oral sex itself to be a form of risk reduction and are probably already reluctant (as are many adults) to discuss oral sex openly or to use dental dams or condoms. Many practitioners feel they have gotten very good at talking about penetrative risk, but that they now need to hone their skills at communicating with their young clients about other types of sexual activities—and to do so they need more information.

Qualitative and quantitative data on sexual behaviors other than intercourse are clearly needed to close the gaps in knowledge about practices that may expose young people to emotional and physical harm. Surveys have not yet been undertaken that would yield more useful data on the broad range of sexual behaviors young people might be engaging in. If such surveys are conducted and reveal that only a small percentage of adolescents are involved, "then we need not be alarmed," according to Laura Stepp, the *Washington Post* reporter who wrote some of the first stories on oral sex. "But if it's a considerable proportion, then we need to get out there with megaphones."[67]

References

1. DiMauro D, *Sexuality Research in the United States: An Assessment of the Social and Behavioral Sciences,* New York: Social Science Research Council, 1995.
2. U.S. Congressional Record—Senate, Apr. 2, 1992, pp. S 4737 and S 4758.
3. Ibid., p. 4737.

4. Lewin T, Teen-agers alter sexual practices, thinking risks will be avoided, *New York Times,* Apr. 5, 1997.

5. Stepp LS, Parents are alarmed by an unsettling new fad in middle schools: oral sex, *Washington Post,* July 8, 1999, p. A1; and Stepp LS, Talking to kids about sexual limits, *Washington Post,* July 8, 1999, p. C4.

6. Franks L, The sex lives of your children, *Talk Magazine,* February 2000, pp. 102–107 & 157.

7. Jarrell A, The face of teenage sex grows younger, *New York Times,* April 2, 2000.

8. Mundy L, Young teens and sex: sex & sensibility, *Washington Post Magazine,* July 16, 2000, pp. 16-21,   29-34.

9. Toomey K, Division of Public Health, Georgia Department of Human Resources, Atlanta, GA, personal communication, Aug. 23, 2000.

10. Rosenthal S, Children's Hospital Medical Center, Cincinnati, OH, personal communication, Sept. 5, 2000.

11. Haffner D, personal communication, Oct. 4, 2000.

12. Tolman D, Wellesley Center for Research on Women, Wellesley, MA, personal communication, Aug. 18, 2000.

13. Hitchcock P, Sexually Transmitted Diseases Branch, National Institute of Allergy and Infectious Diseases, Bethesda, MD, personal communication, Aug. 21, 2000.

14. Edwards S and Carne C, Oral sex and the transmission of viral STIs, *Sexually Transmitted Infections,* 1998, 74(1):6-10.

15. Edwards S and Carne C, Oral sex and the transmission of non-viral STIs, *Sexually Transmitted Infections,* 1998, 74(2):95-100.

16. Dominguez L, Planned Parenthood of New Mexico, Albuquerque, NM, personal communication, Sept. 7, 2000.

17. Schnare SM, Seattle, WA, personal communication, Oct. 26, 2000.

18. Hitchcock P, 2000, op. cit. (see reference 13).

19. Dominguez L, 2000, op. cit. (see reference 16).

20. Toomey K, 2000, op. cit. (see reference 9).

21. Ibid.

22. Roffman D, The Park School, Baltimore, MD, personal communication, Oct. 12, 2000.

23. Brown S, National Campaign to Prevent Teen Pregnancy, Washington, DC, personal communication, Oct. 6, 2000.

24. Haffner D, 2000, op. cit. (see reference 11).

25. Dominguez L, 2000, op. cit. (see reference 16).

26. Rosenthal S, 2000, op cit. (see reference 10).

27. Coles R and Stokes G, *Sex and the American Teenager,* New York: Harper and Row, 1985.

28. Kirby D, ETR Associates, Santa Cruz, CA, personal communication, Sept. 12, 2000.

29. Coles R and Stokes G, 1985, op cit. (see reference 27).

30. Cobb JC, Nonprocreative sexuality as an alternative to contraception, in *Advances in Planned Parenthood, Vol. VIII, Proceedings of the Tenth Annual Meeting of the American Association of Planned Parenthood Physicians,* Princeton, NJ: Excerpta Medica, 1973.

31. Smith EA and Udry R, Coital and non-coital sexual behavior of white and black adolescents, *American Journal of Public Health,* 1985, 75(10):1200-1203.

32. Newcomer SF and Udry JR, Oral sex in an adolescent population, *Archives of Sexual Behavior,* 1985, 14(1):41-46.

33. Werner-Wilson RJ, Are virgins at risk for contracting HIV/AIDS? *Journal of HIV/AIDS Prevention & Education for Adolescents & Children,* 1998, 2(3/4):63-71.

34. Schwartz IM, Sexual activity prior to coitus initiation: a comparison between males and females, *Archives of Sexual Behavior,* 1999, 28(1):63-69.

35. Schuster MA, UCLA/RAND Center for Adolescent Health Promotion, Santa Monica, CA, personal communication, Sept. 13, 2000; and Koplewicz H, Department of Pediatric Psychiatry, New York University School of Medicine, personal communication, July 18, 2000.

36. Schuster MA, Bell RM and Kanouse DE, The sexual practices of adolescent virgins: genital sexual activities of high school students who have never had vaginal intercourse, *American Journal of Public Health,* 1996, 86(11):1570-1576.

37. Koplewicz H, 2000, op. cit. (see reference 35).

38. Gates GJ and Sonenstein FL, Heterosexual genital sexual activity among adolescent males: 1988 and 1995, *Family Planning Perspectives,* 2000, 32(6):295-297 & 304.

39. Weed S, Institute for Research and Evaluation, Salt Lake City, UT, personal communication, Oct. 24, 2000.

40. Gallup short subjects, *The Gallup Poll Monthly,* No. 396, Sept. 1998, Survey GP 9809035, Sept. 21, 1998, Q. 15, p. 47.

41. Blum R, Adolescent Health Program, University of Minnesota, Minneapolis, MN, personal communication, Aug. 8, 2000.

42. Sanders SA and Reinisch JM, Would you say you "had sex" if . . . ?, *Journal of the American Medical Association,* 1999, 281(3):275–277.

43. Bogart L et al., Is it "sex"?: college students' interpretations of sexual behavior terminology, *Journal of Sex Research,* 2000, 37(2): 108–116.

44. Cecil H et al., Classifying a person as a sex partner, unpublished manuscript, University of Alabama at Birmingham, School of Public Health, 2000.

45. News release, *Seventeen* News: National survey conducted by *Seventeen* finds that more than half of teens ages 15-19 have engaged in oral sex, Feb. 28, 2000.

46. Birnbaum C, The love & sex survey 2000, *Twist,* Oct./Nov. 2000, pp. 54-56.

47. Klaus T, Legacy Resource Group, Carlisle, IA, personal communication, Sept. 21, 2000.

48. Bell HA, Just because you see their privates doesn't mean you're not a virgin: adolescents' understanding of sexual terminology, unpublished thesis, Iowa State University, Ames, IA, 2000.

49. Weed S, 2000, op. cit. (see reference 39).

50. Horan PF, Phillips J and Hagan NE, The meaning of abstinence for college students, *Journal of HIV/AIDS Prevention & Education for Adolescents & Children,* 1998, 2(2):51-66.

51. Mercer JG, Defining and teaching abstinence: an e-mail survey of health educators, unpublished thesis, North Carolina State University, Raleigh, NC, 1999.

52. Pfau S, *Abstinence Education in the States: Implementation of the 1996 Abstinence Education Law,* Washington, DC: Association of Maternal & Child Health Programs, 1999.

53. Section 912, (2)(A)-(H), Public Law 104-193, Welfare Act, 104th Congress, Aug. 22, 1996.

54. Devaney B, Mathematic Policy Research, Inc., Princeton, NJ, personal communication, Aug. 22, 2000.

55. Klaus T, 2000, op. cit. (see reference 47).

56. Weed S, 2000, op. cit. (see reference 39).

57. Stephens A, Focus on the Family, Colorado Springs, CO, personal communication, Sept. 9, 2000.

58. Sullivan K, Project Reality, Golf, IL, personal communication, Nov. 6, 2000.

59. Schuster MA, 2000, op. cit. (see reference 35).

60. Darroch JD and Singh S, *Why Is Teenage Pregnancy Declining? The Roles of Abstinence, Sexual Activity and Contraceptive Use,* Occasional Report No. 1, New York: Alan Guttmacher Institute, 1999; and Jones JM et al., *The Declines in Adolescent Pregnancy, Birth and Abortion Rates in the 1990s: What Factors Are Responsible?* Fanwood, NJ: Consortium of State Physicians Resource Councils, 1999.

61. Brown S, 2000, op cit. (see reference 23).

62. Maynard R, Mathematica Policy Research, Inc., Princeton, NJ, personal communication, Sept. 22, 2000.

63. Brown S, 2000, op cit. (see reference 23).

64. Weed S, 2000, op cit. (see reference 39).

65. Abma J, Reproductive Statistics Branch, National Center for Health Statistics, Hyattsville, MD, personal communication, Oct. 11, 2000.

66. Toomey K, 2000, op. cit. (see reference 9).

67. Stepp LS, *Washington Post,* Washington, DC, personal communication, Oct. 11, 2000.

Section

Sexuality Education

A Case for Offering Comprehensive Sexuality Education in the Schools

CHAPTER 9

John P. Elia, Ph.D.

This case for sexuality education challenges conventional assumptions about sexuality and its relationship to gender, children's sexuality and the students' role in developing the curriculum. In laying out this case for sexuality education it may be helpful to review and articulate at this point the concepts upon which these assumptions will be challenged.

One conventional assumption about sexuality is that it is basically physical and that its purpose is reproduction. While sexuality obviously includes the physical and reproductive dimensions, it also has psychological, socio-cultural, and political aspects that are equally as important. The psychological dimensions consists of the emotional and mental states that shape and reflect sexual desire, experience, and meaning. The socio-cultural level consists of norms often phrased as religion and rituals, which prescribe what is acceptable sexual behavior. The politics of sexuality consist of the rules of sexual conduct often phrases as laws either derived from nature or human made, which often have their roots in religious doctrine. This expanded view of sexuality questions the assumption that human sexuality in modern times has been devoted primarily to procreation. Today sexuality is enjoyed for its own pleasure and it is often tied to romance, bonding, communication, adventure, and excitement.

This case for sexuality education challenges the notion that gender and sexuality are interrelated phenomena. This case for sexuality education argues against the reduction of gender to biological sex. While biological sex is a matter of femaleness and maleness, gender is multidimensional. It has psychological aspects. For example, gender self-identity based on internal notions of one's femininity and masculinity. There are socio-cultural norms in terms of expected behaviors of boys and girls and men and women. Also, there are political aspects of gender, which include the differential treatment in economic and political power allotted to men and women.

This expanded notion of gender relates to our expanded notion of sexuality. If our sexuality includes desire, the distinctions of desire in heterosexuality, homosexuality, and bisexuality are made in terms of gender manifestations of prospective partners: varying degrees of femininity and masculinity, and even androgyny are desired in sexual partners. This transcends sexual preference. The rules for sexual contact and performance are often phrased in terms of gender with the men expected to be the initiators and orchestrators of sexual encounters, while women have been traditionally cast in more passive roles. As the gender roles are being redefined and expanded, women have the opportunity to take control of their bodies and sexual encounters. By separating sexuality from gender, as is so often done, we limit the variability of gender and sexual expression.

In this case for sexuality education we are challenging the belief that children are in fact not sexual and not interested in learning about sexuality in the broadest sense, which includes but is not limited to their own sexual subjectivity and meaning at any given point in their development. If we assume, contrary to conventional thinking, that children are experiencing their sexuality throughout their childhood and teenage years and constructing meanings (Bruner, 1996), then the question is "Do schools have a responsibility to help them understand and shape these meanings and apply them to their experiences?" Furthermore, today students are growing up in a sexual culture that on one hand appears to be obsessed with sexuality as depicted in television programs, movies, and magazines, and on the other hand revives a sexual purity movement. Do schools have a responsibility to expose the hypocrisy and irrationality, and allow students the opportunity to think through the contradictions with which they are confronted? One obstacle that must be overcome is the stigmatizing as sexual predators of teachers who courageously raise and address these questions.

When what needs to be taught is out of step with socio-cultural norms, then the issue of who formulates the curriculum and of what it should consist become critical political issues. This case for sexuality education challenges the traditional notion that the curriculum be constructed chiefly by adults who represent the wisdom and the knowledge of the past with which children should be socialized and educated (Arnstine, 1995).

Traditionally it has been believed that sexuality should be kept private and not be a public matter. A cultural norm prohibits making personal sexual experiences and preferences public. This is an issue that has been confronted in the gay, lesbian, bisexual, and transgender movement—popularly known as the Queer Movement—as coming out, in which one discloses publicly one's sexual preferences. The case for sexuality education is based on the assumption that unless people have the opportunity to reveal and describe their sexuality, the variability that exists in sexual behavior, fantasy, desire, and attitudes cannot become part of the popular discourse. On the contrary, students will try to constrict themselves to fit into traditional categories instead of developing their sexuality in ways that could lead to personal fulfillment.

In this conception of sexuality education, the basic subject matter of the curriculum should be the children's own stories of their sexual experiences and desires, and their own interpretation of these. The adult's role is to illuminate those experiences by drawing from the lives and thoughts of the men and women of the past who faced similar issues, and constructed their own meanings. The sexual information contained in much historical biography has been censored either through poor scholarship, or by the biographers subscribing to the view of not publicly revealing the details of the subjects' private lives.

Now that we have outlined the main issues and the breadth with which this case for sexuality education is going to be argued, we will turn next to the case itself.

Among the many contributions of gay, lesbian, and bisexual studies and feminist studies was the questioning of the popular view that sexuality is a monolithic, identifiable, and palpable thing. Sexuality and gender are understood and defined within socio-historical contexts, and are therefore constantly evolving. Before discussing sexuality education, we will explore the concept and characteristics of sexuality more specifically than we have thus far. Then, we will examine various traditional notions and practices of sexuality education, the necessity of moving beyond these traditional notions and practices, a philosophical approach to education that accommodates a responsible treatment of sexuality within a school setting, and the characteristics of a program of sexuality education that would be more inclusive and responsive to students' personal and educational needs than the traditional courses. Next, we will explore why sexuality education should be undertaken in the schools. Finally, a discussion of the characteristics essential to teachers in sexuality education will be explored.

Characteristics of Sexuality

Gay, lesbian, and bisexual studies and feminist studies have questioned traditional notions of sexuality and gender. At first glance, "definitions" of sexuality appeared to have eluded gay, lesbian, bisexual, and feminist scholars. Individuals such as Michel Foucault and Jeffrey Weeks, for example, speak of the "discourses" and "languages" of sexuality without ever providing even a modicum of a concrete definition of "sexuality." One could criticize them and others for not operationalizing what they mean (even broadly) by sexuality. They would probably argue that there is no strict or definitive definition of sexuality, and that its meaning depends on particular socio-historical contexts.

The traditional or standard definitions of sexuality hardly capture the complexity of the topic. For instance, if we consult *The American Heritage Dictionary*, it defines "sexual" as:

> 1. Pertaining to, affecting, or characteristic of sex, the sexes, or the sex organs and their functions. 2. Having a sex or sexual organs. 3. Implying or symbolizing erotic desires or activity. 4. Pertaining to or designating reproduction involving the union of male or female gametes (1976, p. 1188).

This dictionary defines "sexuality" as: (1) The condition of being characterized and distinguished by sex. (2) Concern or preoccupation with sex. (3) The quality of possessing a sexual character or potency (p. 1188).

While it is convenient and expedient to confine one's conception of sexuality to a dictionary definition, it is inadequate for arriving at a satisfactory characterization of sexuality for discussing sexuality education. In many ways, what is defined as "sexual" is "in the eye of the beholder." There is *no* cut-and-dried definition. We need to examine a notion of sexuality that is more definitive than what Foucault and Weeks propose, but is more broadly conceived than the dictionary definition quoted above.

A broad view of human sexuality captures the breadth of experiences people consider to be sexual. Bruess and Greenberg (1988) break sexuality down into four dimensions, *viz.,* (1) ethical, (2) cultural, (3) biological, and (4) psychological aspects. The *ethical* arena include ideals, religious beliefs, moral opinions, and values. *Cultural* aspect of sexuality are: customs, laws, sanctions, and institutions. *Biological* dimensions are: reproduction, fertility control, sexual arousal and response, and physical appearance. *Psychological* components are emotions, motivation, expressiveness, learned attitudes, and behavior. But while Bruess and Greenberg provide a multitude of dimensions that may be connected in some way to sexuality, they fail to provide us with a tangible notion of sexuality itself.

In a philosophical essay that does not take for granted its readers' assumptions of what is meant by "sexuality," Alan Goldman (1977/1991) points out that the concept itself needs to be understood and explored. He states that sexual desire or behavior[1] (sexuality in general) should not be viewed categorically as having orgasm as an ultimate goal or end. Often sexuality is characterized as involving orgasm as a necessary ingredient to serve as some sort of testimonial that "it" was not only in fact a sexual act, but also "the real thing." This view artificially reduces sexuality and robs it of its richness and diversity.

The assumption that sexuality is a "means to an end" (orgasm) is problematic for a number of reasons. It necessarily discounts types of sexuality that do not conclude in orgasm. Also, holding such an assumption may lead one to seek orgasm with such energy and effort that the aesthetic value of the sexual process is lost. In essence, sexuality cannot be characterized as the presence of orgasm. Finally, it makes the assumption that sexuality is a physical and observable practice.

In an essay, "Sexual Behavior: Another position," Janice Moulton (1976/1991) makes the case that sexuality transcends the physical, as she states that seduction, flirtation, courtship, and even the anticipation of a date or sexual contact can not only be considered to be a part of sexuality, but also these experiences of anticipation can be more sexually gratifying than the physical experiences themselves.

Sexuality is a general concept of which many things are a part.[2] Sexual behaviors range from a seductive wink of any eye, to genital-genital or oral-genital contact, to autoeroticism. The psychological aspect of sexuality includes sexual desires, sexual fantasies, sexual dreams, and sexual motives. Also in this realm are how one defines oneself sexually, including her or his sexual identity, and how one perceives oneself sexually in general (and other aspects as outlined above by Bruess and Greenberg, 1988). Besides the behavioral, psychological, ethical, and cultural aspects of sexuality, we cannot forget to mention bio-medical aspects of sexuality, such as sexual health issues ranging from contraception practices and sexually transmitted disease prevention to genital self-exams and breast self-exams. Sexuality is a part of nearly every aspect of human existence.

In a thoroughly argued philosophical essay, "The Limits of Sexuality," Stephen David Ross (1984/1991) argues that sexuality has no limits, and that we construct the meanings of "it" in general, and more specifically what "it" means to us. Espousing an even more radical view, he suggests that sexuality cannot be separated from the rest of life. For example, he asserts that

> The range of sexuality, in our culture especially, is practically without limits: we ar assaulted on all sides by sexual images, in television and film, but also in daily experience, our clothing, size and weight, even what we eat and put under our arms, are permeated with sexual significance . . . The pervasiveness of sexuality suggests that it is not a matter of degree, but it is a characteristic of being human, at least a characteristic way in which we are human, p. 163.

He notes that "[s]exuality is not simply a physical, biological, or bodily condition for us, for it permeates even our highest spiritual activities—literature and art, even mathematics—for we characterize men and women by their different intellectual capacities" (p. 164).

Literature does a wonderful job of illustrating the varying degrees of subtlety of sexuality. In her book on lesbianism, JoAnn Loulan (1987) recounts an experience of one of the characters in her book:

> Remember the first time . . . the first time you felt that flush of love for a woman. For me it was for Mrs. McAndrews in second grade. I would just sit and stare for hours. She was tall, with tightly curled grey hair, and beautiful smooth skin. I was in heaven. That's lesbian magic (p. 32).

Edith Wharton (1918) in her novel, *Summer,* describes a scene depicting female sexuality:

> Since the day before, she had known exactly what she would feel if Harney should take her in his arms: the melting of palm into palm and mouth onto mouth, and the long flame burning from head to foot (p. 106).

An example of male homosexuality is depicted by E. M. Forster (1914) in his *Maurice.*

> He would not deceive himself so much. He would not—and this was the test—pretend to care about women when the only sex that attracted him was his own. He loved men and had always loved them. He longed to embrace them and mingle his being with theirs . . ." (p. 62).

The examples above illustrate how individuals express their sexualities and interpret them in a variety of ways and contexts. Clearly, sexuality is highly individualistic and subjective.

The Sexuality Information and Education Council of the United States (SIECUS) maintains that "sexuality" encompasses "the sexual knowledge, beliefs, feelings, attitudes, values, intentions, and behaviors of individuals" (Barthalow-Koch, 1992, p. 253; see also SIECUS, 1990).

Some expressions of sexuality are clearly recognized while others are not so clearly delineated. Among the obvious expressions of sexuality are masturbation, genital-genital contact, and oral-genital contact. Among the ones that are not so clear-cut are massage, kissing, holding hands, and so on. One could say that any expression that creates physiological and psychological responses that manifest "a bodily desire for one's or another's body" can be characterized as sexual. This can be seen as a form of tension, which can be acted upon by oneself or with others, or not at all.

Sexuality can be manifested and acted upon in numerous ways with various outcomes, ranging from sexual stirring to a "full-blown orgasm." To acknowledge the complexity of sexuality and to facilitate further discussion about it, it is useful to turn to Ludwig Wittgenstein's (1953/1968) *Philosophical Investigations.* He claims that, contrary to Plato's views, words have neither static nor monolithic meanings. Wittgenstein maintains that the meaning of a word lies in its use, and that since most words have a variety of uses, no *one* use necessarily has more legitimacy or veracity than another. Commenting on Wittgenstein's view on language games, T. Z. Lavine (1984) says, "There is no essence which these uses have in common; there are only similarities, which Wittgenstein describes as 'family resemblances,' among the various uses of a word, 'a complicated network or similarities overlapping and crisscrossing' " (p. 406).

Wittgenstein is enormously helpful when we try to characterize sexuality. For example, a gynecologist and urologist are sure to speak differently about what constitutes sexual behavior compared to two relatively unsophisticated teenagers, who, by the way, would use a different language than professional sexuality educators use to discuss such matters. An analytic philosopher who had an opportunity to listen to various groups struggle to characterize sexual behavior would notice "family resemblances" in the various terms used. Wittgenstein does not find fault with groups of people for not universalizing language to mean this or that; insofar as various groups develop their own language "games" with rules that are functional for a given group, there is no assumption that one group's mode of communication is necessarily inferior to another group's.

In a Wittgensteinian sense, when referring to what constitutes sexuality, gynecologists and urologists would often refer to sexual behavior in relation to genitalia, including reproductive health issues. Sexuality is viewed by these professionals as a mechanical activity in relationship to health issues and reproduction. Teenagers, when referring to sexuality, often reduce it to sexual intercourse. For example, many teenagers claim that they have not been sexual, because they have not engaged in sexual intercourse; therefore, they can, and often do, claim virginal status. Professional sexuality educators, unlike the gynecologists, urologists, and teenagers, are likely to view sexuality much more broadly, encompassing not only various sexual activities, but also erotic feelings, relationships, values, and various forms of discourse. These various conceptions of sexuality and the ways of communicating about it are no more valid in one compared to the next. It is simply a matter of the functionality of language and its usage within groups that remains the most important element, according to Wittgenstein. The significance of this is that sexuality is conceived differently rom one group to the next, and this, as we shall see later, has serious implications for sexuality education.

Wittgenstein's conceptions and theories of language help to point out the complexities of sexuality. While Foucault and Weeks refer to various discourses and languages of sexuality in general, which assumes that people in a given geographical area within a particular socio-historical context understand and speak a "universal language of sexuality," Wittgenstein assumes no universal or static form of language. This has tremendous implications for the original question raised in this chapter: "What is sexuality?" As noted above, according to Wittgenstein, different groups use different languages, and that language is dynamic, malleable, with no "hard-and-fast" rules of usage. This necessarily means that as language develops, changes, and is used in different ways, different conceptions of sexuality are developed. This in turn creates innumerable meanings for sexuality, and again, has implications for sexuality education.

Given Wittgenstein's analysis of language, particularly the notion that language is dynamic, necessarily means that there will be various meanings of sexuality. Therefore, sexuality encompasses many things, including actions, events, and thoughts. It cannot be treated as a monolithic entity if the true complexity and multidimensional aspects of sexuality are to be explored. There are things sexually speaking that most people would agree are indeed sexual (e.g., genital-genital intercourse, oral-genital contact, oral-anal contact, genital-anal contact, masturbation, or a deep, passionate kiss, and so on). However, there are plenty of other aspects of sexuality that are less obvious but just as significant to many people such as sexual innuendos, nuances in intimate/sexual communication, issues of sexual consent, and so on). Less obvious forms of sexuality often go unexplored in most sexuality education settings. They need to be explored not only to flesh out sexuality conceptually but also to encourage individuals to acquire a sophisticated understanding of sexuality. As will be explored shortly, traditional sexuality education provides a negatively skewed and superficial knowledge of sexuality. Ideally, a comprehensive approach to sexuality education will provide individuals with a multifaceted and an urbane understanding of sexuality that will ultimately enhance their lives.

Sexuality education must accommodate many aspects of sexuality, including those aspects that have shifting meanings. To provide some focus, let us turn to the work of Bruess and Greenberg (1988). As noted earlier in this chapter, they break sexuality into four dimensions (*viz.,* ethical, cultural, biological, and psychological). Moreover, they recommend that sexuality education deal broadly with a multitude of attitudes, beliefs, behaviors, and relationships. More specific recommendations will be presented later. The main point is that sexuality education will be successful only if it is more inclusive than traditional, narrow conceptions of sexuality.

One might ask, "Why does the success of sexuality education depend on going beyond traditional, narrow conceptions of sexuality?" First, as we will discover in more detail later, traditional conceptions of sexuality do not address its multidimensionality. Second, beyond reproductive sexuality, sexuality has been studied and portrayed from a disease perspective; at least a balanced viewpoint should be offered. Third, while many individuals fit the sexual norm, many others do not. They need to be represented and their invisibility needs to be shattered. Fourth, the traditional, narrow view of sexuality is limiting and very prescriptive. Affording individuals a diverse and broad knowledge base will likely assist them in making better-informed sexual decisions, and could potentially enrich their sexual relationships.

Traditional Notions and Practices of Sex Education

Sexuality education has never enjoyed much of a priority in American primary and secondary schools. When it has existed, it has not reflected the complexity of the topic. Sex education began in the United States during the late-nineteenth and early-twentieth centuries to combat sexually transmitted disease (STDs) and to instill sexual morality and propriety in the young. The legacy of educating students about the bio-medical and hygienic aspects of sexuality has survived up to the present. Most sex education classes at the secondary level are housed in health education or biological sciences. Health educators and biology teachers are saddled with the responsibility of teaching sex education; there are neither specific classes on sexuality education, nor specially trained sexuality educators.

In years past, it was considered inappropriate to educate pupils about sexuality in coeducational settings. At that time, sexuality education was foisted onto physical education teachers, not because they had special training, but because this was one of the only times during the school day when students were segregated by sex in gym class (Tyack and Hansot, 1992). Having gym teachers teach sexuality education not only symbolically linked sexuality solely to the physical aspects of life but also actually reinforced the notion that sexuality was a physical thing, ignoring the psychological, socio-cultural, and ethical dimensions of sexuality.

Early in this century, scare tactics were employed to teach proper sexual behavior and uphold moral standards. There was a preoccupation with sexually transmitted diseases (STDs) (then referred to as venereal diseases). It was common for teachers to show students slides of the most horrific manifestations of various venereal diseases, attempting to scare students into abstinence, and restrict sexual behaviors to acts of procreation within the confines of the marital bedroom. There are striking similarities of sex education in the past with current sexuality education practices. In addition, by deploying scare tactics and extolling the virtues of abstinence, schools continue to try to control adolescents' sexuality rather than affirm it. The possibility of contracting sexually transmitted diseases is constantly hanging over the heads of students: much of sexuality education today is nothing more than a warning about sexuality's myriad dangers, ranging from sexual abuse and rape to death.

Both the overt curriculum and the hidden sexuality education curriculum from the primary grades through secondary schools teach that sexuality is essentially dangerous. In the primary grades, children are taught about "good touch" and "bad touch." Essentially they learn about child sexual abuse. Along the same lines that sexuality is portrayed as dangerous, Jonathan Silin (1995), a noted educator and HIV/AIDS educational consultant, reports that in elementary schools children are learning about HIV/AIDS only in the context of health studies, devoid of any sociocultural considerations. The focus is mostly on how HIV/AIDS *is* contracted, and relatively little information is offered about how it is *not* contracted. However, abstinence is usually mentioned as a preventative measure. What is learned about sexuality, excluding strictly reproductive sexuality (the biological facts), is that it is an unacceptable and a mysterious topic.

To illustrate this point further, Silin describes and analyzes the HIV/AIDS elementary school curriculum outlined in The New York State Aids Instructional Guide, developed by the New York State Education Department in 1987. He notes that

> [M]any districts adopted it [the AIDS Instructional Guide] *in toto* as the curriculum in order to save time and avoid controversy. This is an interesting political document, with its community review panels to assure decency, its denial of the sexual realities of teenagers' lives, and its careful attention to parents' right to withdraw their children from lessons dealing with HIV prevention (p. 62).

Admittedly, schools as they presently exist need to save time, and parents need to be afforded the right to remove their child(ren) from what they believe are inappropriate educational experiences. But assuring "decency," whatever this means, and denying the sexual realities of students, conveys the message that sex is dangerous or bad. Astutely avoiding a topic whether as an effort to be decent or to avoid sexual realities, sends a loud and clear anti-sexual message.

HIV/AIDS education, although very necessary, connects sexuality with disease. Some states have mandated HIV/AIDS education. As we know, Silin is critical about HIV/AIDS education having such a health focus; this creates sexophobia. To offer students a broader perspective and to avoid a sex-negative trap, this epidemic should be taught using a broader, interdisciplinary perspective, and should not be used as a tool to propagate scare tactics and create unwarranted fear.

At the secondary level, sexuality education focuses on sexually transmitted diseases (STDs) with a special emphasis on HIV/AIDS, as an attempt, in part, to reinforce the virtues of abstinence. Also, the coverage of sexual harassment and date rape is common (Haffner, 1992). All that can go wrong with sexuality is emphasized in the majority of sexuality education curricula. Sexuality education is commonly provided in physical education, health education, and biology classes. Most sexuality education is reduced to a unit within these classes. At best, students receive a few weeks of instruction annually. Some sexuality education ". . . 'courses' are limited to a lecture of an hour or two" (Hacker, 1981, p. 207).

What is taught is usually limited to the biological aspects of human sexuality. Sol Gordon (1979) refers to this educational practice as "the relentless pursuit of the fallopian tubes." The picture about what constitutes sexuality education is quite clear. The "plumbing," "mechanical," and disease aspects constitute the curriculum. This reduces sexuality to a physical phenomenon, ignoring many other facets of sexuality such as learning about interpersonal communication, building self-esteem, developing intimate relationships, and examining values. Some might argue that these aspects can be taught in other curricula. Indeed, they could be offered independently of sexuality education. However, they would likely be taught devoid of any sexuality contexts. Being that sexuality is so central to most of our lives, the above-mentioned facets of sexuality need addressing in addition to the "plumbing" aspects of sexual functioning.

Students have received many other messages from this limited perspective of sexuality. Although it may never be articulated by sexuality educators, students leave the classroom with an understanding that heterosexuality is more revered and is simply better than other sexual identities. Discussions about bisexuality and homosexuality are often missing. Essentially, this conveys the message that bisexuals, gays, and lesbians are not "fully sexual human beings" (Ellis, 1984), or to the contrary, that they are overly sexual and hardly need mentioning. When bisexuality and homosexuality are discussed, only a very short amount of time is allotted. Nearly all of the time is spent on heterosexuality. Often students are taught with the assumption that they will eventually settle down into a heterosexually based, monogamous, nuclear family, and produce children (Haffner, 1992). Traditional sexuality education programs seldom question traditional gender roles, sexism, and basic assumptions about traditional views of sexuality in general.

Although most sexuality education courses teach the physiological, mechanical aspects of sexuality, Haffner (1992) notes that in some courses ". . . the hidden curriculum teaches teenagers that in order to be popular, one has to be attractive, physically fit and able-bodied, heterosexual, conform to gender-role expectations, and dress according to school norms" (p. vii). Much of the current curricula give students the impression that sexual expression is reserved for adults and if minors engage in such activities they are "playing with fire." The idea of the fluidity of sexual expression, the language of sexual intimacy, and the creativity of human sexual response is sorely missing in traditional sexuality education programs (Sears, 1992).

Moving Beyond Traditional Notions and Practices of Sexuality Education

To provide students with adequate and responsible sexuality education, curricular efforts should be reconceptualized and made far more inclusive than ever before. As we have already explored, traditional notions have reduced sexuality to a mechanical, physical act and are narrowly conceived. Additionally, sexuality education in the past tended to be and still appears to be socially and educationally irresponsible, not to mention authoritarian.

Traditional sexuality education is socially irresponsible, in part, because it fails to address sexual issues of individuals who identify as non-heterosexuals and do not plan on getting traditionally married or assuming parental responsibilities. It also ignores issues of ethnic diversity. Most sexuality education today assumes a monolithic understanding of sexuality and sexual relationships, ignoring values, customs, and practices of people from various cultural contexts. In other words, because the biological and health aspects of sexuality comprise the majority of sexuality education, sexuality is grossly oversimplified. In the process of biologizing sexuality to the point of viewing "it" as a readily identifiable physical manifestation, the philosophical, psychological, and socio-cultural aspects of sexuality go unexamined. Its social irresponsibility is also revealed in its assumption that sexual interaction occurs only among able-bodied adults; the disabled (differently abled individuals) are ignored and are relegated to being sexually invisible (see Chapter 13 in this volume). How must these students who do not fit into "the norm" (in terms of sexual identity, physical ability, and ethnicity) feel when passed over? Surely they must feel invisible, inferior, defective, wrong, perverse, and even downright weird!

Inevitably, sexuality education involves addressing some aspects of gender. Issues of gender are not treated responsibly either. A number of scholars of sexuality education have noted that nearly all forms of sexuality education fail to challenge traditional gender role stereotypes, which allow patriarchal practices to continue. This in turn helps keep women socially and economically oppressed, treated as second-class citizens. How socially responsible is this? Sexuality education must address issues of gender because sexual behaviors, expectations, and even the initiation of potentially romantic involvements are gender based. Our society has expectations of females and males in general, and along sexual lines as well. An examination of gender roles, then, becomes a major aspect of sexuality education. Again, gender undergirds and shapes sexual relationships.

Current sexuality education efforts are educationally inadequate and irresponsible as well. Given the fact that so few hours are devoted to sexuality education, not to mention that only a finite number of topics are included (e.g., abstinence, sexually transmitted diseases, HIV/AIDS), it is simply impossible to provide an adequate, appropriate, effective, and responsible education. The educational net must be cast more broadly, and this will require a more substantive treatment. A unit in a general biology class will not do! A few hours in a health and safety course, in which sexuality education competes for coverage along with driver's education, drug education, and nutrition, are inadequate.

Some individuals might argue that sexuality education is adequate, appropriate, responsible, and effective even given its minor role in the curriculum. Many people think this is all of the time that it should be afforded: a unit in a health or biology class is perfectly acceptable. After all, it is a sensitive topic and teachers are already overburdened, not to mention that there is not too much to teach regarding sexuality, anyway. This is a popular point of view. This is absolutely true if all we want to do is reproduce the idea that sexuality can be boiled down to a few biological facts along with some precautions about how to avoid sexually transmitted diseases. This could be accomplished in a few weeks! However, if comprehensive sexuality education is desired, not only does much more need to be included but also the way sexuality education is conceptualized and taught needs revamping to include an interdisciplinary approach in which students are taught to discover sexual issues in a broader context as opposed to what has traditionally occurred. This will be argued in more detail later in this chapter.

To return to the idea that public schooling endorses authoritarian measures, it can be said that most teachers run their classrooms like prisons; students are treated like inmates (Illich, 1970). Donald Arnstine (1995), a philosopher of education, speaks cogently about this aspect of the school system, as he writes

> . . . the system's purpose is to support and help maintain the status quo of our dominant social institutions, which are hierarchical, authoritarian, and unequal, competitive, racist, sexist, and homophobic. It achieves this purpose by keeping the young in school under adult surveillance as long as possible . . . (p. 183).

Supporting Arnstine's observations, Jerry Farber (1969), a critic of schooling practices, avers

> In fact, for most of your school life, it doesn't make that much difference what subject you're taught. The real lesson is the method. The medium in school truly is the message. And the medium is, above all, coercive. You're forced to attend. The subjects are required. You have to do homework. You must observe school rules. And throughout, you're bullied into docility and submissiveness (p. 61).

It stands to reason that because most teachers have not had any formal education in human sexuality studies, and because teachers, too, are victims of the general societal "sexophobia/erotophobia," they tend to be controlling of their students. Also, because sexuality is such a sensitive and controversial topic, sexuality educators are more vulnerable to school administrative and community criticism—including the school board—than, say, art, English, history, science, or social studies teachers. The apprehension and fear on the part of those attempting to teach sexuality education create an even more authoritarian atmosphere than in "mainstream" classrooms. Some teachers try to avoid controversy personally, even to the extent of inviting guest speakers from various organizations such as a local department of public health, Planned Parenthood, or other organizations. Often these invited speakers give bland lectures so as not to upset the school board and local community. Students frequently hear about the medical aspects of sexuality, while coverage of other important aspects is foregone. The genuine interests of the students is not taken into consideration. Students get lectured to by an "outsider" who is neither familiar with the students' needs nor their personalities.

Maximizing Sexuality Education: A Compatible Philosophy of Education

The traditional approach outlined above not only prevents a worthwhile educational experience from occurring but is also the antithesis of an educational process that teaches democratic ideals. It does not prepare students for democratic involvement in society, and it discourages, active, participative citizenship. The traditional educational process reduces students to passive learners who, during the course of their twelve years of mandatory attendance, develop much learned helplessness and even apathy about the "education" that is served up in school (Farber, 1969; Goodlad, 1984). John Goodlad, a noted author in the field of education, observes in his landmark work, *A Place Called School* (1984), that when interviewing students about their experiences in school their feelings were ". . . far from either enthusiastic or full of dislike . . . virtually all of the indices fell off toward the negative side with upward progression through the grades" (p. 232). In another passage, Goodlad (1984) observes "[w]hether we looked at how teachers related to students or how students related to teachers, the overwhelming impression was one of affective neutrality—a relationship neither abrasive nor joyous" (p. 110). Again, we see the apathetic nature of students' relationships with their teachers.

Along traditional educational lines, working alone as a self-sufficient being is encouraged and rewarded (Arnstine, 1995; Goodlad, 1984). This is absurd, given that "true" self-sufficiency is a myth and is logically impossible. We all need others to get along in life. We need some people for moral and emotional support. We need others to be able to share ideas and thus become better thinkers. Some people meet our erotic and sexual needs. And there are those we help, which, in part, gives us a sense of self-worth and self-esteem (self-efficacy) and a reason to be in this world. Some individuals transcend any one of the above categories and perform a multitude of functions. The point is that schools, as they currently function, encourage students to become socially disabled. Given that life can be conceived of as social interactions of one sort or another, it is immoral and unethical for schools to encourage silence, isolation, and "self-sufficiency." Goodlad (1984) points out that after getting "snapshots" of more than 1,000 classrooms, he observed that more or less students were sitting quietly in rows and disconnected from each other. Jonathan Kozol (1991), a prominent author of several works on the grave conditions of schooling and childhood, registers his concern for how children ". . . seem not just lacking in important, useful information that would help them to achieve their dreams, but, in a far more drastic sense, cut off and disconnected from the outside world" (p. 70). It is clear that this type of atmosphere does not promote social interaction. What is likely to result from this kind of experience is that students will be ill-equipped socially to work with others to solve problems both in and out of school, and to relate to others in general. Therefore, it is reasonable to reach the conclusion that schools are promoting—although unwittingly—social disability.

In addition, schools encourage "authority addiction," in which students become overly dependent on teachers who play extraordinarily authoritarian roles. Goodlad (1984) notes that "[o]ur students perceived their teachers to be in charge of the classroom and, on average, perceived themselves to be doing what the teacher told or expected them to do" (p. 110). Students learn very early that the "name of the game" is to please teachers at all costs. The students' views, genuine interests, and needs often take a back seat, and are supplanted with a pre-established, rigid curriculum, which is often far removed from the concerns and lives of the students. Most of the school day is devoted to socialization and not education (Arnstine, 1995). Students spend at least a dozen years in school in an environment that is "artificial" and foreign to the world in which they will find themselves for the rest of their lives, a world that is heavily dependent on the human relationships that develop from social interaction, assistance to and from others, cooperative problem solving, shared governance, etc.

The chief aim of schooling ought to be fostering social, intellectual, and personal growth. A good example of this is the "whole-child concept" of education. According to Ornstein and Levine (1993) this educational approach proposed that ". . . schools had to be concerned with the growth and development of the entire child, not just with certain mental aspects of the child's growth" (p. 500). This is not possible unless schools change radically. While it is unrealistic to move entirely into a progressive, Deweyan educational mode (described later in this chapter), there should at least be a serious attempt to devote a significant part of the school day to allow students of various abilities, backgrounds, and interests to interact and work conjointly on projects or topics that interest them. This would be a step in the right direction. After all, most public schools are heterogeneous in terms of race and ethnicity, religious backgrounds, socio-economic classes, intellectual and physical abilities, sexual preferences, interests, and so on. Arnstine (1996) notes that diversity is a necessary condition for learning, and that it is an important element of a democratic education.

It makes sense that a society such as ours, that at least "pays lip service" to being democratic, ought to run its public educational system on democratic ideals. The spirit of such an educational enterprise ought to pay serious attention to and embrace a philosophy that deals with representation, dissent, controversy, justice, fairness, respect for diversity, freedom of speech, equality, choice, consent and so on. Nel Noddings (1992) notes that

> To achieve a democracy we must try things out, evaluate them without personal prejudice, revise them if they are found wanting, and decide what to do next through a process of reasoned consensus or compromise in which authority of expertise is consulted but not allowed to impose its views with no discussion of how, why, and on what grounds (pp. 164–165).

According to James Sears (1992) "[t]he educator has an important role in a democratic society: to encourage intellectual flexibility, to foster analytical thought, and to expand tolerance" (pp. 147–148). But professional educators at the primary, secondary, and even post-secondary levels have failed to fulfill the role that Noddings (1992) and Sears (1992) outline above both in the standard curriculum and in sexuality education. John Goodlad (1990) points out that in teacher education programs the ". . . heavy dominance of lecturing by teacher education faculty (and the resulting passivity on the part of the students) allows little opportunity for critical, independent thinking to flourish among teachers in training" (p. 185). Teachers are often well-intentioned about encouraging their students to think critically and independently, and work cooperatively, but the reality is a far cry from what teachers proclaim to want for their students.

A requisite approach to moving beyond traditional notions of sexuality education is to articulate a philosophy of education that accommodates the complexities of this educational enterprise. An appropriate philosophy of education would be one that is compatible with and espouses democratic ideals. James Sears (1992) asserts that ". . . [p]ublic schools in a democratic society are a marketplace for ideas. 'Access to ideas,' as Justice Brennan wrote, 'prepares students for active and effective participation in the pluralistic, often contentious society in which they will soon be adult members' " (p. 147 as quoted in Dutile, 1986). It is important that a practical and socially responsible philosophy of education be a foundation for a responsive and solid sexuality education curriculum.

Many modern philosophies of education come from traditions of idealism, realism, analytic philosophy, humanism, existentialism, and pragmatism.[3] Of these, pragmatism is the most promising for moving away from traditional methods of sexuality education (and schooling in general for that matter) and moving toward a democratic educational process. Born out of pragmatism during the first half of this century (1900–1950), the progressive education movement was led by John Dewey, George Counts, Harold Rugg, and William Heard Kilpatrick (Stevens and Wood, 1992). While progressive educators did not argue for a specific and preplanned curriculum, they all agreed that fostering democratic ideals in education was imperative.

According to progressive educators, the school should concern itself with children's experiences. This idea conflicted with traditionalists[4] such as Arthur Bestor, James Conant, and Admiral H. G. Rickover, who believed that students ought primarily to learn "the basics," colloquially referred to as the three R's. This mode of education relies quite heavily on memorization and recitation, and is more or less an "industrial model of education" whereby schooling is to prepare students for life and work. Current educational programs like "Goals 2000" and "Back to the Basics" best exemplify the traditionalists' philosophy. The traditional approach to education relies heavily on teachers as authoritarians whose primary responsibility is imparting ready-made bodies of knowledge to students, while they sit passively "at attention" receiving and trying to make sense of facts and data. Attention is seldom paid to relevance (if any) of course work to students' lives.

Progressive educators oppose such educational methods. They view employment possibilities as a secondary, if not a tertiary, aim of schooling. These educators encourage students toward self-governance, and are child-centered or society-centered. In fact, progressive educators were heavily influenced by developmental psychologists: G. Stanley Hall and Arnold Gesell sensitized progressive educators to the importance of child development, readiness, and motivation in a learning environment. This environment should be sensitive to children's needs and interests.

Although many individuals could be identified with the progressive education movement, we shall focus on one of the most prominent American philosophers of education and an exemplar of pragmatism and progressive education, John Dewey. His philosophy of education can offer much to creating a sensible form of sexuality education in the schools. We have already learned of how shallow, ineffective, and irresponsible past and current sexuality education efforts have been. Dewey and his followers would disapprove of how schooling is conducted. Schools today are wedded to the traditional approach to education, and sexuality education has been no exception.

In *Experience and Education* (1938), John Dewey asserted that the teacher's chief task is to organize meaningful classroom experiences that emerge from children's environments. Dewey believed that ". . . the rise of what is called new education and progressive schools is of itself a product of discontent with traditional education" (p. 18). He notes ". . . [t]he main purpose or objective is to prepare the young for future responsibilities and for success in life, by means of acquisition of organized bodies of information and prepared forms of skill which comprehend the material of instruction" (p. 18). When speaking about students in the context of traditional methods of instruction, Dewey maintains "[s]ince the subject-matter as well as standards of proper conduct are handed down from the past, the attitude of pupils must, upon the whole, be one of docility, receptivity, and obedience" (p. 18). Dewey opposed traditional, authoritative education. Dewey emphasized that education necessarily needed to focus on social activities ". . . and that the school was a social agency that helped shape human character and behavior" (Ornstein and Levine, 1993, p. 140). Rather than preparing students (the "young" or "immature," as Dewey referred to them) for adult life, their immediate interests and needs needed to be tended to for personal growth to take place. Nel Noddings (1992) characterizes Dewey's conceptions of education by stating:

> [f]or Dewey education . . . is a constructive achievement. It is not a matter of absorbing something already laid out, tried and true. It is a matter of tying things out with the valued help of experts (teachers), of evaluating, revising, comparing, sharing, communicating, constructing, choosing. Strictly speaking, there is no end product—no ideally educated person—but a diverse host of persons showing signs of increasing growth" (p. 165).

Many have mistakenly understood Dewey's recommendations to mean aimless, haphazard, and chaotic classroom activities. This is not true. What Dewey advocated was teachers allowing students to be socially active beings, and facilitating and guiding them through experiences. Dewey believed that individuals are curious about their world and want to explore it. In doing so, according to Dewey, individuals ultimately encounter problems that need to be solved. If the situation that creates the problem for the individual is of genuine interest she or he will be fully invested (intrinsically motivated) to use intelligent measures to solve the problem (Dewey, 1916). Dewey believed that people with common concerns and interests should work together to solve problems. This is an active approach to gaining knowledge. He believed that knowledge was not good just for its own sake. Rather, gaining knowledge through educative experiences was "good" insofar as it served some type of instrumental process and facilitated personal and social growth.

To Dewey the school is a microcosm of the larger society. It brings the young together, an opportunity for social participation in testing their ideas. The school is a socio-cultural laboratory where students can use the scientific method to solve problems and become reflective and active thinkers (Dewey, 1900/1902, 1916, and 1938; Ornstein and Levine, 1993). In this setting the individual is free to express and test ideas and beliefs no matter how controversial. Everything is subject to critical inquiry, even the curriculum. In fact, Dewey advocated that students and teachers work conjointly to create a "curriculum."

Dewey did not favor obliterating authority altogether. The traditional authoritarian model of the teacher is transformed so that the teacher is viewed as the "senior" member in a group who assists students with refining their questions and their conceptions of their areas of inquiry, rather than as a teacher inculcating previously organized bodies of knowledge into the heads of students. Dewey was convinced that so long as teachers used their authority in a coercive or inhumane way, genuine inquiry would be blocked. Dewey opposed this. Stevens and Wood (1992), attempting to articulate Dewey's views, write "[t]he teacher's task is to order and organize meaningful classroom experiences that draw from the child's environment and utilize information from the academic disciplines" (p. 293). Students use an interdisciplinary approach, methodologies and information from many academic disciplines for solving particular problems. These experiences then become educative ones.

An example of engagement in a Deweyan educative experience is sexual harassment. This topic is sensitive and not likely to be raised—and should not be addressed as an isolated issue—in a classroom without a broader socio-cultural context. A sexuality educator could put this issue in a broad social context by facilitating a discussion on gender. One way to accomplish this is to have students view an MTV program, and ask them to observe how females and males are portrayed. Asking students to break into small groups of four to six members, a teacher could ask them to discuss similarities between what society expects of males and females gender-wise and what MTV portrays. Students will undoubtedly enumerate traditional gender role stereotypes encouraged by our society. They are likely to communicate that males are encouraged to be strong, uncommunicative, unemotional, sexually active, competent, intelligent, authoritarian, and dominant. Students are likely to assert that females are supposed to be weak, communicative, emotional, sexually abstemious, incompetent, intellectually dull, powerless, and submissive.[5]

Following the discussion of gender stereotypes, the sexuality educator could engage students in discussion of how such attitudes are displayed in their lives, both in and out of school. To explore these issues thoroughly, several institutions might be examined. For example, analyses of the educational, medical, political, and religious institutions are needed to show how these entities perpetuate traditional gender role stereotypes. The various forms of media (particularly the advertising industry) also need to be examined critically.

After this discussion, students might be encouraged to see the relationship between the institutionalization of traditional gender role stereotypes and how people relate to one another. At this point, students, by their comments and questions, are likely to reveal an interest in a particular aspect of this issue (e.g., communication patterns between men and women, women and women, and men and men, violence, date or acquaintance rape, sexual harassment, or other aspects). Drawing from the students' observations and experiences, the teacher might encourage students to focus on how gender stereotypes negatively influence interpersonal and work relationships, even to the extent of being precursors to sexual harassment.

Sexual harassment is an important social issue relevant to nearly everyone. Dewey believed that ". . . the school must represent present life—life as real and vital to the child as that which he [or she] carries on at home, in the neighborhood, or on the playground" (Dworkin, 1959, p. 22). Dewey would agree that relationships are paramount to the educative experience. Most people want to date and become romantically and sexually involved. Aspects of dating and sexual etiquette would pique the interest of most students. The teacher, whether in a classroom, workshop, or other type of forum, could spark the interest of the students even further by a discussion. Students could examine such topics as consent, violence, inappropriate sexual advances, and how all of these issues are portrayed in the media. Students could begin to see connections between these aspects of daily life and how they influence social relations, not only on a personal, more immediate level but also on a more general community and societal level.

An exploration of issues surrounding sexual harassment should go beyond discussion and move into various educative activities. With the guidance of a teacher or counselor, students could involve themselves in a variety of activities in school and out in the community. One idea would be to encourage students to examine how men and women are pictured in the media and report on how these depictions might perpetuate sexual harassment and sexism. This would involve students going beyond the confines of the school and examining various types of media: advertising, newspaper articles, music, art, and so on. This would provide students with an opportunity to critique traditional representations of men and women. Students could organize panel discussions and debates with community members and professionals. Another idea would be for students to produce a school play or an in-class skit depicting traditional roles of men and women, and then provide "correctives" in the production to illustrate alternatives to traditional, patriarchal practices. The performance might begin by showing societal attitudes on men and women in general, and then portray a couple becoming intimate (either realistically or symbolically), and show how a situation could lead to sexual harassment. Equally as important, the performance could illustrate "healthy" attitudes and behaviors that would illuminate the importance of equality, consent, and effective communication not only to prevent sexual harassment in and out of intimate relationships but also to create satisfying and fulfilling relationships.

Sexuality education, like other courses of study, suffers from censorship, dilution of material and information, and outright bigotry. In many cases, teachers are told what they can and cannot teach because it is an area of contested values. Many are forbidden to teach about birth control, homosexuality, and masturbation, just to list a few of the prohibited topics. Furthermore, if students desire to ask questions or pursue issues that fall outside of the purview of what is permitted in the curriculum, their inquiries are usually ignored summarily or pushed aside, thus not taken seriously.

What Sexuality Education Ought to Include

Sexuality has always been and will continue to be a controversial topic. Its contentiousness has resulted in public schools' having avoided giving it a solid position in the curriculum. Also, sexuality education has not been viewed as part of an "academic" curriculum. In fact, not only have school boards and other policy-making entities not even so much as hinted about having sexuality education enjoy a curricular priority but they have actively resisted providing responsible sexuality education.[6] As already mentioned, not to offer a subject or discuss a topic because it is controversial is antithetical to democratic ideals. If for no other reason than this, sexuality education, along with all of the other "unmentionables," deserves coverage, discussion, and exploration!

Upholding democratic ideals is not the only reason for offering sexuality education. It is only one among many reasons for offering such a program of study. Before we go on to explore arguments for why a rational sexuality education ought to have a prominent place in the schools, we need to examine what we are referring to as "responsible or rational sexuality education." What does it include?

First, is gender education. This is tied to sexuality education in the sense that people usually[7] fall into two categories—females and males—based on biological sex. Based on the notion of opposite sex, there ought to be an exploration of assumptions about gender and gender role stereotypes. It is important to discuss various aspects of gender, ranging from sexism to the notion that females and males are opposites. Many scholars raise questions about the social construction of the binary notion of opposite sex. Even the issue of how girls are treated differently from boys in school settings is a worthwhile topic.[8] Transgender individuals—cross dressers and transsexuals—exist in and out of schools. Practices and lifestyles of those who do not conform to traditional gender role stereotypes (in everything from mannerisms to dress) ought to be critically examined, if for no other reason than to expose the hegemony and consequences of traditional notions of gender.

Conceptions of gender and how the socialization process influences how we relate to one another are in need of much examination.[9] Also, the ways that gender is portrayed in the media deserve attention and close, critical scrutiny.

Intimate and sexual relationships need to be explored in a sexuality education program. This includes such aspects as barriers to forming relationships, initiating relationships, sexual decision making, conflict resolution, sexual consent, communication about sexual matters (from perceptions to individual preferences and limits) deserve coverage. Additionally, assumptions about what constitutes a "valid" relationship need to be explored. In a pluralistic society, students ought to know the numerous forms of sexual relationships, for example, monogamous, non-monogamous, bisexual, heterosexual, homosexual, open, and closed relationships.

While it is important to learn how to relate to others in sexual situations, it is also important to learn about oneself, sexually speaking. This is often done by exploring not only one's thoughts about sexual matters but also exploring one's body by autoeroticism or masturbation. Statistically, many people masturbate. The old myths about physical illness (e.g., going blind, etc.) and bodily changes (e.g., growing hair on the palms of hands, etc.) persist. This creates many questions and much anxiety among adolescents. Also, it would be beneficial to discuss people's private sexual fantasies and that they are common.

Students ought to be prepared for the physical changes they will experience as they enter and go through puberty and their adolescent years. Girls ought to be prepared emotionally and intellectually for menstruation. This issue should be addressed responsibly and sensitively, unlike some of the horror stories about the ways that girls learn about their menstrual cycles. For example, Crooks and Baur (1996) report that, according to one study, "43% of women reported feeling confused, frightened, panicky, or ill when they started their first period, and one-third of the women . . . did not know about menstruation before they began to menstruate . . ." (p. 99). Some young women are told that they are going to bleed to death, that they have the curse, and other such myths. Young men are not any better-informed about menstruation. Sexuality education needs to be inclusive. It needs to address the biological, mechanical aspects of sexuality and at the same time consider their socio-cultural considerations. The main point is that it should be done intelligently and sensibly.

The issue of sexual diversity ought to be addressed in sexuality education. This includes the disabled, those suffering from various medical conditions, or recent sufferers of spinal cord injuries. Injured or disabled individuals are discounted sexually. They are sexually invisible. Many perceive them to be sexless or asexual with no interest in having sexually fulfilling relationships. This myth needs to be exploded, and sexuality education is an appropriate forum to examine these issues.

Sexual invisibility is a major problem. Those who do not fit the typical conception of what is considered "normal" are invisible. Bisexuals, gays, and lesbians are often either ignored or bashed! Even though thousands upon thousands of bisexuals, gays, and lesbians have made societal contributions (literary prominence, historical recognition, scientific advancements, etc.), their sexual preferences continue to be ignored in the traditional curriculum. One might argue that if one is studying achievements of prominent writers, artists, and historical figures, there is no reason to discuss their sexual preferences. But it is of paramount importance that their sexualities be known. To the extent that their works reflect and are a part of their sexuality, this provides us with a sense of the lenses through which they viewed and related to the world. Most importantly, these significant people can serve as role models for bisexual, gay, and lesbian people. Famous people like Leonardo Da Vinci and Michelangelo have a "more complete" visibility in the curriculum. When literature is taught at the high school level (and more than occasionally at the college and university level) the fact that James Baldwin, E. M. Forster, Audre Lorde, Mary Renault, Gore Vidal, and Walt Whitman were other than heterosexual is never explored, not to mention that the homosexually significant overtones of their work remain unexamined.

We also need to consider that many bisexual, gay, lesbian, and questioning youth are being verbally, emotionally, and physically assaulted in the schools (Elia, 1993/1994).[10] Homophobia is rampant and needs to be addressed. The whole issue of the marginalization and subsequent discrimination against non-heterosexuals needs serious attention in the schools.

Along with the fulfilling and pleasurable aspects of sexuality are the potential consequences of "unprotected" sexual behavior. Sexually transmitted disease (STD) prevention and contraception are part of sexuality education. Traditionally, scare tactics have been the primary educational modality. Along similar medical lines, boys ought to be taught to do testicular self-examinations and girls should learn how to perform monthly breast self-examinations. Young males between the ages of fifteen and thirty-five are at the highest risk for testicular cancer (Crooks and Baur, 1996). Women, both younger and older, run risks of breast cancer, depending on genetics and life style (Boston Women's Health Book Collective, 1992). Also, young women ought to learn about the importance of annual Pap smears and detection of cervical cancer. Female and male adolescents should be encouraged to look after their sexual health.

Sexuality education programs should explore sexual dysfunctions and demystify them. Whether a lack of lubrication or absence of orgasm in women or a premature ejaculation or erectile difficulty in men, these issues deserve exploration.[11] Also, an examination of inhibited sexual desire (ISD), a common sexual complaint, deserves attention. The etiologies of these dysfunctions need close examination so people can either prevent or manage sexual difficulties and have fulfilling sex lives.

The media now commonly report on issues of sexual harassment, not only in and out of the workplace, but also in the schools.[12] Akin to sexual harassment, as a form of sexual violence, are sexual coercion and rape. These very serious issues focus attention on the issue of sexual consent. Because these behaviors are illegal, it is important that students become acquainted with sex and the law. Furthermore, in some states various sexual behaviors are illegal under the sodomy laws.

Even though the issues mentioned above are crucial and should be integral to any "comprehensive sexuality education" program,[13] such an endeavor ought to be derived from student interest coupled with guidance from a sexuality educator no matter in what forum (e.g., a sexuality education class, a class from standard curriculum [biology, English, history, and social studies, etc.], after-school program, and so on). This is in keeping with the philosophical underpinnings of progressive education. Moving into a completely "student-centered" approach may not be possible now, given the constraints of today's classroom, but students and teachers could work out a curriculum in which students could pursue what they find most interesting and personally relevant. If sexuality education has any chance of being successful, we must pay attention to and respect the students' curiosities, interests, hopes, fears, and needs.

As to what and how sexuality education ought to be taught, considerable attention must be paid to the underlying philosophy of instruction. To date, most sexuality education teachers have used the *"disease model,"* otherwise known as the *"crisis intervention approach"* (Biehr, 1989). That is, whenever a problem is perceived societally, such as the rise in the rate of teenage pregnancies or an increased incidence of sexually transmitted diseases, there is often a concerted effort to eradicate such problems. For everyone involved in this process, from policy makers and school administrators, to teachers and even the students themselves, the message is quite clear. Sexuality is problematic and unhealthy. An alternative to this traditional approach is what has come to be known as the *health promotion model,* which emphasizes that sexuality can be part of a health and rewarding life rather than educating to prevent disease (Carroll and Wolpe, 1996).

Why Should Sexuality Education Be Taught in the Schools?

There are many reasons why sexuality education belongs in the schools. As we explored earlier, it is a way of putting our democratic ideals to work. This by no means suggests that we use a democratic educational framework to justify an "academic free-for-all," or an "anything goes" approach. It is important that students are respected and not coerced into revealing private things that would create embarrassment or injury to their reputations. Insofar as students feel uncomfortable with sexuality education, they should be permitted to opt out at points of discomfort. No student should ever be held prisoner in a classroom; this is counterproductive and even injurious. Sexuality education is so controversial that it has been stultified by those who oppose it. It is important to note that because of its controversial nature, sexuality education has existed in some schools only on a superficial level, and is usually abstinence-based. Less than ten percent of children (kindergarten through high school) in the nation receive so-called comprehensive sexuality education (SIECUS, 1994 & 1996; Haffner, 1992; Hacker, 1981).

It does not matter whether it is sexuality education, drug education, or other aspects of the guidance curriculum that are viewed as disputatious. That a topic is controversial is no justification to avoid it. Avoiding sexuality education altogether or diluting it to encompass only a superficial lesson in reproductive anatomy and physiology is restrictive and a form of censorship! The reality, however, is that many individuals are skeptical about and deeply opposed to opening up sexuality education and making it more far reaching and more inclusive than traditional measures. They often voice concerns about issues of the violation of privacy and the potentially harmful effects of teachers abusing authority in such a deeply contested area as sexuality education. Additionally, many people believe that because students—the immature—want to please their teachers and are easily influenced by adults who are symbols of authority, it is downright dangerous to include, as part of the regular curriculum, aspects of personal lives, as "subject matter" to be learned. In part, this explains why sexuality education has been reduced to studying biological factors and disease aspects of sexuality. Lessons are seen as "objective," value free, and therefore non-controversial.

Let us examine these concerns more closely. One major concern is that sexuality education is not academic. It is true that it is not part of the traditional subject matter curriculum; however, it is an academic enterprise. Studying sexuality can involve a number of disciplines from anthropology to zoology. In primary and secondary schools nearly every subject can be used to examine countless aspects of sexuality. It has been argued elsewhere in this chapter that sexuality education can add personal relevance to subjects that lack personal appeal, and therefore could potentially make them more intrinsically valuable and rewarding.

The issue of privacy is of paramount concern. Many believe that students need to be afforded privacy, and anything that violates this is egregiously inappropriate. This sounds good and safe, but it can also be used as a rhetorical device to create distance between teachers and students, and students from their peers. The fact that students should not be violated is undisputable! This issue, however, is not clear-cut. As we have already seen, schools have suffered tremendously from being impersonal and lacking in human interaction. It can be argued that for schooling to provide the best, most optimal education, students need to be personally connected with one another and their teachers. Personal relevance and social interaction are key ingredients for the making of a solid educational experience (Dewey, 1916; Arnstine, 1995; Goodlad, 1984; Farber, 1969).

Working conjointly and getting acquainted with others necessarily erodes privacy somewhat. This does not mean that students and teachers need to "reveal all" or have a "no holds barred" policy regarding the disclosure of the innermost aspects of lives. What it does mean is that people build trusting relationships, discover shared interests, personalize the topic under consideration, and work toward discovering relevance and meaning. If students work together and with their teachers, not only is their present experience going to be higher in quality (compared to traditional pedagogical practices) but also they are going to be better suited to work with others outside of the school setting.

Another major concern is that teachers could abuse their authority when dealing with such a controversial subject as sexuality education. Indeed, this is a valid concern. But teachers could abuse their authority while teaching any subject. Nothing is inherently "dangerous" about sexuality education. Teachers could abuse their power and authority anytime. When a principal hires a teacher, he or she does so with the understanding that this person can be trusted as a professional.

Censorship is one of the most significant threats to sexuality education. In response to this, sexuality education expert Peter Scales (1981) notes that

> The trend toward censorship has created a climate that may be influencing our children as well. A study of Who's Who American high school students, the top few percent in the country, revealed a couple of years ago that two-thirds *favor* censorship, about the same proportion that opposed it ten years earlier [sic.]. Our First Amendment freedoms, the freedom of speech and the freedom of and from religion, are under siege; but Gallup reported in 1980 that 75% of adult Americans don't even know what the First Amendment is! How can they be alarmed at the threat being posed to it today by new Right militants in their guise as patriots and protectors of the family? (p. 301).

Censorship is a direct threat to democracy, and we cannot afford to promote censorship in the schools. The open and the hidden curriculum both suggest to children that it is acceptable to endorse censorship. Pretty soon it becomes perfectly acceptable and *de rigueur*. Censorship creates ill-informed citizens who often become neither active nor critical thinkers. Censorship constitutes a major threat to freedom. It directly hinders academic freedom in the classroom. It is another reason why the information given to children remains "prefabricated" and "canned." When sexuality education is taught, it remains highly controlled. Choice, both at the level of the teacher and of the student, is a moot point: There is none. Being able to choose is an important aspect of a democratic education (Arnstine, 1995).

Choice ought to exist on two levels. First, it is important to have available opportunities for students to study sexuality. Second, students should be able, at least to some degree, to choose aspects of sexuality that they find relevant to their lives, or topics they find intriguing. It could even be possible that there not be a specific course on sexuality education. Rather, students enrolling in courses such as biology, English literature, history, psychology, or social studies could pursue topics in human sexuality that interest them. They could undertake such projects with teachers' guidance. Whether or not a specific course is offered, students should be afforded some choice of studies. For this to exist, the school board, school administrators, teachers, counselors, librarians, and parents or guardians need to support freedom of inquiry and encourage students to undertake projects or have experiences that would have real value for them and would be high quality as well.[14] This falls under the rubric of freedom of inquiry, which is at the heart of democratic ideals. In many ways it is the opposite of censorship, which, as Scales suggests, is infiltrating our educational system at an ever-quickening pace, and is threatening our freedom at the Constitutional level.

Another reason why a broadly based sexuality education should be taught is to foster the quality of life for students and individuals in general. As we have learned, sexuality runs through the very fabric of social life. It is important to help students become sexually self-aware, as they explore their own sexuality and develop relationships that are both intimate and sexual. Many believe that students are not or should not be sexual. But many students engage in sexual relationships, whether people believe they should or not. If children or adolescents are not sexual, why do more than one million unintended teenage pregnancies occur annually in the United States (Carroll and Wolpe, 1996)? Furthermore, studies indicate that forty percent of ninth-graders and forty-five percent of tenth-graders have engaged in sexual intercourse, and once they have engaged in this activity, they are likely to repeat the experience (see Kelly, 1994, p. 149).

Psychologists and counselors agree that sexually intimate relationships are one of the most important and cherished aspects of our lives. According to a classic study, approximately ninety percent of nine-to eleven-year-olds have individuals they considered special "boyfriends" and "girlfriends" (Kelly, 1994). Kelly (1994) note that "Eighty-five percent of adolescents report having had a boyfriend or girlfriend . . ." (p. 148). Yet few people receive education in the area of sex and relationships. Also, we must not forget that sexual pleasure adds immeasurably to the quality of interpersonal relationships. Many people are astonished to find out that only thirty percent of women achieve orgasms strictly by penis-vagina intercourse. Usually, some type of clitoral stimulation is necessary. Also, many males ejaculate more quickly than they wish. These issues need to be brought out into the open to maximize the happiness and the functionality of relationships. People have a right to learn about their bodily responses and sexuality in general. "Healthy," well-functioning relationships add immeasurably to the quality of life, and this should be an integral part of schooling.

Sexuality education should occur early in the primary grades, and it should always strive to be age appropriate. For instance, it would be hardly appropriate to discuss the intricacies of sexual communication or sexually transmitted diseases prevention techniques with first- or second-graders. Likewise, it would be inappropriate to teach solely basic, fundamental information (e.g., that bodies can feel good when touched, boys have penises and girls have vulvas, bodies change when children grow older, people can experience different types of love, individuals and families have different sexual values, or communication can occur in many different ways and is essential for relationship development) to high school juniors or seniors. These subjects should be handled very broadly and simply in the primary grades, and then become more specific and sophisticated in middle and high school.

In 1996, the Sex Information and Education Council of the United States (SIECUS) published its second edition of *Guidelines for Comprehensive Sexuality Education.* Essentially it recommends that sexuality education be broken into six categories: (1) human development;

(2) relationships; (3) personal skills; (4) sexual behavior; (5) sexual health; and (6) society and culture. SIECUS recommends that children from five through eighteen years of age become educated in each of these areas in an age-appropriate fashion. For example, SIECUS (1996) breaks age-appropriate materials into four levels: (1) middle childhood, ages five through eight; (2) preadolescence, ages nine through twelve; (3) early adolescence, ages twelve through fifteen; and (4) adolescence, ages fifteen through eighteen.

As we have already discovered earlier, sexuality is extremely complicated. However, to illustrate how a sexuality educator might provide age-appropriate information, the topics of masturbation and shared sexual behavior will be outlined in terms of SIECUS' recommendations. The following developmental messages are recommended by SIECUS for information on masturbation:

LEVEL 1 (for five- to eight-year-olds):
Touching and rubbing one's own genitals to feel good is called masturbation.
Some boys and girls masturbate and others do not.
Masturbation should be done in a private place.

LEVEL 2 (for nine- to twelve-year-olds):
Masturbation is often the first way a person experiences sexual pleasure.
Many boys and girls begin to masturbate for sexual pleasure during puberty.
Some boys and girls never masturbate.
Masturbation does not cause physical or mental harm.
Some families and religions oppose masturbation.

LEVEL 3 (for thirteen- to fifteen-year-olds):
How often a person masturbates varies for every individual.
A person worried about masturbation might talk to a trusted adult.
Most people have masturbated at some time in their lives.
Masturbation, either alone or with a partner, is one way a person can enjoy and express her or his sexuality without risking pregnancy or an STD/HIV.
Many negative myths exist about masturbation.
A few boys engage in a very dangerous and sometimes fatal form of masturbation that involves limiting their air supply.

LEVEL 4 (for fifteen- through eighteen-year-olds)
People who are single, married, or in committed relationship may masturbate.
Masturbation may be an important part of a couple's sexual relationship (pp. 34–35).

The following developmental messages about shared sexual behavior are recommended by SIECUS (1996):

LEVEL 1
Adults often kiss, hug, touch, and engage in other sexual behavior with one another to show caring and to share sexual pleasure.

LEVEL 2

People have different ways to share sexual pleasure with one another.

Being sexual with another person usually involves more than sexual intercourse.

LEVEL 3

When two people express their sexual feelings together, they usually give and receive pleasure.

Sexual relationships are enhanced when two people communicate with each other about what forms of sexual behavior they like or dislike.

Sexual relationships can be more fulfilling in a loving relationship.

Being sexual with another person usually involves different sexual behaviors.

A person has the right to refuse any sexual behavior.

Some sexual expressions are prohibited by law and disapproved of by certain religions and families.

People with disabilities have sexual feelings and the same need as all people for love, affection, and physical intimacy.

LEVEL 4

For most people, sharing a sexual experience with a partner is a satisfying way to express sexuality.

Couples and individuals need to decide how to express their sexual feelings.

Some sexual behaviors shared by partners include kissing, touching, talking, caressing, massage, sharing erotic literature or art, bathing/showering together, and oral, vaginal, or anal intercourse.

Many sexual behaviors that are pleasurable do not put an individual at risk of an unintended pregnancy or STD/HIV.

Individuals are responsible for their own sexual pleasure (p. 35).

The above criteria illustrate that various and even "sensitive" topics can be addressed responsibly to all school-age children as long as age appropriateness is taken into consideration. While SIECUS provides guidelines for age-appropriate sexuality education, it is important to use them intelligently. That is, these guidelines should be viewed as a rough estimate of children's and adolescents' readiness to receive certain kinds of information, and not an absolute, ironclad directive. SIECUS' developmental levels are generalizations, and would be appropriate for most students. But countless students are either quite advanced or slower than peers in their age cohort. Therefore, educators have to use these "cookie cutter" age-appropriate recommendations with caution and care. Again, it is important that teachers get to know their students individually, and approach education with students' interests and needs in mind, and always be vigilant about the relevance that materials have to the lives of students.

In a philosophical essay on sex education, John Passmore (1980) writes that literature teachers are often inspired and encouraged to teach students the love of literature. He poses the question: "Why are teachers in general not encouraged to teach students the love of other people?" He suggests that sexuality education should be taught to destroy myths about sexuality, to assist students in making decisions about their sexuality, and finally, to prepare them ". . . for love, with its joys, its responsibilities" (p. 32). His three recommendations for sexuality education fall under the general rubric of loving and caring about oneself and others: This is the primary message Passmore offers his readers.

Not only could skills be acquired to manage intimate/sexual relationships but also many of the skills learned are likely to be "transferable" to other aspects of one's life. For example, communication and conflict resolution techniques can be applied to all of one's relationships with employers, friends, relatives, lovers/sex partners, and others. This is only one of many examples of how sexuality education is directly relevant to one's life in general.

Additionally, sexuality education could be expected to help reduce the incidence of sexual harassment, sexual coercion, and rape. These crimes are far too common to be ignored in the education of the young: statistically, one in four women will be raped (Crooks and Baur, 1996). This statistic is conservative, given that the report rate is low. The report rate is low, in part because approximately eight-five percent of rapes are date rapes or acquaintance rapes, and the individuals who get raped are reluctant to press criminal charges against "significant others." Sexuality education could be enormously helpful in making clear the issues associated with sexual consent, and could be instrumental in teaching rape prevention.

Since sexuality is an important aspect of most people's lives, sexuality education would be beneficial in promoting positive mental and physical health. Many people feel negatively about sexuality because of how it has been portrayed by religious and bio-medical writers. It is a sad fact that many people do not accept their own sexual thoughts, fantasies, and practices. Conversations about sexuality occur behind closed doors in a secretive fashion, and in many cases, sexual partners do not even discuss sexual matters. Sexuality education would be instrumental in "normalizing" and depathologizing sexuality. Without sexuality education many people will likely continue to feel bad about their own sexuality and about sexuality in general.

Sexuality education could serve as a major vehicle to control the spread of sexually transmitted diseases. Also, it would be helpful in informing females and males alike about the importance of monthly examinations to detect cancers and other medical problems. Let us examine an example of a current issue in female sexual health. Several television commercials advertise a variety of fruit-scented douches (e.g., apple, raspberry, cinnamon, peach, etc.). Already ashamed of their genitalia and natural body odor, many women buy such products. This is deleterious on two levels. On a mental health level, this simply reproduces and feeds into how bad many women feel about themselves and their sexuality. It perpetuates the notion that women's genitalia are defective, odious, even odoriferous, and somehow simply not okay. On a physical health level, these products are detrimental to women's sexual health. Douching disrupts the natural ecology (including pH) of the vagina. Helpful bacteria, such as lactobacilli, are washed away, thereby increasing the risk of yeast infections. Some cervical cancers have been linked to douching practices. This is not common knowledge. Sexuality education could examine some of these advertisements, practices, and underlying attitudes about sexuality to protect individuals from mental distress and physical ailments. A critical examination of these kinds of things is crucial, and sexuality education would be best suited to handle such concerns.

Perhaps the best reason for teaching sexuality education in the schools is because it is likely to be relevant to the students' lives. So much of what is taught in schools today is not only presented unimaginatively but is also disconnected from the lives of the students. Sexuality will capture the interest of students because of its centrality to most of their lives. Most students want to date or carry on some type of romantic involvement. Numerous surveys have indicated that most adolescents desire sexuality education (Carroll and Wolpe, 1996; Crooks and Baur, 1996).

Sexuality education, because of its personal appeal, could lead to more fruitful ways of studying subject matter. Studying history to remember heroes, battles, and significant dates for their own sake has bored and tormented students for decades. But if a student became interested in studying the history of sexuality in the United States, he or she would gain an appreciation for history in general, and would gain much insight about the history of sexuality. Otherwise, a student might not consider history as a topic worth pursuing. A good novel offers insight into the history of some sexual practices, laws, and mores. Knowledge gleaned from a good novel or an engaging piece of fiction, for that matter, would be interesting and useful for students. Sexuality education could be used as a hub or connection to study subjects from creative writing and English literature to zoology. Students would likely attach personal meaning and intrinsic value to the education they receive. The educational experience becomes a high-quality one.

Sexuality education in the schools would necessarily have to address various sexual lifestyles, sexual values and belief systems, and the numerous forms of sexual expression. Because of the vast differences that can be found with differing viewpoints held by the students, this form of education would be an effective vehicle to study and to practice democratic ideals. There would be controversy, dissent, debate, questioning, and so on. Students would be afforded a firsthand experience of what it means to be in a pluralistic society and work out problems and concerns in a socially rich environment. To pretend that these differences do not exist is unfair to the students, who will eventually find themselves outside the school walls with individuals who have a variety of beliefs and practices regarding sexual and social relationships. Also, to ignore such differences is unfair to the students who differ from the "norm," for they will remain invisible and unappreciated.

Much prejudice is directed at those who do not display "normal" sexual or gender behaviors. Bisexuals, gays, lesbians, or those who simply do not fit the typical gender role stereotypes are discriminated against in the schools. Physical and verbal abuse are directed at these sexual and gender "misfits." Sexuality education could address discrimination, and encourage at least tolerance if not acceptance of these people by using a democratic educational framework, emphasizing such qualities as justice, equity, freedom for all, and protection of minority rights. This becomes another opportunity to explore the nature of democracy.

Jan Steutel and Ben Spiecker (1996), philosophers of education, suggest that *good* sex ought to be both the aim of sexuality education and a chief reason why it ought to be offered. They refer to "*good*" in two ways: in the moral and non-moral senses of the term. In the moral sense of "*good*" they refer to the types of sexuality that can withstand moral criticism. In other words, such issues as consent, keeping one's integrity intact, and being mindful of one's and others' physical and emotional well-being are a part of morally *good* sex. On the other side, the non-moral sense of "*good*" has to do with the pleasurable, gratifying, and generally enjoyable sexual encounters that lead to being fulfilled ". . . in a flourishing life" (p. 2). These writers argue forcefully both the moral and non-moral aspects of *good* sex need to be integral in sexuality education to lead a moral/ethical sexual life coupled with one that takes sexual pleasure into account in aiming at personal growth and happiness.

No matter how many arguments one offers about why sexuality education should be offered in the schools, the question arises, Why should the schools, rather than some other agency, shoulder this responsibility? Here is why the common or public school is the best and most reasonable site for such an educational enterprise. First, the public school system reaches nearly all children. Other agencies such as Planned Parenthood cannot possibly offer all children a responsible sexuality education. Most children do not come into contact with such organizations. Nearly all children find themselves in public classrooms five days a week for twelve years.

The quality of instruction in schools is another concern. In the schools we find certified, credentialed professional educators. However, to date very few teachers are prepared to deal with sexuality. There needs to be a concerted effort to train teachers in this area. Despite the lack of teacher training in this area, schools have professionally trained educators; other community agencies do not offer this kind of quality of instruction. However, some individuals claim that sexuality education has no business being in schools or in any other agencies and should be addressed in the privacy of the home.

Many children and adolescents end up learning about sexuality on the streets, resulting in incorrect and inadequate information.[15] Another source of inadequate information is the mass media; one study reports that adolescents view between 1,900 and 2,400 sexually related images annually on television (Brown, Childers, and Waszak, 1990). Many of these messages are contradictory and confusing. Yet these minors have no real way of discussing the meanings and implications of the images they see with anyone other than friends, who know little more than they do. What usually results is the perpetuation of misinformation.

Characteristics Essential to Teachers in Sexuality Education

Now that a case for sexuality education in the public schools has been made, it is important to turn to an exploration of various characteristics that sexuality educators should possess. It takes a special kind of teacher to teach sexuality education effectively and intelligently. According to Malfetti and Rubin's (1967) study, "Sex Education: Who's Teaching the Teachers?," they list six desirable characteristics of sexuality educators. Among them are: (1) *acceptance of human sexuality*, which includes a positive regard for one's own sexuality, and being accepting and respectful of others' sexualities; (2) *respect for youth*, including but not limited to treating students with dignity, addressing their questions and concerns warmly, honestly, openly, sensitively, and clearly. This also includes building a trustful relationship with students; (3) *ability to communicate*, which includes the ability to not only discuss sensitive and potentially embarrassing topics but also to communicate the genuineness with which one is treating their concerns, interests, and questions; (4) *empathy*, which includes putting one "in the shoes of students" in an effort to understand fully students' experiences. This also includes availability to students, being sensitive to the needs of students, and a desire to assist students, etc.; (5) *non-authoritarian teaching techniques*, which includes utilizing a non-threatening teaching style. It is important that sexuality educators approach their students warmly and compassionately; and (6) *knowledgeable about sexuality*, including not only factual knowledge but also an appreciation of the interdisciplinary nature of human sexuality studies, and ability to facilitate student learning in an interdisciplinary fashion. Also, sexuality educators should be cognizant of community resources as they will undoubtedly be of use to students much of the time.[16]

In light of our previous discussion of embracing democratic ideals in schooling, it is extremely important that sexuality educators do not shy away from sensitive or controversial topics. To the extent possible, teachers need to defend their rights and students' rights to pursue unconventional or unpopular areas of inquiry. Academic freedom needs to be used to ensure a worthwhile educational process. If educators and school administrators are not willing to embrace this kind of education—to the extent possible, even if it involves "pushing the envelope" a little here and there—then old, authoritarian, and conventional educational techniques will prevail. Thus, fruitful and effective sexuality education will be precluded. We cannot afford to reproduce the standard, old-fashioned educational techniques if we are to provide students with a relevant, meaningful, rich, and exciting educational experience.

Debate rages about whether or not any form of sexuality education belongs in the schools, let alone who ought to be teaching it. This has been hotly contested for many decades.

Notes

1. Alan Goldman uses the terms "sexual desire" and "sexual behavior" throughout his essay, and makes the point that these aspects of sexuality cannot be seen in terms of "means to an end." I have taken the liberty of mentioning "sexuality" in its broadest sense (including but not limited to sexual desire and behavior) to point out that sexuality is more complicated than a means to an end. In other words, sexuality is not always manifested in orgasm, a physical process, and so on. Sexuality can be

experienced as an aesthetic experience without any goal or end in mind. For example, someone might fantasize about another person and enjoy the experience for the experience alone. The fantasizer, for example, might not even want to be in physical contact with the object of her or his fantasy.

2. For a philosophical analysis of what constitutes sexuality, see for example, Alan Soble's (ed.) *The Philosophy of Sex: Contemporary Readings.* 2nd ed. Savage: Rowman & Littlefield Publishers, 1991. Especially see section II of this volume, which focuses on "analyzing the sexual." The authors in this collection of essays respond to one another's arguments, ultimately illustrating just how vast and ubiquitous sexuality is. For another work that treats the "nature" of sexuality, see Robert Baker and Frederick Elliston's (eds.) *Philosophy and Sex.* Buffalo: Prometheus Books, 1984. The introduction of this volume is useful and treats the semantics of sexuality. Yet another volume, although less helpful, that covers this topic is Russell Vannoy's *Six Without Love: A Philosophical Exploration.* Buffalo: Prometheus Books, 1980. Chapters Three and Four explore various aspects of sexuality.

3. For a thorough coverage of these various philosophies of education, see Edward J. Power's *Philosophy of Education: Studies in Philosophies, Schooling, and Educational Policies* (Prospect Heights; Waveland Press, 1982). Specifically, see chapters Three and Four for a brief but comprehensive treatment. Also, see Nel Noddings' *Philosophy of Education.* Boulder: Westview Press, 1995, *passim.*

4. When I refer to "traditionalists," "the traditionalists' philosophy of education," or "traditional approaches to schooling," I am specifically referring to the brand of schooling that has existed for about a century: the type of schooling that stresses the learning and mastery of "the basic subjects." In some educational circles it is referred to as "a liberal education." It focuses heavily upon memorization and recitation of facts, independent of student interests. For a few works that cogently characterize this form of schooling, consult Donald Arnstine's *Democracy and the Arts of Schooling* (Albany: State University of New York Press, 1995), *passim,* and Joel Spring's *American Education: An Introduction to Social and Political Aspects* (5th ed. New York and London: Longman Publishers, 1991) Chapters One and Nine, and *passim.* For a treatment of how the traditional curriculum and school culture in general silences students and fosters deep competition (and no cooperation) among students, see John Goodlad's *A Place Called School: Prospects for the Future* (New York: McGraw Hill, 1984). For a recent work that supports "the traditional approach" see E. D. Hirsch's *Cultural Literacy: What Every American Needs to Know* (Boston: Houghton Mifflin Company, 1987).

5. For a detailed analysis about attitudes and stereotypes regarding gender in schools, see Myra Sadker and David Sadker's *Failing at Fairness: How Our Schools Cheat Girls* (New York: Simon and Schuster, 1994). It makes perfectly good sense that students and members of North American society at large would have traditionally based

attitudes and expectations regarding gender given how we are saturated and bombarded with how females and males are expected to behave. From mainstream advertising to major motion pictures, with very few exceptions, we are reminded of how we should carry ourselves gender-wise. How about sexism and homophobia in and out of schools? These are gender-based forms of prejudice. Students could readily identify "appropriate" characteristics of females and males. We all know the drill. Some of us follow suit and others of us do not. And we also know that those who do not uphold traditional gender roles are punished covertly and overtly.

6. By "responsible sexuality education" I am referring to a brand of sexuality education that far surpasses the diluted, censorious, and mechanical (the "plumbing aspects") forms that supposedly represent "sexuality education." When one hears about this school district or that district offering sexuality education, what often will be learned about such programs is that they are "bare bones," offering nothing more than a watered-down version of reproductive physiology, a censored Planned Parenthood lecture, and some moral bolstering to "remain" abstinent.

7. I use the word "usually" because some individuals are known to be intersexed, in that they possess female and male genitalia. Although this phenomenon is rare, I want to avoid any gross generalizations.

8. For a thorough and up-to-date analysis of the ubiquity of sexism in the schools, see Myra and David Sadker's *Failing at Fairness: How Our Schools Cheat Girls* (New York: Touchstone Books, 1995).

9. For a discussion about how sexuality education can include information about gender issues and about how sexuality education is an appropriate venue to explore these issues, see Christine LaCerva's essay, "Talking about Talking about Sex: The Organization of Possibilities" (pp. 124–138), and Susan Shurberg Klein's essay "Commentary: Why We Should Care about Gender and Sexuality in Education" (pp. 171–180): both of these pieces appear in James Sears's (ed.) *Sexuality and the Curriculum: The Politics and Practices of Sexuality Education.* (New York: Teachers College, Columbia University Press, 1992). A work that examines anti-sex rhetoric surrounding sexuality education and how it negatively impacts adolescent females is Michelle Fine's "Sexuality, Schooling, and Adolescent Females: The Missing Discourse of Desire." *Harvard Educational Review* 58 (1), (February 1988): 29–53.

10. For accounts of homophobia in high school settings, see *The High School Journal* 77 (1 & 2), (1993/1994). This is a special issue on the gay teenager. There are many articles within this volume that deal almost exclusively with the manifestations of homophobia.

11. I only mentioned a few examples of female and male sexual dysfunctions to make a point: that these types of sexual difficulties warrant examination and discussion. For an extensive treatment of sexual dysfunctions, consult Helen Singer Kaplan's *New Sex Therapy: Active Treatment of Sexual Dysfunctions* (New York: Brunner/Maze.,

1974) and Bernie Zilbergeld's *The New Male Sexuality* (New York: Bantam Books, 1992).

12. For a detailed description of sexual harassment among students see Katherine Selligman's article, "Boys Join List of the Sexually Harassed" in the *San Francisco Examiner* (November 17, 1996, pp. A1 and A16). This is only one article among many recent accounts that raise this concern.

13. The term "comprehensive sexuality education" was coined in the 1950s in Sweden to refer to an educational process that went beyond the coverage of sexually transmitted diseases and reproductive anatomy and physiology. "Comprehensive sexuality education" encompasses the bio-medical, psychological, and socio-cultural aspects of sexuality.

14. For an explication and examples of high-quality experiences, see Donald Arnstine's *Democracy and the Arts of School* (Albany: State University of New York Press, 1995) Chapter Four.

15. Most children learn incorrect information about sexuality from their friends. For more information on this, see Robert Crooks and Karla Baur's *Our Sexuality* (6th ed. Pacific Grove: Brooks/Cole Publishers, 1996), p. 379. They cite many studies that corroborate their claim about adolescents' acquisition of faulty sexual knowledge.

16. Anne M. Juhasz's "Characteristics Essential to Teachers in Sex Education" *The Journal of School Health* 40 (1), (January 1970): 17–19 was consulted, and was enormously helpful in fleshing out this section of this chapter.

Bibliography

Arnstine, Donald. *Democracy and the Arts of Schooling.* Albany: State University of New York Press, 1995.

———. "Diversity: A Necessary Condition for Learning." A paper presented at the California Association for the Philosophy of Education (CAPE) Meeting, Sacramento, CA. October 25, 1996.

Baker, Robert., and Elliston, Frederick (eds.). *Philosophy and Sex.* Buffalo: Prometheus Books, 1984.

Barthalow-Koch, Patricia. "Integrating Cognitive, Affective, and Behavioral Approaches into Learning Experiences for Sexuality Education." In James Sears's (ed.) *Sexuality and the Curriculum: The Politics and Practices of Sexuality Education.* New York: Teachers College, Columbia University Press, 1992: 253–266.

Biehr, B. Problem Sexual Behaviors in School-Aged Children and Youth." *Theory into Practice* 28 (1989): 221–226.

Boston Women's Health Book Collective. *The New Our Bodies Ourselves: A Book By and For Women.* New York: Touchstone Books, 1992.

Brown, J. D., Childers, K. W., and Waszak, C. S. "Television and Adolescent Sexuality." *Journal of Adolescent Health Care* 11 (1), (1990): 62–70.

Bruess, Clint E., and Greenberg, Jerold S. *Sexuality Education: Theory and Practice*. 2nd ed. New York: MacMillan Publishers, 1988.

Bruner, Jerome. *The Culture of Education*. Cambridge: Harvard University Press, 1996.

Carroll, Janell L., and Wolpe, Paul R. *Sexuality and Gender in Society*. New York: HarperCollins, 1996.

Crooks, Robert., and Baur, Karla. *Our Sexuality*. 6th ed. Pacific Grove: Brooks/Cole Publishers, 1996.

Dewey, John. *The School and Society and The Child and the Curriculum*. Chicago: University of Chicago Press, 1900/1902.

————. *Democracy and Education*. New York: Macmillan, 1916.

————. *Experience and Education*. New York and London: Collier Macmillan Publishers, 1938.

Dutile, F. *Sex, Schools, and the Law*. Springfield: Thomas Publishers, 1986.

Dworkin, Martin S. *Dewey on Education: Selections*. New York: Teachers College, Columbia University Press, 1959.

Elia, John P. "Homophobia in the High School: A Problem in Need of a Resolution." *The High School Journal 77* (1 & 2), (1993/1994): 177–185.

Ellis, M. "Eliminating Our Heterosexist Approaches to Sex Education." *Journal of Sex Education and Therapy* 10 (1984): 61–63.

Farber, Jerry. *The Student as Nigger*. New York: Contact, 1969.

Fine, Michelle. "Sexuality, Schooling, and Adolescent Females: The Missing Discourse of Desire." *Harvard Educational Review* 58 (1), (February, 1988): 29–53.

Forster, E. M. *Maurice*. New York and London: W.W. Norton, 1971 (Originally published in 1914).

Goldman, Alan. "Plain Sex." In Alan Soble's (ed.) *The Philosophy of Sex: Contemporary Readings*. 2nd ed. Savage: Littlefield Adams Quality Paperbacks, 1991: 73–92.

Goodlad, John I. *A Place Called School: Prospects for the Future*. New York: McGraw Hill, 1984.

————. *Teachers for Our Nation's Schools*. San Francisco: Jossey-Bass Publishers, 1990.

Gordon, Sol. "Coming to Terms with Your Own Sexuality First." *The Journal of School Health* 49 (5), (1979): 247–250.

Hacker, Sylvia S. "It Isn't Sex Education Unless . . ." *The Journal of School Health* 51 (4), (April 1981): 207–210.

Haffner, Debra W. "Foreword: Sexuality Education in Policy and Practice." In James Sears's (ed.) *Sexuality and the Curriculum: The Politics and Practices of Sexuality Education*. New York: Teachers College, Columbia University Press, 1992: vii–viii.

Hirsch, E. D. *Cultural Literacy: What Every American Needs to Know*. Boston: Houghton Mifflin Company, 1987.

Illich, Ivan. *Deschooling Society*. New York: Harper Colophon Books, 1970.

Juhasz, Anne M. "Characters Essential to Teachers in Sex Education." *The Journal of School Health* 40 (1), (January 1970): 17–19.

Kaplan, Helen Singer. *The New Sex Therapy: Active Treatment of Sexual Dysfunction*. New York: Brunner/Mazel, 1974.

Kelly, Gary F. *Sexuality Today: The Human Perspective*. 4th ed. Sluice Dock and Guilford: The Dushkin Publishing Group, 1994.

Klein, Susan Shurberg. "Commentary: Why Should We Care about Gender and Sexuality in Education?" In James Sears's (ed.) *Sexuality and the Curriculum: The Politics and Practices of Sexuality Education*. New York: Teachers College, Columbia University Press, 1992: 171–180.

Kozol, Jonathan. *Savage Inequalities: Children in America's Schools.* New York: Crown Publishing Group, 1991.

LaCerva, Christine. "Talking about Talking about Sex: The Organization of Possibilities." In James Sears's (ed.) *Sexuality and the Curriculum: The Politics and Practices of Sexuality Education.* New York: Teachers College, Columbia University Press, 1992: 124–138.

Lavine, T. Z. *From Socrates to Sartre: The Philosophic Quest.* New York: Bantam Books, 1984.

Loulan, JoAnn. *Lesbian Passion: Loving Ourselves and Each Other.* San Francisco: Spinsters/Aunt Lute, 1987.

Malfetti, James L., and Rubin, Arlene M. "Sex Education: Who Ought to Be Teaching the Teachers?" *Teachers College Record* (December 1967): 213–222.

Moulton, Janice. "Sexual Behavior: Another Position." In Alan Soble's (ed.). *The Philosophy of Sex: Contemporary Readings.* 2nd ed. Savage: Littlefield Adams Quality Paperbacks, 1991: 63–72.

Noddings, Nel. *The Challenge to Care in Schools.* New York: Teaches College, Columbia University press, 1992.

———. *The Philosophy of Education.* Boulder: Westview Press, 1995.

Ornstein, Allan C., and Levine, Daniel U. Foundations of Education. 5rh ed. Boston: Houghton Mifflin Company, 1993.

Passmore, John. "Sex Education." *The New Republic,* October 4, 1980, pp. 27–32.

Power, Edward J. *Philosophy of Education: Studies in Philosophies, Schooling, and Educational Policies.* Prospect Heights; Waveland Press, 1982.

Ross, Stephen David. "The Limits of Sexuality." In Alan Soble's (ed.) *The Philosophy of Sex: Contemporary Readings.* 2nd ed. Savage: Littlefield Adams Quality Paperbacks, 1991: 159–178.

Sadker, Myra., and Sadker, David. *Failing at Fairness: How Our Schools Cheat Girls.* New York: Touchstone Books, 1994.

Scales, Peter. "The New Opposition to Sex Education." *The Journal of School Health* (April 1981): 300–304.

Sears, James T. "Dilemmas and Possibilities of Sexuality Education: Reproducing the Body Politic." In James Sears's (ed.) *Sexuality and the Curriculum: The Politics and Practices of Sexuality Education.* New York: Teachers College, Columbia University Press, 1992: 7–33.

———. "The Impact of Culture and Ideology on the Construction of Gender and Sexual Identities: Developing a Critically Based Sexuality Curriculum." In James Sears's (ed.) *Sexuality and the Curriculum: The Politics and Practices of Sexuality Education.* New York: Teachers College, Columbia University Press, 1992: 139–156.

Selligan, Katherine. "Boys Join List of the Sexually Harassed." *San Francisco Examiner,* 17 November 1996, sec. A, pp. 1 and 16.

Sexuality Information and Education Council of the United States (SIECUS). "Position Statement 1990." *SIECUS Report* 4 (4), (1990): 10–12.

———. *SIECUS Fact Sheet # 3 on Comprehensive Sexuality Education and the Schools: Issues and Answers.* New York: Sexuality Information and Education Council of the United States, 1994.

———. *Guidelines for Comprehensive Sexuality Education: Kindergarten–12th Grade.* 2nd ed. New York: National Guidelines Task Force of the Sexuality Information and Education Council of the United States, 1996.

Silin, Jonathan G. *Sex, Death, and the Education of Children: Our Passion for Ignorance in the Age of AIDS.* New York: Teachers College, Columbia University press, 1995.

Spring, Joel. *American Education: An Introduction to Social and Political Aspects.* 5th ed. New York and London: Longman Publishers, 1991.

Steutel, Jan., and Spieker, Ben. "Good Sex as the Aim of Sexual Education." Paper presented at the *Annual Meeting of the Philosophy of Education Society,* Houston, Texas. March 29, 1996.

Stevens, Edward., and Wood, George H. *Justice, Ideology, and Education: An Introduction to the Social Foundations of Education.* 2nd ed. New York: McGraw Hill, 1992.

The American Heritage Dictionary of the English Language. (New College Edition). Boston: Houghton Mifflin Company, 1976.

The High School Journal 77 (1 & 2), (1993/1994).

Tyack, David B., and Hansot, Elisabeth. *Learning Together: A History of Coeducation in American Public Schools.* New York: Russell Sage Foundation, 1992.

Vannoy, Russell. *Sex Without Love: A Philosophical Exploration.* Buffalo: Prometheus Books, 1980.

Wharton, Edith. *Summer.* New York: Perennial Library/Harper & Row, 1979 (Originally published in 1918).

Wittgenstein, Ludwig. *Philosophical Investigations.* Translated by G. E. M. Anscombe. Oxford: Basil Blackwell, 1953/1968.

Zilbergeld, Bernie. *The New Male Sexuality.* New York: Bantam Books, 1992.

Facts in Brief: Sexuality Education

Alan Guttmacher Institute

CHAPTER

Sex and Pregnancy Among Teenagers

- By their 18th birthday, 6 in 10 teenage women and nearly 7 in 10 teenage men have had sexual intercourse.
- A sexually active teenager who does not use contraception has a 90% chance of becoming pregnant within a year.
- Of the approximately 950,000 teenage pregnancies that occur each year, more than 3 in 4 are unintended. Over 1/4 of these pregnancies end in abortion.
- The pregnancy rate among U.S. women aged 15–19 has declined steadily—from 117 pregnancies per 1,000 women in1990 to 93 per 1,000 women in 1997. Analysis of the teenage pregnancy rate decline between 1988 and 1995 found that approximately 1/4 of the decline was due to delayed onset of sexual intercourse among teenagers, while 3/4 was due to the increased use of highly effective and long-acting contraceptive methods among sexually experienced teenagers.
- Despite the decline, the United States continues to have one of the highest teenage pregnancy rates in the developed world—twice as high as those in England, Wales or Canada and nine times as high as rates in the Netherlands and Japan.
- Every year, roughly 4 million new sexually transmitted disease (STD) infections occur among teenagers in the United States. Compared with rates among teens in other developed countries, rates of gonorrhea and chlamydia among U.S. teenagers are extremely high.
- Though teenagers in the United States have levels of sexual activity similar to their Canadian, English, French and Swedish peers, they are more likely to have shorter and more sporadic sexual relationships and less likely to use contraception.

The Alan Guttmacher Institute (AGI), *Sexual and Reproductive Health: Women and Men, Facts in Brief,* New York: AGI, 2002, http://alanguttmacher.org

Local Sexuality Education Policy

- More than 2 out of 3 public school districts have a policy to teach sexuality education. The remaining 33% of districts leave policy decisions up to individual schools or teachers.
- 86% of the public school districts that have a policy to teach sexuality education require that abstinence be promoted. 35% require abstinence to be taught as the *only option* for unmarried people and either prohibit the discussion of contraception altogether or limit discussion to its ineffectiveness. The other 51% have a policy to teach abstinence as the *preferred option* for teens and permit discussion of contraception as an effective means of preventing pregnancy and STDs.
- Only 14% of public school districts with a policy to teach sexuality education address abstinence as *one option* in a broader educational program to prepare adolescents to become sexually healthy adults.
- Over 1/2 of the districts in the South with a policy to teach sexuality education have an abstinence-only policy, compared with 20% of such districts in the Northeast.

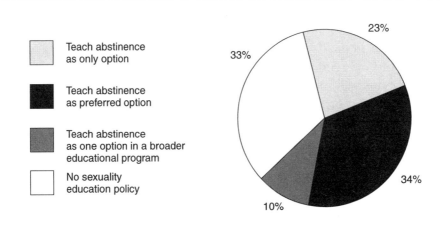

chart a
Sex Education Policies

Most school districts promote abstinence.

Teach abstinence as only option

Teach abstinence as preferred option

Teach abstinence as one option in a broader educational program

No sexuality education policy

23%

33%

34%

10%

Source: Landry DJ, Kaeser L and Richard CL, Abstinence promotion and the provision of information about contraception in public school district sexuality education policies, *Family Planning Perspectives*, 1999, 31 (6)280–286.

- While most states require schools to teach sexuality education, STD education or both, many also give local policymakers wide latitude in crafting their own policies. The latest information on state-level policies is available at www.guttmacher.org/pubs/spib_SSEP.pdf.

Sexuality Education in the Classroom

- Sexuality education teachers are more likely to focus on abstinence and less likely to provide students with information on birth control, how to obtain contraceptive services, sexual orientation and abortion than they were 15 years ago.
- The proportion of sexuality education teachers who taught abstinence as the only way to prevent pregnancy and STDs increased from 1 in 50 in 1988 to 1 in 4 in 1999.
- The overwhelming majority of sexuality education teachers believe that by the end of the 7th grade, students should have been taught about puberty, how HIV is

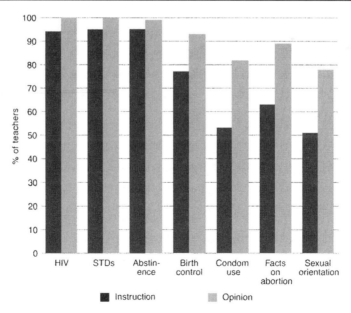

chart b
Thinking vs. Doing

There is a large gap between what teachers think should be taught and what they teach when it comes to birth control, abortion and sexual orientation.

Source: Darroch JE, Landry DJ and Sing S, Changing emphasis in sexuality education in U.S. public secondary schools, 1988–1999, *Family Planning Perspectives, 2000, 32(5):204–211 & 265.*

transmitted, STDs, how to resist peer pressure to have sex, implications of teenage parenthood, abstinence from intercourse, dating, sexual abuse and nonsexual ways to show affection.

- The majority of teachers believe that topics such as birth control methods and how to obtain them, the correct way to use a condom, sexual orientation, and factual and ethical information about abortion should also be taught by the end of the 12th grade. These topics are currently being taught less often and later than teachers think they should be.
- More than 9 in 10 teachers believe that students should be taught about contraception, but 1 in 4 are prohibited from doing so.
- 1 in 5 teachers believe that restrictions imposed on sexuality education are preventing them from meeting their students' needs.
- The majority of Americans favor more comprehensive sexuality education over abstinence-only education.
- At least 3/4 of parents say that in addition to abstinence, sexuality education should cover how to use condoms and other forms of birth control, abortion, sexual orientation, pressures to have sex and the emotional consequences of having sex.
- At least 40% of students report that topics such as STDs and HIV, birth control, how to use and where to obtain birth control, and how to handle pressure to have sex either were not covered in their most recent sexuality education course or were not covered sufficiently.

Government Support of Abstinence-Only Education

- There are currently 3 federal programs dedicated to funding restrictive abstinence-only education—section 510 of the Social Security Act, the Adolescent Family Life Act's teenage pregnancy prevention component, and the Special Projects of Regional and National Significance program (SPRANS)—with total annual funding of $102 million for FY 2002.
- Federal law establishes a stringent 8-point definition o "abstinence-only education" that requires programs to teach that sexual activity outside of marriage is wrong and harmful—for people of any age—and prohibits them from advocating contraceptive use or discussing contraceptive methods except to emphasize their failure rates.
- There is currently no federal program dedicated to supporting comprehensive sexuality education that teaches young people about both abstinence and contraception.
- Despite years of evaluation in this area, there is no evidence to date that abstinence-only education delays teenage sexual activity. Moreover, recent research shows that abstinence-only strategies may deter contraceptive use among sexually active teenagers, increasing their risk of unintended pregnancy and STDs.

- Evidence shows that comprehensive sexuality education programs that provide information about both abstinence and contraception can help delay the onset of sexual activity in teenagers, reduce their number of sexual partners and increase contraceptive use when they become sexually active. These findings were underscored in *Call to Action to Promote Sexual Health and Responsible Sexual Behavior,* issued by former Surgeon General David Satcher in June 2001.

Sources of Data

The data in this fact sheet are the most current available. Most of the data are from research conducted by The Alan Guttmacher Institute (AGI) and published in:

Why is Teenage Pregnancy Declining? The Roles of Abstinence, Sexual Activity and Contraceptive Use; Teenage Sexual and Reproductive Behavior in Developed Countries: Can More Progress Be Made?; and the peer-reviewed journal *Perspectives on Sexual and Reproductive Health* (formerly *Family Planning Perspectives*).

Additional sources include the Kaiser Family Foundation and the National Campaign to Prevent Teen Pregnancy.

Issues and Answers: Fact Sheet on Sexuality Education

SIECUS

CHAPTER

Sexuality education is the lifelong process of building a strong foundation for sexual health. It takes place daily in homes, schools, faith-based institutions, and through the media. Even though this topic is often discussed, myths and misunderstandings persist. This fact sheet is designed to clarify this issue for parents, educators, health care professionals, policymakers, the media, and others so they can understand the complexities and importance of sexuality education.

Learning about Sexuality

Issue: What is sexuality education?
Answer: Sexuality education is a lifelong process of acquiring information and forming attitudes, beliefs, and values. It includes sexual development, reproductive health, interpersonal relationships, affection, intimacy, body image, and gender roles.

Sexuality education addresses the biological, sociocultural, psychological, and spiritual dimensions of sexuality from the cognitive domain (information); the affective domain (feelings, values, and attitudes); and the behavioral domain (communication and decision-making skills).[1]

Issue: Where do young people learn about sexuality?
Answer: Sexuality education begins at home. Parents and caregivers are—and ought to be—the primary sexuality educators of their children. Teachable moments—opportunities to discuss sexuality issues with children—occur on a daily basis.

From the moment of birth, children learn about love, touch, and relationships. Infants and toddlers learn about sexuality when their parents talk to them, dress them, show affection, play with them, and teach them the names of the parts of their bodies. As children grow, they continue to receive messages about sexual behaviors, attitudes, and values from their families and within their social environment.

Some parents and caregivers are comfortable discussing sexuality issues with their kids. others feel anxious about providing too much information or embarrassed about not knowing answers to questions that are asked. Honest, open communication between parents and children—through childhood, the pre-teen years, adolescence, and young adulthood—can help lay the foundation for young people to mature into sexually healthy adults.

Young people also learn about sexuality from other sources. These include friends, teachers, neighbors, television, music, books, advertisements, toys, and the Internet. They also frequently learn through planned opportunities in faith communities, community-based agencies, and schools.

Education in the Home

Issue: Are parents and children comfortable discussing sexuality?
Answer: Research has shown that parents and children have a wide range of comfort levels when it comes to discussing sexuality. However, children consistently report wanting to receive information about sexuality from their parents.

- In one study of 687 students in grades 9 through 12, 36% said they wanted to talk to their parents about sex. Of the 405 parents surveyed for this study, 58% felt that their teens wanted to talk to them about sex.[2]
- A study of 374 parents of students in grades 7 through 12 found that 65% were "somewhat comfortable" or "very comfortable" talking to their teens about sexuality.[3]
- *Talking with Kids about Tough Issues,* a study released in 2001 by the Kaiser Family Foundation, Nickelodeon, and Children Now, surveyed 1,249 parents of children 8 to 15 years of age and 823 children in that age group. The study found that 32% of children were "very comfortable" and 45% were "kind of comfortable" talking to the parents about puberty; 42% were "very comfortable" and 45% "kind of comfortable" talking to their parents about HIV/AIDS; 27% were "very comfortable" and 49% were "kind of comfortable" talking to their parents about the basics of sexual reproduction; and 43% were "very comfortable" and 38% were "kind of comfortable" talking with their parents about what it means to be gay.[4]

Issue: Are parents talking to their children about sexuality?
Answer: Research shows that parents and children do discuss numerous issues related to sexuality, but that the frequency of these discussions and the topics covered vary.

- In a study published by the *Journal of School Health,* almost all parents (94%) reported that they had talked to their teens about sexuality. However, only 9% believed that most parents adequately communicated with their teens about sexuality.[5]
- *Talking with Kids about Tough Issues* found that 65% of parents reported talking to their children about puberty, 59% about the basic facts of sexual reproduction, 55% about HIV or AIDS, and 52% about what it means to be gay.[6]
- In addition, among respondents in that study whose children were between the ages of 12 and 15, 49% discussed how to know when he/she is ready to have a sexual relationship, 54% discussed how to handle pressure to have sex, and 32% discussed what kinds of birth control are available and where to get them.[7]
- In another study, parents report speaking "a great deal" with their children about STDs (40%), dating relationships (37%), and not having sexual intercourse until marriage (36%). In contrast, the parents reported that they spoke to their children "not at all" about masturbation (39%), prostitution (42%), pornography (40%), and abortion (34%).[8]
- It is important to note that parents and children do not always agree about the content or frequency of these conversations. In *Talking with Kids about Tough Issues,* 59% of 8 to 11 year olds whose parents say they talked to them about HIV/AIDS do not recall the conversation, nor do 39% of 8 to 11 year olds whose parents say they talked to them about the basics of sexual reproduction, or 36% of 8 to 11 year olds whose parents say they talked to them about puberty.[9]
- In another study, 98% of parents felt they had communicated with their teens about alcohol use, drug use, and sex while only 76% of teens said these discussions took place.[10]

Issue: Is adult-child communication about sexuality effective?
Answer: Teens consistently rank their parents as one of their primary sources of information on sexuality issues and studies have shown that adult-child communication can decrease sexual risk behaviors.

- *Talking with Kids about Tough Issues* found that 58% of children said they learned "a lot" about sex, "treating people who are different," drugs, alcohol, and violence from their mothers, 38% from their fathers, and 32% from other people in their families.[11]
- A 1999 study released by the kaiser Family Foundation found that 59% of adolescents 10 to 12 years of age and 45% of adolescents 13 to 15 years of age said that they personally learned the "most" about sexuality from their parents.[12]
- A study published in the *Journal of Adolescent Research* found that parent-teen discussions about condoms were related to greater condom use at last intercourse, greater lifetime condom use, and greater consistent condom use.[13]

- In addition, a study of the role of adult mentors found that youth who reported having a mentor were significantly less likely to have had sexual intercourse with more than one partner in the six months prior to the study than their peers who reported not having an adult mentor.[14]

School-Based Education

Issue: What are the goals of school-based sexuality education?
Answer: School-based sexuality education complements and augments the sexuality education children receive from their families, religious and community groups, and health care professionals. The primary goal of school-based sexuality education is to help young people build a foundation as they mature into sexually healthy adults. Such programs respect the diversity of values and beliefs represented in the community.

Sexuality education seeks to assist young people in understanding a positive view of sexuality, provide them with information and skills about taking care of their sexual health, and help them make sound decisions now and in the future.

Comprehensive sexuality education has four main goals:

- to provide accurate information about human sexuality
- to provide an opportunity for young people to develop and understand their values, attitude,s and beliefs about sexuality
- to help young people develop relationships and interpersonal skills, and
- to help young people exercise responsibility regarding sexual relationships, including addressing abstinence, pressures to become prematurely involved in sexual intercourse, and the use of contraception and other sexual health measures.[15]

Issue: How do school-based programs differ?
Answer: Schools and communities are responsible for developing their own curricula and programs regarding sexuality education. The following terms and definitions provide a basic understanding of the sexuality education programs currently offered in schools and communities.

- **Comprehensive sexuality education.** Sexuality education programs that start in kindergarten and continue through twelfth grade. These programs include information on a broad set of topics and provide students with opportunities to develop skills and learn factual information.
- **Abstinence-based.** HIV-prevention and sexuality education programs which emphasize abstinence. They also include information about non-coital sexual behavior, contraception, and disease prevention methods. These programs are also referred to as *abstinence-plus* or *abstinence-centered.*

- **Abstinence-only.** HIV-prevention and sexuality education programs which emphasize abstinence from all sexual behaviors. They do not include any information about contraception or disease prevention methods.
- **Abstinence-only-until-marriage.** HIV-prevention and sexuality education programs which emphasize abstinence from all sexual behaviors outside of marriage. They do not include information about contraception or disease-prevention methods. They typically present marriage as the only morally correct context for sexual activity.

Issue What do comprehensive programs ideally include?
Answer: The National Guidelines Task Force, composed of representatives from 15 national organizations, schools, and universities, identified six key concept areas that should be part of any comprehensive sexuality education program: human development, relationships, personal skills, sexual behavior, sexual health, and society and culture.

The Task Force published the *Guidelines for Comprehensive Sexuality Education,* which include information on teaching 36 sexuality-related topics in an age-appropriate manner.[16]
Issue: What does school-based sexuality education include?
Answer: The content of sexuality education varies depending on the community and the age of the students in the programs. Recent studies provide some insight into what is taught in America's classroom today.

- In a national survey released by the Kaiser Family Foundation, 61% of teachers and 58% of principals reported that their school takes a comprehensive approach to sexuality education, described as teaching young people that they should wait to engage in sexual behavior but that they should practice "safer sex" and use birth control if they do not. In contrast, 33% of teachers and 34% of principals described their school's main message as abstinence-only-until-marriage.[17]
- In the same survey, teachers reported covering the following topics in their most recent sexuality education course: HIV/AIDS (985), abstinence (97%), STDs (96%), and the basics of reproduction (88%), birth control (74%), abortion (46%), and sexual orientation and homosexuality (44%).[18]
- The Centers for Disease Control and Prevention's (CDC's) Division of Adolescent and School Health has published *School Health Education Profiles* (SHEP) which summarizes results from 35 state surveys and 13 local surveys conducted among representative samples of school principals and health education coordinators. SHEP found that 97% of health education courses required by states included information about HIV prevention, 94% included information about STD prevention, and 85% included information about pregnancy prevention.[19]
- Among those schools that required HIV education, 99% taught about HIV infection and transmission, 76% taught about condom efficacy, and 48% taught how to use condoms correctly.[20]

- In addition, 95% of health education courses required by states taught skills to help students resist social pressures, 97% taught decision-making skills, and 90% taught communication skills.[21]

Research on Education

Issue: Are comprehensive sexuality education programs that teach students about both abstinence and contraception effective?

Answer: Numerous studies and evaluations published in peer-reviewed literature suggest that comprehensive sexuality education is an effective strategy to help young people delay involvement in sexual intercourse. Research has also concluded that these programs do not hasten the onset of sexual intercourse, do not increase the frequency of sexual intercourse, and do not increase the number of partners of sexually active teens.

- **Emerging Answers: Research Findings on Programs to Reduce Teen Pregnancy,** a report released in 2001 by The National Campaign to Prevent Teen Pregnancy, identified successful teenage pregnancy prevention initiatives, including five sexuality/HIV education programs, two community service programs, and one intensive program that combined sexuality education, health care, and activities such as tutoring. *Emerging Answers* concluded that sexuality and HIV education programs do not hasten sexual activity, that education about abstinence and contraception are compatible rather than in conflict with each other, and that making condoms available does not increase sexual behavior.[22]
- **No Easy Answers,** a report commissioned in 1997 by The National Campaign to Prevent Teen Pregnancy, reviewed both sexuality and HIV education programs. The report concluded that skills-based sexuality education—those programs that, among other things, teach contraceptive use and communications skills—can delay the onset of sexual intercourse or reduce the frequency of sexual intercourse, reduce the number of sexual partners, and increase the use of condoms and other contraception. The review concluded that sexuality and HIV education curricula that discuss abstinence and contraception do not hasten the onset of intercourse, do not increase the frequency of intercourse, and to not increase the number of sexual partners.[23]
- **UNAIDS, Sexual Health Education Does Lead to Safer Sexual Behavior-UNAIDS Review,** commissioned in 1997 by the Joint United Nations Programme on HIV/AIDS (UNAIDS), examined 68 reports on sexuality education from France, Mexico, Switzerland, Thailand, the United Kingdom, the United States, and various Nordic countries. It found 22 studies that reported that HIV and/or sexual health education either delayed the onset of sexual activity, reduced the number of sexual partners, or reduced unplanned pregnancy and STD rates. It also found that education

about sexual health and/or HIV does not encourage increased sexual activity. The authors concluded that quality sexual health programs helped delay first intercourse and protect sexually-active youth from pregnancy and STD's, including HIV.[24]

Issue: What are the characteristics of effective programs?
Answer: Research has shown that effective programs share a number of common characteristics. These characteristics was developed by Doug Kirby, Ph.D, author of both *Emerging Answers* and *No Easy Answers*.
Effective programs:

- focus narrowly on reducing one or more sexual behaviors that lead to unintended pregnancy or STDs/HIV infection
- are based on theoretical approaches that have been successful in influencing other health-related risky behaviors
- give a clear message by continually reinforcing a clear stance on particular behaviors
- provide basic, accurate information about the risks of unprotected intercourse and methods of avoiding unprotected intercourse
- include activities that address social pressures associated with sexual behavior
- provide modeling and the practice of communication, negotiation, and refusal skills
- incorporate behavioral goals, teaching methods, and materials that are appropriate to the age, sexual experience, and culture of the students
- last a sufficient length of time to complete important activities adequately
- select teachers or peers who believe in the program they are implementing and then provide training for those individuals[25]

Issue: Are abstinence-only-until-marriage programs effective?
Answer: To date, no published studies of abstinence-only programs have found consistent and significant program effects on delaying the onset of intercourse.

- The National Campaign to Prevent Teen Pregnancy's report titled *Emerging Answers: Research Findings on Programs to Reduce Teen Pregnancy* identifies successful teenage pregnancy-prevention initiatives but indicates that none are abstinence-only programs. The report indicates that evidence is not conclusive about such programs but that, thus far, the information is "not encouraging." In fact, the report states that none of the evaluated abstinence-only programs "showed an overall positive effect on sexual behavior, nor did they affect contraceptive use among sexually active participants."[26]
- Of the previous studies of abstinence-only programs, none have found consistent and significant program effects on delaying intercourse. At least one has provided strong evidence the program did not delay the onset of intercourse.
- Proponents of abstinence-only-until-marriage programs often conduct their own in-house evaluations and cite them as proof that their programs are effective. Outside

experts have found, however, that these evaluations are inadequate, methodologically unsound, or inconclusive based on methodological limitations.[27]

- The CDC's *Research to Classroom Project* identifies curricula that have shown evidence of reducing sexual risk behaviors. A recent paper written by the White House Office of National AIDS Policy points out that "none of the curricula on the current list of programs uses an 'abstinence-only' approach."[28]

Issue: Are "Virginity Pledges" effective?

Answer: In recent years, many abstinence programs have begun ton include pledge cards for students to sign promising to remain virgins until they are married. Recent research suggests that under certain conditions these pledges may help some adolescents delay sexual intercourse. For these adolescents, the pledge helped them delay the onset of sexual intercourse for an average of 18 months. The study, however, also found that those young people who took a pledge were less likely to use contraception when they did become sexually active.[29]

Government's Role

Issue: Is there a federal policy on sexuality education?

Answer: There is no federal law or policy requiring sexuality or HIV education. The federal government is explicit in its view that it should not dictate sexuality education or its content in schools. Four federal statutes preclude the federal government from prescribing state and local curriculum standards:

- the Department of Education Organization Act, Section 103a
- the Elementary and Secondary Education Act, Section 14512
- Goals 2000, Section 314(b)
- the General Education Provisions Act, Section 438

Issue: How does the federal government's abstinence-only-until-marriage education program fit in?

Answer: While the federal government does not have a policy about sexuality education and has never taken an official position on the subject, a number of federal programs have been instituted in recent years that provide funding for strict abstinence-only-until-marriage education.

- In 1996, the federal government created an entitlement program, Section 510(b) of Title V of the Social Security Act, that funnels $50 million per year for five years into states for abstinence-only-until-marriage programs. Those that choose to accept Section 510(b) funds must match every four federal dollars with three state-raised dollars and then disperse the funds for educational activities.
- Programs that accept the Section 510(b) funds must adhere to the following strict definition of "abstinence education":

a. has as its exclusive purpose, teaching the social, psychological, and health gains to be realized by abstaining from sexual activity;

b. teaches abstinence from sexual activity outside marriage as the expected standard for all school age children;

c. teaches that abstinence from sexual activity is the only certain way to avoid out-of-wedlock pregnancy, sexually transmitted diseases, and other associated health problems;

d. teaches that a mutually faithful monogamous relationship in the context of marriage is the expected standard of human sexual activity;

e. teaches that sexual activity outside of the context of marriage is likely to have harmful psychological and physical effects;

f. teaches that bearing children out of wedlock is likely to have harmful consequences for the child, the child's parents, and society;

g. teaches young people how to reject sexual advances and how alcohol and drug use increase vulnerability to sexual advances; and

h. teaches the importance of attaining self-sufficiency before engaging in sexual activity.

- Funding for abstinence-only-until-marriage education has increased nearly 3,000% since this federal entitlement program was created in 1996.[30] The federal government has since approved an additional 50 million dollars of funding for abstinence-only-until-marriage programs. Although these funds are not part of Section 510(b), programs must conform to the strict eight-point definition. In addition, these new funds are awarded directly to state and local organizations by the Maternal and Child Health Bureau through a competitive grant process instead of through state block grants as is the case for Section 510(b) funds.

Issue: Do state governments have policies on sexuality education?
Answer: States vary in their approach to sexuality education. Some mandate that schools provide sexuality education, others mandate that schools provide STD and/or HIV/AIDS education, and others mandate both. Some states make no mandates at all while others make recommendations.

Among states that mandate sexuality education and/or STD and/or HIV/AIDS education, some include specific requirements or restrictions on the content of these courses while others leave these decisions to local communities.

Even in those states where sexuality education is not mandated, certain requirements and restrictions are sometimes placed on those schools that opt to teach either sexuality education or STD and/or HIV/AIDS education.

There is a lack of uniformity in language used by states to enact mandates. This makes categorization difficult. For more information, contact your state legislature.

SEXUALITY EDUCATION MANDATES

- Nineteen states, including the District of Columbia, require schools to provide sexuality education. (DE, DC, GA, IL, IA, KS, KY, MD, MN, NV, NJ, NC, RI, SC, TN, UT, VT, WV, WY)
- Thirty-two states do not require schools o provide sexuality education. (AL, AK, AZ, AR, CA, CO, CT, FL, HI, ID, IN, LA, ME, MA, MI, MS, MO, MT, NE, NH, NM, NY, ND, OH, OK, OR, PA, SD, TX, VA, WA, WI)[31]

  Content requirements. Regarding sexuality education, content requirements for abstinence and contraception were examined. Many states also have mandates for the inclusion or prohibition of other information, such as information on puberty and sexual orientation.

- Of the 19 states that require schools to provide sexuality education, three (IL, KY, UT) require schools that teach sexuality education to teach abstinence but do not require that they teach about contraception.

- Of the 19 states that require schools to provide sexuality education, nine (DE, GA, NJ, NC, RI, SC, TN, VT, WV) require schools that teach abstinence to also teach about contraception.

- Of the 32 states that do not require schools to provide sexuality education, 11 (AL, AZ, CO, FL, IN, LA, MI, MS, OK, SD, TX) require that curricula, when taught, must include information about abstinence but not about contraception. Of those 11 states, six (AL, FL, IN, LA, MS, TX) require that curricula, when taught, must include abstinence-only-until-marriage education.

- Of the 32 states that do not require schools to provide sexuality education, five (CA, HI, MO, OR, VA) require that curricula, when taught, must provide information about abstinence and contraception. Of these five, three (CA, MO, VA) specify abstinence-only-until-marriage education.[32]

STD/HIV EDUCATION MANDATES

- Thirty-six states, including the District of Columbia, require schools to provide STD, HIV, and/or AIDS education. (AL, CA, CT, DE, DC, FL, GA, IL, IN, IA, KS, KY, MD, MI, MN, MO, NV, NH, NJ, NM, NY, NC, ND, OH, OK, OR, PA, RI, SC, TN, UT, VT, WA, WV, WI, WY)
- Fifteen states do not require schools to provide STD, HIV, and/or AIDS education. (AK, AZ, AR, CO, HI, ID, LA, ME, MA, MS, MT, NE, SD, TX, VA)[33]

  Content requirements. For STD and/or HIV/AIDS education, content requirements for abstinence and prevention methods were examined.

- Of the 36 states that require schools to provide STD, HIV, and/or AIDS education, two (IN, OH) require that such education also teach abstinence-only-until-marriage but do not require information about prevention methods.

- Of the 36 states that require schools to provide STD, HIV, and/or AIDS education, 24 (AL, CA, DE, FL, GA, IL, KY, MI, MN, MO, NJ, NM, NY, NC, OK, OR, PA, RI, SC, TN, UT, VT, WA, WV) require that such education also teach about abstinence and methods of prevention. Of these 24 states, 12 (AL, CA, FL, GA, IL, MN, MO, NC, SC, TN, UT, WA) specify abstinence-only-until-marriage education.

- Of the 15 states that do not require schools to provide STD, HIV, and/or AIDS education, four (AZ, LA, MS, TX) require that such education also teach abstinence but not prevention methods. Of these four, three (LA, MS, and TX) specify abstinence-only-until-marriage.

- Of the 15 states that do not require schools to provide STD, HIV, and/or AIDS education, two (HI, VA) require that such programs, if taught, must also teach abstinence and methods of prevention. Virginia specifies abstinence-only-until-marriage[34]

Support for Comprehensive Sexuality Education

Issue: Do parents, teachers, and students support it?
Answer: Recent research shows that parents, teachers, and students consistently support sexuality education and that they want more rather than fewer topics included in these classes.

- A 2000 study released by the Kaiser Family Foundation found that virtually all parents, teachers, principals, and students want some form of sexuality education taught in secondary school, and all overwhelmingly support teaching high school students a broad range of topics including birth control and safe sex. For middle and junior high school students, support is more divided; about half or more of students, parents, teachers, and principals favor teaching all aspects of sexuality education.[35]

- Parents surveyed wanted sexuality education to teach the following topics and skills: HIV/AIDS and other STDs (98%), the basics of reproduction and birth control (90%), how to deal with the pressure to have sex and emotional issues and consequences of being sexually active (94%); how to talk with a partner about birth control and STDs (88%); how to use condoms (85%); how to use and where to get other birth control (84%); abortion (79%); and sexual orientation and homosexuality (76%).[36]

- A third of parents (33%) said they wanted their children to learn abstinence as the only option until marriage. However, many of the same parents also wanted their children to learn preventative skills such as how to use condoms and other birth control methods.[37]
- In addition, nearly three-quarters of parents (74%) said that they wanted schools to present issues in a "balanced" way that represented different views in society.[38]
- When asked what they wanted to learn more about, students who had already had sexuality education classes named the following: knowing how to deal with the emotional consequences of being sexually active (46%); knowing how to talk with a partner about birth control and STDs (46%); and knowing how to use or where to obtain birth control (40%).[39]

Issue: Does the public support sexuality education?
Answer: Numerous national polls find overwhelming public support for comprehensive sexuality education.

- A national poll conducted by Hickman-Brown Research, Inc., in 1999 for SIECUS and Advocates for Youth found that 93% of all Americans support the teaching of sexuality education in high schools and 84% support sexuality education in middle/junior high schools.[40]
- A survey conducted by Peter D. Hart Research Associates, Inc., for the Children's Research and Education Institute in 1999 found that 66% of registered voters are in favor of teaching sexuality education in the public elementary schools, 22% are negative about sexuality education in the public elementary schools, and 12% are neutral on the topic.[41]
- A recent Phi Delta Kappa/Gallup Poll, *The Public's Attitudes Toward the Public Schools,* found that 87% of Americans favor including sexuality education in school curricula.[42]

Issue: Do national and government organizations support sexuality education?
Answer: Numerous national and government organizations have expressed support for comprehensive sexuality education.

- Officials at the National Institutes of Health[43], The Institute of Medicine[44], the U.S. Centers for Disease Control and Prevention[45], the White House Office on National AIDS Policy[46], and the Surgeon General's Office[47] have all publicly supported sexuality education programs that included information about abstinence, contraception, and condom use.
- Prominent public health organizations also support comprehensive sexuality education including the American Medical Association[48], the American Academy of Pediatrics[49], the American College of Obstetrics and Gynecology[50], and the Society for Adolescent Medicine.[51]

- In fact, more than 127 mainstream national organizations focusing on young people and health issues including Advocates for Youth, Girls Inc., the National Association for the Advancement of Colored People, and the YWCA of the USA have joined the National Coalition to Support Sexuality Education to assure comprehensive sexuality education for all youth in the United States.

Issue: Is there more information available on these issues.

Answer: SIECUS provides resources and services to help parents, educators, policymakers, the media, and the public understand sexuality education. SIECUS' Web site (www.siecus.org) contains over 1,000 pages of information and links to numerous organizations working in this area. SIECUS also produces fact sheets, bibliographies, and other publications to expand on the information in this fact sheet. contact SIECUS for a publications catalogue. In addition, SIECUS' Mary S. Calderone Library is open to the public for assistance with research.

References

1. National Guidelines Task Force, *Guidelines for Comprehensive Sexuality Education, 2nd Edition,* Kindergarten-12th Grade (New York: Sexuality Information and Education Council of the United States, 1996), p. 3.
2. *Teen Today 2000, Liberty Mutual and Students Against Destructive Decisions/Students Against Drunk Driving* (Boston, MA, Students Against Drunk Driving, 2000).
3. T. R. Jordan, et al., "Rural Parents' Communication with Their Teenagers about Sexual Issues," *Journal of School Health,* vol. 70, no. 8, pp. 338–44.
4. The Henry J. Kaiser Family Foundation, *Talking with Kids about Tough Issues: A National Survey of Parents and Kids, Questionnaire and Detailed Results* (Menlo Park, CA: The Henry J. Kaiser Family Foundation, 2001) pp. 16–17.
5. T. R. Jordan, et al., "Rural Parents Communication with Their Teenagers About Sexual Issues."
6. The Henry J. Kaiser Family Foundation, *Talking with Kids about Tough Issues: A National Survey of Parents and Kids.*
7. Ibid.
8. T. R. Jordan, et al., "Rural Parents Communication with Their Teenagers About Sexual Issues."
9. The Henry J. Kaiser Family Foundation, *Talking with Kids about Tough Issues: A National Survey of Parents and Kids.*
10. *Teen Today 2000, Liberty Mutual and Students Against Destructive Decisions/Students Against Drunk Driving*
11. The Henry J. Kaiser Family Foundation, *Talking with Kids about Tough Issues: A National Survey of Parents and Kids.*

12. Ibid., chart 4.

13. D. Whitaker and K. S. Miller, "Parent-Adolescent Discussions about Sex and Condoms: Impact on Peer Influences of Sexual Risk Behaviors," *Journal of Adolescent Research,* March 2000, vol. 15, no. 2, pp. 251–73.

14. S. R. Beier, et al, "The Potential Role of an Adult Mentor in Influencing High-risk Behaviors in Adolescents," *Archives of Pediatrics & Adolescent Medicine,* April 2000, vol. 154, pp. 327–31.

15. National Guidelines Task Force, Comprehensive Sexuality Education, pp. 3, 5.

16. Ibid. pp. 7–10.

17. The Henry J. Kaiser Family Foundation, Sex Education in America: A View from Inside the Nation's Classrooms, Chart Pack (Menlo Park, CA: The Henry J. Kaiser Family Foundation, 2000), chart 9.

18. Ibid, chart 10.

19. "Characteristics of Health Education Among Secondary Schools—School Health Education Profiles, 1996" *Morbidity and Mortality Weekly Report,* September 11, 1998, vol. 47, no. SS–4, pp. 1–31, table 4.

20. Ibid., table 12.

21. Ibid., p. 5.

22.2 D. Kirby, *Emerging Answers: Research Findings on Programs to Reduce Teen Pregnancy* (The National Campaign to Prevent Teen Pregnancy, May 2001).

23. D. Kirby, *No Easy Answers* (Washington: National Campaign to Prevent Teen Pregnancy, 1997).

24. "Sexual Health Education Does Lead to Safer Sexual Behaviour—UNAIDS Review" Press Release, Joint United Nations Programme on HIV/AIDS, October 22, 1997.

25. D. Kirby, "What Does the Research Say about Sexuality Education/" *Educational Leadership,* Oct. 2000, p. 74.

26. D. Kirby, *Emerging Answers,* "Summary," p. 8.

27. C. Bartels, et. al, *Federally Funded Abstinence-Only Sex Education Programs: A Meta-Evaluation.* Paper presented at the Fifth Biennial Meeting of the Society for Research on Adolescence, San Diego, CA, February 11, 1994; B. Wilcox, et al., Adolescent Abstinence Promotion Programs: An Evaluation of Evaluations. Paper presented at the Annual Meeting of the American Public Health Association, New York, NY, November 18, 1996.

28. Office of National AIDS Policy, The White House, *Youth and HIV/AIDS 2000: A New American Agenda* (Washington, DC: Government Printing Office, 2000), p. 14.

29. P. Bearmen and H. Brueckner, *Executive Summary: Promising the Future,* December 1999 [Who published? Where?]

30. C. Dailard, "Fueled by Campaign Promises, Drive Intensifies to Boost Abstinence-Only Education Funding," *The Guttmacher Report on Public Policy,* vol. 3, no. 2, April 2000.

31. National Abortion and Reproductive Rights Action League Foundation (NARAL), *Who Decides? A State-by-State Review of Abortion and Reproductive Rights* (Washington, DC: NARAL, the NARAL Foundation, January 2001)

32. Ibid.

33. Ibid.

34. Ibid.

35. The Henry J. Kaiser Family Foundation, *Sex Education in America: A View from Inside the Nation's Classrooms,* p. 32.

36. Ibid., chart 12.

37. Ibid., chart 14.

38. Ibid, p. 30.

39. Ibid., chart 15.

40. *SIECUS/Advocates for Youth Survey of Americans' Views on Sexuality Education* (Washington: Sexuality Information and Education Council of the United States and Advocates for Youth, 1999).

41. *Teaching Sex Education in the Public Elementary Schools,* phone survey, Peter D. Hart Research Associates, Inc., February 20–26, 1999.

42. "The 30th Annual Phi Delta Kappa/Gallup Poll of the Public's Attitudes Toward the Public Schools," *Phi Delta Kappan,* September 1998, p. 54.

43. National Institutes of Health, *Consensus Development Conference Statement* (Rockville, MD: The Institutes, 1997).

44. Institute of Medicine, Committee on Prevention and Control of Sexually Transmitted Diseases T. R. Eng, W. T. Butler, editors., *The Hidden Epidemic: Confronting Sexually Transmitted Diseases* (Washington, DC: National Academy Press, 1997).

45. Centers for Disease Control and Prevention, statement of Dr. Lloyd Kolbe, director, Division of Adolescent and School Health, June 1998.

46. Office of National AIDS Policy, The White House, *Youth and HIV/AIDS 2000: A New American Agenda* (Washington, DC: Government Printing Office, 2000).

47. D. Satcher, *The Surgeon General's Call to Action to Promote Sexual Health and Responsible Sexual Behavior* (Washington, DC: U.S. Government Printing Office, 2001).

48. Council on Scientific Affairs, American Medical Association, *Report 7 of the Council on Scientific Affairs: Sexuality Education, Abstinence, and Distribution of Condoms in Schools* (Chicago: American Medical Association, 1999).

49. American Academy of Pediatrics, "Policy statement: Condom Availability for Youth," *Pediatrics,* vol. 95, 1995, pp. 281–85.

50. American College of Obstetrics and Gynecology, *Committee on Adolescent Health Care-Committee Opinion*, 1995.

51. Society for Adolescent Medicine, *Position Statements and Resolutions: Access to Health Care for Adolescents*, March 1992.

Section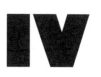

Sexual Preference

The Necessity of Addressing Sexual Identity in the Schools

John P. Elia, Ph.D. [1]

CHAPTER 12

Introduction

Public school personnel nationwide are obsessed with cracking the academic whip to get students prepared to compete globally. The rhetoric used to support such academic rigor usually garners support from the majority. However, we must examine what we lose by continuously supporting such an educational approach. This has meant that curricular programs that fall outside of the "3Rs," are seen as superfluous, and therefore share little if any priority in curricular offerings. Sexuality education is a prime example of a topic that is treated with contempt and suspicion—and is viewed as academically deficient—by most schools nationally.

Due to various political and personal views, offering comprehensive sexuality education[2] in the schools has been an uphill battle. Just two years ago SIECUS' National Guidelines Task Force reported that only five percent of the nation's youth receive comprehensive sexuality education. The majority of students receive information about the "plumbing" aspects of sexual functioning, complete with scare tactics about the possible ills of sexual behavior. Very little time is devoted to discussing issues other than the biological "facts" of sexual functioning. An important area of sexuality education that continues to be grossly ignored is sexual identity.[3] Although our society has a great deal of tension, and personal and social problems surrounding sexual identity, we continue to overlook its importance in schools. In this article I will argue why we can no longer afford to ignore sexual identity. Among some of the major reasons why we must address sexual identity in the schools are to: avoid personal and social harm, build more harmonious relationships and communities, and strengthen a commitment to democratic education.

Avoiding Personal and Social Harm

Specifically regarding the issue of sexual identity, the education process in schools has been unkind, inequitable, and unethical to students. While this sounds like a hyperbolic claim—and maybe even unforgivably rhetorical—at first glance, it can be substantiated. It is no secret that heterosexuality is perceived by many to be better and more noble than bisexuality or homosexuality. If this were not the case then issues about gays and lesbians in the military or policing people's sexuality would be moot points. Discussions of bisexuality and homosexuality are avoided at all costs. And, indeed, there are numerous personal and social costs incurred by not addressing these topics.

Some individuals are likely to argue that it is not crucial to deal with bisexuality and homosexuality in the schools. They might assert that because sexual minorities comprise only a minority of the population it does not make sense to devote attention to these matters. Others might even take a more radical position and suggest that such a coverage "promotes" bisexuality and homosexuality among our youth. Yet others reject the idea on the grounds that it's not the school's job to ameliorate personal or social problems. Some people are unaware that there is an issue at all. Many of these people are not mean or malicious: they just have not given it much thought. They contend that schools should be solely responsible for academic advancement with an emphasis on the 3Rs. They have a narrow view—the prevailing one—of what ought to comprise schooling.

Let's turn to an examination of the arguments outlined above and expose their weaknesses. First is the idea that because only a relatively small percentage of people identify as bisexual, gay, or lesbian (b/g/l) it is not worthwhile to devote attention to sexual identity issues. This argument follows similarly to "the greatest good for the greatest number" line of reasoning. This is problematic on at least two fronts. First, it discounts individuals and their experiences simply because they do not belong to the majority. Second, it assumes that the so-called heterosexual majority would not benefit from such coverage. There has been considerable personal harm done to b/g/l youth by keeping the issues of sexual identity silent in the curriculum. By continuing a heterosexist[4] form of instruction many b/g/l students sit in classrooms feeling isolated, depressed, and anxious. There are numerous data that report that school failure, drug and alcohol abuse, dropout, and attempted suicide and suicide rates are alarmingly high among this population.[5] In terms of the impact of addressing various aspects of sexual identity with heterosexual students, there is much to be gained. Keeping b/g/l issues closeted feeds the mistrust, fear, mysteriousness, and hatred that manifests itself as biphobia or homophobia both among b/g/l individuals and their heterosexual peers.

It is more complicated than the straights pitting themselves against b/g/l people. For example, bisexuals are often misunderstood and held in contempt by heterosexuals and homosexuals alike. There is even a lot of prejudice, misunderstanding, and internecine rivalry between gays and lesbians. We should not assume that there is harmony among sexual minorities simply because they share sexual minority status. Refusing to address issues of sexual identity in the schools fuels much discontent in and out of schools, pits students of all sexual identities against one another creating personal harm and in many cases leading to academic failure.

The position that addressing sexual identity issues "promotes" bisexuality or homosexuality is problematic and troubling. The most likely interpretation of this claim is that by covering such a topic students might be more inclined to experiment with bisexuality and homosexuality, or maybe even adopt these as their sexual identities than they would if the subject were ignored. The above position makes the assumption that it would be wrong for an individual to experiment sexually or choose to live a sexual lifestyle that is fulfilling and satisfying to her or him. It also assumes that such identities can be changed easily. I believe that educators are, in part, charged with responsibility of getting students to think critically about their lives and assisting them with discovering their likes, dislikes, interests, talents, and even limitations. We cannot separate the academic and the personal as rigidly as one might think. Caring about students as individuals must share a high priority if the schools are to be successful.

Many people maintain that it's not the school's responsibility to ameliorate personal and social problems. They maintain that schooling ought to be strictly academically based and that personal and social problems should be solved outside of school. Again, this assumes that the academic can be neatly separated from the personal and social. Even if they could be separated, we need to consider whether or not this is an appropriate approach to schooling. Traditionally, most teachers have taught their subjects without considering the personal and social implications of what and how they teach. A consideration of how materials is relevant to the lives of students is crucial. Let's return to the issue of sexual identity. B/g/l youth are made to feel invisible when topics are taught from a completely heterosexist point of view. How could they obtain personal relevance when educators omit references to b/g/l issues? B/g/l students not only get turned off to what they are supposed to be learning, but also there is personal harm done. Let's not forget about the distressingly high suicide rates among this population. B/g/l students feel discounted and a sense of prejudice against them. Subtle and overt forms of heterosexism, biphobia, and homophobia are not foreign to schools.[6] Social harm is done when people do not feel connected to one another. Not addressing sexual identity issues builds walls, not bridges, and as a result friendships and other personal connections are precluded.

Building More Harmonious Relationships and Communities

It is never easy addressing as delicate of a topic as sexual identity in the schools. If we want schools to be safer places—both emotionally and physically—for our youth, we must grapple openly with sexual identity issues. There is nothing more precious than our relationships with others. To think of the number of caring and working relationships that have been precluded or destroyed due to prejudice is mind-boggling. Just think of the possibilities of having students of various backgrounds working together to solve problems that emerge from their studies and relationships with one another. Jerome Bruner (1996) maintains that "[b]oth adults and children have points of view, and each is encouraged to recognize the other's, though they may not agree" (pp. 56–57). There surely will be uneasiness and even conflict by pulling issues of sexual identity out of the academic closet. But at least the conspiracy of silence will be broken and students will have a chance to discuss issues, air concerns, and be afforded the possibility of relating to one another with some degree of understanding and respect.

The possibility of building solid and harmonious working relationships and friendships with others regardless of their sexual identities can emerge more readily from the schools' commitment to deal openly and directly with various sexual identities both in the academic and personal realms. There is much to be gained by such an educational approach. First, dialogue will undoubtedly occur and students will be able to discuss their similarities and differences in an open, honest, and non-violent fashion. Second, it will enrich the curriculum by including a discussion of b/g/l issues and people who have historically remained largely invisible. Third, it will provide a sense of comfort and visibility to b/g/l youth, thereby helping them feel less invisible, anxious, depressed, and suicidal. Fourth, the possibility exists of helping b/g/l youth build friendships and associations with other b/g/l as well as heterosexual peers.

Building a sense of community in the schools is important. Nel Noddings (1996) declares that "[W]e should try to establish some of the desirable features associated with community: a sense of belonging, of collective concern for each individual, of individual responsibility for the collective good, and appreciation for the rituals and celebrations of the group" (pp. 266–267). It is essential, however, that individuals and their individuality be respected and that the group or community not coerce individuals to buy into a collective identity at the cost of individuality. The United States Bill of Rights speaks of the protection of individual rights against the tyranny of the majority. This concept needs to be adhered to in our schools if we wish to educate our youth in a democratic fashion.

A Commitment to Democratic Education

We have a responsibility to treat all children equitably. It is reprehensible to have a system of schooling that brushes aside and ignores those students who do not represent the cultural norm for the reasons mentioned earlier. To use the words of A. V. Kelly (1995), this ". . . alienate[s] from educational opportunities large numbers of those pupils whose background and cultural origins, social or ethnic, render both the knowledge they are offered and the values implicit in that knowledge inappropriate to the kind of educational experiences they need . . ." (p. 109). A curriculum based on democratic principles aims to be inclusive and suitable for all students no matter what sexual identity, cultural background, and socio-economic class, etc.

There are many democratic principles that schools should promote to encourage people to work and live together as positively and humanely as possible. Some of these principles are: equality, justice, representation, respect, fairness, freedom, choice, and willingness to debate controversial ideas. These principles should be taught across the curriculum. Teaching democratic principles is not a static process. It involves getting students involved with one another to work out their concerns. Raising issues of diverse sexual identities could be a splendid way of enhancing a democratic educational process in our schools. Arnstine (1995) puts it quite well when he says "[d]iversity is a help, not an obstacle, in setting where education is sought" (p. 244).

We live in a pluralistic society. As far as sexual minorities are concerned, the time has come to realize that we can no longer afford to treat some of our youth as though they are invisible and do not matter. Schools have been repugnant and morally reprehensible regarding the lack of care they have given some students. They have turned their backs on many of our nation's youth. Thus, schools, along with some of our other major institutions such as with many forms of organized religion and medicine, have participated in the perpetuation of heterosexism, biphobia and homophobia. This, in turn, has created harm to individuals and has been flagrantly anti-democratic.

Conclusion

Schools are well positioned to be agents of positive educational and social change. Using a democratic framework along with an ethic of caring, schools would be in a powerful position to treat all students equitably and provide them with an environment that not only affirms diversity but also promotes intellectual and personal growth. Also, as indicated earlier, a commitment to democratic education would serve to ameliorate the terrible injustices (which have caused personal and social harm) done to some of our youth and would likely promote more positive human relations. Keeping issues of bisexuality and homosexuality hidden perpetuates misconceptions and prejudice, and ultimately serves to maintain barriers between people. Bridges need to be built, not walls.

Notes

1. Thanks to Mr. Michael Van Dyke for the constructive criticism he offered me as I prepared this article. This work is better as a result of his feedback.
2. Comprehensive sexuality education refers to a broadly based sexuality education that includes but is not limited to a discussion of the bio-medical, ethical, political, psychological, and socio-cultural aspects of sexuality. Comprehensive sexuality education is an effort to treat sexuality in its broadest sense; it is inclusive rather than exclusive. Most sexuality education in the schools is exclusive in that it focuses heavily on the bio-medical aspects of sexuality and ignores many other, equally important aspects of sexuality. For an explication of the concept of comprehensive

sexuality education, see, for example, SIECUS' *Guidelines for Comprehensive Sexuality Education: Kindergarten-12th Grade.* 2nd ed. New York: National Guidelines Task Force of Sexuality Information and Education Council of the United States, 1996.

3. Sexual identity encompasses various aspects of bisexuality, heterosexuality, and homosexuality.

4. Heterosexism refers to the idea that all people are, or should be, heterosexual. Heterosexism is also characterized by the presumption of universalized heterosexuality. In an institutional setting like schools, heterosexism manifests itself as ignoring bisexual, gay, or lesbian (b/g/l) issues or people; topics across the curriculum are taught from a heterosexual point of view, excluding b/g/l issues. For a detailed account of this concept, consult Robert A. Rhoades' *Coming out in College: The Struggle for a Queer Identity* (Westport & London: Bergin & Garvey, 1994), p. 7.

5. For more information (including statistical data) on the alarming rates of attempted and actual suicide of bisexual, gay, lesbian, and youth troubled by or questioning their sexual identity, see Karen Harbeck's (Ed.) *Coming Out of the Classroom Closet: Gay and Lesbian Students, Teachers, and Curricula* (New York: Haworth Press, 1992); specifically, consult the introduction to this volume.

6. This issue is treated extensively in a number of articles in a special issue of *"The High School Journal* (volume 77, numbers 1 and 2, 1993/1994), which is devoted to issues of bisexual, gay, and lesbian youth.

Bibliography

Arnstine, Donald. *Democracy and the Arts of Schooling.* Albany: State University of New York Press, 1995.

Bruner, Jerome. *The Culture of Education.* Cambridge: Harvard University Press, 1996.

Freire, Paulo. *Pedagogy of the Oppressed.* New York: Continuum, 1970.

Kelly, A. V. *Education and Democracy: Principles and Practices.* London: Paul Chapman Publishers, 1995.

Noddings, Nel. *"On Community,"* *Educational Theory,* Summer, 1996.

Sexuality Information and Education Council of the United States. *Guidelines for Comprehensive Sexuality Education: Kindergarten-12th Grade.* 2nd ed. New York: National Guidelines Task Force of the Sexuality Information and Education Council of the United States, 1996.

Mistakes That Heterosexual People Make When Trying to Appear Non-Prejudiced: The View from LGB People

CHAPTER

Terri D. Conley, Ph.D.
Christopher Calhoun, B.A.
Sophia R. Evett, Ph.D.
Patricia G. Devine, Ph.D.

Abstract

In two studies, lesbians, gay men and bisexuals were queried concerning mistakes that well-meaning heterosexual people have made when interacting with them. In qualitative, open-ended research, we determined that the most common mistakes concerned heterosexuals' pointing out that they know someone who is gay, emphasizing their lack of prejudice, and relying on stereotypes about gays. Following up with a quantitative, close-ended questionnaire, we determined that the mistakes respondents experienced most often involved heterosexuals (a) relying on stereotypes and (b) ignoring gay issues; the most annoying mistakes were heterosexuals (a) using subtle prejudicial language and (b) not owning up to their discomfort with gay issues. We used two theoretical perspectives, shared reality theory and the contact hypothesis, to analyze the quantitative responses. Implications for intergroup relationships between heterosexual people and gay people are discussed.

From *Journal of Homosexuality,* Vol. 42(2) 2001 by Terri D. Conley, Ph.D. et al. Copyright (c) 2001 by Haworth Press, Inc. Reprinted by permission.

Keywords

Lesbians, gay men, intergroup relationships, minority perspectives

Research on attitudes toward gay men and lesbians has been a cornerstone of research on the topic of homosexuality for more than two decades. Numerous researchers have documented the extent to which heterosexual people by and large dislike, disapprove of, and are fearful of lesbian, gay, and bisexual (LGB) people (for reviews see Herek, 1994, 1998). However, more recent research has demonstrated the situations in which heterosexuals are likely to be more amenable to gay men and lesbians (Herek & Capitanio, 1996; Herek & Glunt, 1993).

Devine and colleagues (Devine, Monteith, Zuwerink & Elliot, 1991; Devine, Evett, & Vasquez-Suson, 1996) demonstrated that a substantial subset of heterosexuals actually have positive reactions toward lesbians, gay men, and bisexuals, and feel guilt or compunction when they respond negatively toward gay people. Devine et al. (1996) found that these people are likely to be moderately low in prejudice, as measured by standard scales assessing prejudice toward gay people. This group of people would like to behave in non-prejudiced ways, but are not completely successful in doing so. We would expect this group of people to benefit from interacting with gay people, but to be likely to make mistakes in the process of doing so. One way to investigate these mistakes would be to ask heterosexual people what mistakes they have made. However, heterosexuals may not be aware of the mistakes they are making. Therefore, we took the alternative approach of seeking out information about these mistakes from the recipients of the mistake behaviors: gay and lesbian people themselves. Although this is a one-sided analysis of mistakes that heterosexuals make, this project provides the often overlooked perspective of LGB people.

This is an important approach, we believe, because what has been missing in the study of intergroup relationships between LGB people and heterosexuals is a response from the gay people themselves. A great amount of information has been learned about how heterosexuals feel about gay people. Much less has been learned about how gay people react to heterosexuals' hostility, or their attempts to be friendly, helpful, or to appear non-prejudiced. In this paper, we present qualitative and quantitative data addressing this question. Specifically, we were interested in what types of mistakes heterosexuals make when they are trying to appear non-prejudiced. We wanted to view such mistakes in the eyes of the people who are recipients of this behavior: LGB people themselves.

There are obviously a great number of "mistakes" that people make when they are being overtly hostile or prejudiced towards gay men and lesbians. However, for our purposes, we are interested in the types of mistakes that are made by people who would like to portray themselves as non-prejudiced. Throughout the project, we did not precisely define the term "mistakes" for the participants in the study, but rather asked generally about mistakes and allowed respondents to define mistakes for themselves. We were especially interested in how heterosexuals respond to gay people when they are trying to be non-prejudiced, but are not quite sure of how to do it. We specified this goal in the questions that we posed for the respondents.

Study 1

In this study, we sought LGB people's open-ended responses to a question about mistakes that heterosexual people make. Respondents were recruited from a mid-sized community and were asked a series of open-ended questions. The question that we will focus on for the purposes of this paper concerns their reports of mistakes that heterosexuals make when trying to appear non-prejudiced. Of course, listing mistakes is not the same as being bothered by mistakes, and does not necessarily reflect the extent to which people have experienced mistakes. However, we view this study as a first attempt to examine LGB reactions to heterosexuals' mistakes.

Method

RESPONDENTS

Participants in the study were respondents to flyers that expressed a need for LGB people to participate in a study focusing on "interactions between homosexuals and heterosexuals." Respondents were offered $7.00 for completing the questionnaires. Fifty women and 47 men participated in the study. The overall mean age for the sample was 28.5. Almost all of the sample (95%) was White.

MEASURES

Respondents answered questions about basic demographic information (e.g., age, gender, level of education, years identified as gay, lesbian or bisexual) and answered several questions about interactions with heterosexual people that will not be addressed here (see Conley, Devine, Rabow, & Evett, in press). Participants read a description of well-intentioned, but nervous people, and were asked "What are the most common mistakes people make if they are trying to show you that they are not prejudiced?": Participants were provided with blank lines on which to write their open-ended responses to the questions. The responses were coded as described in the coding section.

PROCEDURE

Respondents completed questionnaires in groups, or, if requested, in private. They were allowed to spend as much time as necessary to complete the questionnaire; most respondents finished within one hour.

CODING

Development of a coding scheme. A coding scheme was developed to fully capture the responses to the open-ended question. Two coders independently read the responses to each of the questions several times. After developing familiarity with the entire body of responses for each question, the two coders independently identified common themes in the open-ended responses to the question about mistakes. Themes to be used in the coding protocol were determined by agreement between coders, and in the event of discrepancies (i.e., one coder identified a theme and the other did not) the theme was discussed until consensus was reached about whether or not it should be incorporated into the coding scheme (see Backstrom & Hursh-Cesar, 1981). The themes that respondents identified are listed in Table 1.

Coding of responses. Each coder rated each response for the 11 mistake categories in Table 1. The responses from each participant could contain many mistake categories (hence, the percentages in Table 1 do not add up to 100). Coders read the response and then, for each mistake category, the response was coded "0" if the mistake was not mentioned and "1" if it was mentioned. Percentage agreement between coders was .91. In all cases, a third coder resolved discrepancies.

Results and Discussion

The LGB people in this study had no problem identifying common mistakes that heterosexuals make when trying to portray themselves as unprejudiced. Eight-seven percent of respondents reported at least one mistake that fell within the coding scheme. The most common response concerned heterosexuals needing to state that they know another gay person: over one-third of the respondents reported that heterosexuals point out that have an acquaintance who is gay. For example:

> [They say,] "I know someone who is gay." Who cares? So do I.

> They always know of someone who's gay, and say that "They are really nice and have a steady job." Like we wouldn't?

> [They tell] me that "my best friend's sister is," or, "someone at work is" or "I used to know a nice person who was." This type of bull shit bores me.

An alternate version of this issue concerns the assumption that any two given gay people will be romantically interested in each other. Thus, some respondents expressed frustration with heterosexual people who continually play "matchmaker" with their gay acquaintances.

> They continually try to set you up with their other gay friends!!

These assumptions related to the phenomenon known in social psychological theory as out-group homogeneity (e.g., Brewer, Dull, & Lui, 1981). The assumption is that all gay people are alike and thus would be compatible relationship partners with one another. A related assumption is that there is a much smaller community of gay people than actually exists.

TABLE I   Reported Common Mistakes That People Make When Trying to Show That They Are Not Prejudiced

Category of Response	%	Example of Response
• **Stating that they know another gay person:** Stating that they know another gay person, and expecting that the respondent would know and/or want to date this person	34.0	"Saying this like, 'I have a cousin in New York City who's gay. His name's John Smith. Do you know him?"
• **Pointing out that they are not prejudiced:** Stating that they do not disapprove of homosexuality, or that they are not prejudiced	25.8	"(Saying) 'I'm fine with you being gay' Gee, thanks! Also saying 'I don't care if you are gay' kind of twists my gut."
• **Relying on stereotypes:** Making statements based on stereotypes about gays and lesbians	23.7	"They think lesbians want to be men. They think in terms of butch and femme roles. They think the gays they see in parades (flamboyant drag queens, dykes on bikes) are representative of the whole community."
• **Being overcautious:** Trying *too* hard, overcompensating; being overzealous in their attempts to portray themselves as non-prejudiced	20.6	"(Displaying too much) 'happiness' or accommodating me to the point where I feel like a child."
• **Not owning up to discomfort:** Being hypocritical, not owning up to their discomfort with issues related to homosexuality	18.6	"Trying to act very sexually sophisticated and blase about (me being gay) when secretly they are freaking out."
• **Using subtle prejudicial language**	15.5	"They use words like 'normal' when talking about heterosexuality."
• **Asking inappropriate or too many questions:** Asking inappropriate questions (e.g., about sexuality or personal topics), or too many questions	12.4	"Asking prying questions—seeming to be curious but really just being obnoxious: 'What do you do in bed?' 'What do you do with another guy?' "
• **Ignoring gay issues:** Ignoring the topic of homosexuality completely, failing to acknowledge an individual's gay/lesbian identity	11.3	"Out of embarrassment, they avoid saying anything about my gayness or my sexuality, my lifestyle. It's as if the main component of my life becomes invisible."
• **Acting gay:** Trying to be part of the "ingroup"; acting like they are attracted to members of the same sex	8.2	" 'Checking out' people of the same sex. It's like they're trying to impress me by acting 'like' me and talking' about girls being 'cute' when they are really into dating men. It's offensive 'cause it's like, I'm fine with them liking men, they don't have to 'act' with men."
• **No mistakes:** There really are no mistakes if an individual is well-intentioned	7.2	"I can't really label anything a mistake. Everyone gets points for trying."

They say "I have a cousin in New York City who's gay. His name's John Smith. Do you know him?"

The second most common response involves making explicit statements about their *lack* of prejudice with regard to homosexuality. The LGB individuals in this sample reported that heterosexuals who were not sure of their feelings about homosexuality can be distinguished by their explicit statements of acceptance. Representative comments include:

The simple statement of "it doesn't matter to me" shows the least sensitivity. They are usually lying, and if they truly cared they would realize the implications and comment as truthfully as they can.

They announce that "you people should be able to do whatever you want" which implies that it's an issue of whether they should "allow anything" or not.

They say "Wow. How cool." Queerness is not a fad!

[They say] "I'm fine with you being gay." Gee thanks! Also saying, "I don't care if you are gay" kind of twists my gut. I just imagine what it must be like for a black person to hear "I don't care if you are black." It feels really wrong.

This sampling of responses shows that, when it comes to relationships between different groups, the road to hell can be paved with good intentions. These explicit expressions of tolerance often seem to have the ironic effect of making an individual appear even more prejudiced.

Another common mistake is one which would probably be most expected given research on heterosexual people's attitude toward gay men and lesbians. Many of the respondents reported that heterosexual people respond to them in ways that reflect views of them as perverted, bizarre, or otherwise stereotypical. Almost a quarter of respondents listed this type of mistake. For example:

[They indicate] that they would like to go to a gay bar with me. Translation: can we go to the zoo and see all the animals?

Assuming that gay and lesbian people wish to be the opposite sex is offensive to most of us.

[They] assume a bad experience in childhood made me "this way."

One time a woman (a good friend) let me know that she absolutely didn't care that I was gay. In fact she had a lot of gay male friends but I was her first gay woman friend. She then went on to say that this would be sort of an adventure to watch our relationships grow and watch herself react. It was almost like that this was my life—calling it an adventure took something from me. I'm not sure what, but it was like—"wait a second—this isn't an adventure! This is my life! Why is being my friend going to be an adventure for you?!"

They think lesbians want to be men. They think in terms of butch and femme roles. They think the gays they see in parades (flamboyant drag queens, dykes on bikes) are representative of the whole community.

I know a couple people at work who jokingly call me a "pervert"—I don't consider them true friends, but don't say anything either way because I don't want them to be enemies either. But my feelings get hurt repeatedly and I don't want to show myself as vulnerable by saying that it hurts when they joke around or tease me.

These quotes illustrate how, even among well-meaning people, cultural knowledge of the stereotypes appear to hamper their interpersonal relationships with members of this culturally stigmatized group.

Some of the mistakes that LGB people in this sample reported contradicted each other. For example, 18% of respondents considered *Overemphasizing homosexuality* to be a mistake, yet on the other hand, 11% of respondents reported that *Ignoring gay issues* is a mistake. Thus, it does appear that in some sense, heterosexual people may be walking a very fine line between acceptable and unacceptable treatments of the topic. This tightrope may be made thinner by the general suspiciousness that minority group members, including gay people, have of majority group members (Conley, Devine, Rabow & Evett, in press): people who have been stigmatized for long periods of time by heterosexual people may come to expect prejudicial treatment, even if the heterosexual people are well-meaning.

Although we specifically asked respondents to list mistakes, there were a few (7%) of respondents who noted that they appreciated people's well-meaning attempts at behaving in a non-prejudicial way. For example:

I don't feel right about being too picky. Anyone who genuinely wants me to know that they are not prejudiced, as long as they are not being patronizing, gets plenty of patience and compassion from me.

Really, it's hard to make any mistakes in an effort toward being compassionate! I'd rather have a person fumble in being unprejudiced than be homophobic.

This study provides preliminary evidence about the types of mistakes that LGB people encounter. In the next study we assessed the frequency of these types of mistakes, how bothered LGB people are by heterosexuals' mistakes, and we explored the correlates of participants' experiences and reactions to these mistakes.

Study 2

This study serves as a more detailed investigation of the findings demonstrated in Study 1. In this study, we created a close-ended questionnaire based on the open-ended responses from Study 1. In this questionnaire, we asked respondents both how often they had experienced the various mistakes revealed in Study 1 and how much such mistakes bothered them. This questionnaire was completed by bisexual, lesbian and gay respondents.

THEORETICAL PERSPECTIVES

Shared reality theory and contact theory may contribute to our understanding of how lesbian, gay and bisexual people might perceive heterosexuals' mistakes. We used these two theoretical perspectives to derive hypotheses about the types of responses we expected to receive.

Shared reality theory. Shared reality theory (Hardin & Higgins, 1996: Hardin & Conley, 2001) presumes that shared beliefs, or shared understandings of a situation, form the basis of relationships, and that relationships do not survive without social validation. Conversely, beliefs are more likely to exist to the extent that they are validated in important relationships.

There are several different ways to share beliefs about gay issues. For example, a heterosexual person may a) know that an individual is LGB or b) both know and be supportive of the fact that an individual is LGB. Likewise, an LGB person could try to share reality with heterosexual people by showing that they are LGB through their appearance, or by actively promoting gay perspectives. Because the current statements on shared reality theory do not make distinctions between these specific types of shared realities, we utilize a variety of interpretations of shared reality in the generation of our hypotheses. Specifically, we have four measures of shared reality, each reflecting a slightly different type of shared experience. These include: (1) *The need to educate heterosexuals.* To the extent that LGB people endorse the need to share their beliefs about gay issues with heterosexual people, they should be less bothered by mistakes of heterosexual people. That is, their desire to develop shared reality with heterosexual people suggests an openness to more positive relationships with this group. (2) *The ability to distinguish between heterosexual people who are high or low in prejudice.* To the extent that LGB people believe that they are able to recognize the prejudice level of heterosexuals (i.e., to recognize heterosexuals' perception of gay people), based on shared reality we predict that they should be more tolerant of the mistakes of heterosexual people. Thus, if LGB people believe they share reality with heterosexual people, they should be more likely to have positive relationships than people who find heterosexuals' attitudes inscrutable. (3) *Family support.* According to shared reality, family support should be particularly important in the extent to which mistakes bother LGB people. Family support indicates that important people in an LGB individual's life are aware of her or his sexual orientation, and also approve of the individual's sexual identity. Therefore, to the extent an individual has greater family support, we expect that she or he will be less bothered by the mistakes of heterosexual people. Because their identities are supported in their important relationships they should be less threatened by challenges to their identities. (4) *The extent to which others know the individual is LGB by his or her appearance.* To the extent that LGB people feel that others know they are gay or bisexual, we would expect that they would be less bothered by mistakes made by well-intentioned heterosexual people. That is, we assume that their willingness to share their identity with heterosexual people indicates a desire for closer relationships with heterosexuals. This desire should be reflected in more tolerance for heterosexuals' mistakes.

Contact hypothesis. The original contact hypothesis (Allport, 1954) and more recent conceptualizations of it (e.g., Stephan, 1987) have proposed that under the correct circumstances, contact will reduce hostility, prejudice, and stereotypes, and improve intergroup interactions. The original contact hypothesis was based on the idea of contact under ideal circumstances. More recent research on the contact hypothesis has focused on factors that establish when contact works and when it does not (Stephan, 1987).

In contrast to the marginally successful findings surrounding intergroup interactions among members of different ethnic groups, more promising effects of contact have been demonstrated in heterosexuals' attitudes toward gay people (Herek & Glunt, 1993; Herek & Capitanio, 1996). Results support the idea that heterosexuals who have had more interpersonal contact with gay men and lesbians are more likely to have positive attitudes toward homosexuality. Herek and Capitanio (1996) suggested that contact may be more effective in reducing prejudice toward gay people because homosexuality is a "concealable stigma." Therefore, heterosexuals may be able to interact with gay people without letting the stigma of homosexuality influence their impressions. Then, once they have developed a positive impression of the gay person, knowledge of that individual's homosexuality may cause them to evaluate other gay people more positively.

It is more difficult to predict the effects of contact for LGB individuals' reactions to heterosexual people. After all, most LGB people have substantial contact with heterosexual people every day. Therefore, there is probably little variance in the amount of contact that gay and lesbian people have had with heterosexuals. However, they may not have the kind of positive contact necessary to promote positive intergroup relationships. For the purposes of this paper, we focus on fear of negative evaluation from heterosexual people, and positive contact experiences with heterosexual people who are aware of the respondents' sexual orientation. Of course, this is not a direct test of the original contact hypothesis, because the original hypothesis was not designed with members of minority groups in mind. However, although this is not an exact rendition of the contact hypothesis, we reasoned that this is a reasonable working model of how the contact hypothesis, would work among members of minority groups.

In our attempts to extrapolate from the majority-group focused version of the contact hypothesis that predominates, we included a measure of past contact and a measure of expected future contact experiences in our questionnaire to tap into the spirit of the contact hypothesis. For past contact, we asked participants the extent to which they had experienced positive contact with heterosexual people, with regard to future contact, we asked participants about the extent to which they expected that they would be viewed negatively by others who are aware of their sexual orientation. To the extent that participants expect more positive reactions from heterosexuals, they should be more accepting of their mistakes. That is, they will probably be likely to interpret heterosexuals' mistakes more benignly and have a greater desire to continue contact, which will make them more tolerant of mistakes.

We will draw upon each of these theoretical perspectives. However, we note that these perspectives do not necessarily present competing nor mutually exclusive hypotheses. Some of the hypotheses we associate with shared reality theory could be viewed as having been derived from the contact hypotheses, and vice versa. For our purposes, we believe it sufficient to say that these perspectives together can be used to derive the particular set of predictors contained in our analyses.

Method

RESPONDENTS AND PROCEDURE

Respondents in the study were recruited through friendship networks of experimenters in Los Angeles and in central Wisconsin (no differences were detected between the two sets of respondents based on geographic area). They completed a brief, anonymous, questionnaire and were not compensated for their participation. Thirty-six women and 30 men participated in the study. The overall mean age for the sample was 31.4. The sample was 57% White, 22% Latina/o, 11% Asian American and 6% African American (the remainder of respondents were either from other ethnicities or declined to state their ethnicities).

MEASURES

In the beginning of the questionnaire, respondents were asked to think about mistakes that heterosexual people make when trying to appear unprejudiced. Next, they were presented with what we described as "potential mistakes." These included nine mistakes from the first study and others that we felt may be important even though they were not mentioned by participants in the first study. Our phrasings of the "potential mistakes" in the questionnaire were as follows: (1) *Pointing out that they are not prejudiced:* Heterosexual people have explicitly stated that they do not approve of homosexuality, or that they are not prejudiced. (2) *Focusing on the topic of homosexuality:* Heterosexual people have focused too much on the topic of homosexuality, seeming to assume it is the most important aspect of your life, or talked about the subject too much. (3) *Ignoring gay issues:* Heterosexual people have ignored the topic of homosexuality, failing to acknowledge your bisexual/lesbian/gay identity. (4) *Relying on stereotypes:* Heterosexual people who are trying to be non-prejudiced have made statements based on stereotypes of gays and lesbians. (5) *Asking inappropriate or too many questions:* Heterosexual people have asked inappropriate questions (e.g., about sexuality or personal topics), or too many questions. (6) *Using subtle prejudicial language:* Heterosexual people have used subtle prejudicial language (e.g., "you people" or "I tolerate gays") while professing acceptance of gay men and lesbians. (7) *Stating they know another gay person:* Heterosexual people have stated that they know another gay person and expected that you would know and/or want to date this person (i.e., heterosexuals assumed a very small gay community). (8) *Not owning up to discomfort:* Heterosexual people have been hypocritical: have not owned up to their discomfort with issues related to homosexuality. They have acted as if they accept homosexuality when it becomes obvious that they do not. (9) *Acting gay:* Heterosexual people have tried to be part of the "ingroup," have tried to act like they are really a part of the gay community when they are around you. (For example, discussing their attraction to or affection for members of the same sex, using gay community terminology). Two additional mistakes that had been added after informally eliciting responses from gay people in the Los Angeles area were also included. These mistakes were (1) *Indicating that they would not have known the respondent is gay:* Heterosexual people express surprise when you diverge from stereotypically "gay" or "lesbian" behavior (in terms of your dress, for example, or your hobbies and interests), or state that they "wouldn't have known" you were gay. (2) *Treating respondent as an LGB representative:* Heterosexual people treat you as a representative or spokesperson for the LGB community, not as just an individual. For each mistake, respondents were asked (a) How often have you experienced this? and (b) How much does this potential mistake anger or annoy you? They responded to question (a) on a five-point scale ranging from 0 (Never) to 4 (Daily). Likewise, they responded to question (b) on a five-point scale ranging from 0 (Not at all) to 4 (Extremely). Additionally, respondents were asked to indicate the extent to which they agreed with the statement "There really are no 'mistakes' if a heterosexual individual is truly well-intentioned."

Then they were asked basic demographic questions (age, gender, and ethnicity) and were asked about their identification with regard to sexual orientation. They were also asked how "out" they are and responded on a five-point scale ranging from 0 (Not at all out) to 4 (Almost completely out). Finally, they were given nine statements based on shared reality theory and the contact hypothesis and asked to indicate their agreement or disagreement with each of the statements.

Measures related to the contact hypothesis. Three dependent variables addressed different aspects of contact. First, respondents' agreement with the item "People would like me less if they knew I was gay/lesbian/bisexual" was assessed. Participants also indicated agreement with the items "My work/school performance would be evaluated more harshly if people knew that I am LGB" and "I have had predominantly positive experiences with heterosexuals who are aware of my sexual orientation." These items were measured using seven-point Likert scales ranging from "strongly disagree" to "strongly agree."

Measures related to shared reality theory. Shared reality items tapped into the degree to which the respondents felt that (1) heterosexuals could tell that they were lesbian or gay from their appearance, (2) LGB people have a responsibility to educate heterosexuals about homosexuality, and (3) they can tell whether heterosexuals are high or low in prejudice toward LGB people when they meet them. Also included was a question about whether their families were supportive of their gay identity.

Results and Discussion

Mean ratings of how often respondents had experienced each mistake, and how much each mistake angered or annoyed respondents are included in Table 2.

EXPERIENCE WITH MISTAKES

A series of hierarchical regression analyses were conducted on each of the nine outcome variables concerning the extent to which respondents experienced the mistakes. Although these analyses do not directly address our theoretical hypotheses, which address LGB people's tolerance for mistakes, they do provide us with correlates of participants' experiences with these mistakes. In all of our analyses, gender, age, and level of "outness" were entered in the first step. We reasoned that these factors could independently contribute to participants'

TABLE 2 Most Common and Most Annoying Mistakes Reported on Close-Ended Questionnaire in Study 2

Most Common Mistakes (M)	Most Annoying Mistakes (M)
Relying on stereotypes (1.87)	Using subtle prejudicial language (2.17)
Ignoring gay issues (1.64)	Not owning up to discomfort (2.15)
Not owning up to discomfort (1.58)	Relying on stereotypes (2.03)
Focusing on the topic of homosexuality (1.54)	Ignoring gay issues (1.82)
Indicating they would not have known respondent is gay (1.52)	Focusing on the topic of homosexuality (1.49)
Pointing out that they are not prejudiced (1.52)	Indicating they would not have known respondent is gay (1.44)
Using subtle prejudicial language (1.34)	Indicating that they know someone else who is gay (1.33)
Treating respondent as an LGB representative (1.33)	Treating respondent as an LGB representative (1.33)
Asking inappropriate, or too many questions (1.24)	Asking inappropriate, or too many questions (1.25)
Indicating that they know someone else who is gay (1.19)	Pointing out that they are not prejudiced (1.22)
Acting gay (0.94)	Acting gay (1.11)

responses to our questions, and that these factors should be partialled out in order to best determine the effects of our theoretical predictions. Next, the six theoretical predictor variables of interest were entered. The results of these analyses are presented in Table 3.

TABLE 3 Significant Predictors of Extent to Which Participants Experienced Mistakes in Study 2

	B	df	t	p
Relying on stereotypes				
STEP 1				
Age	−.32	(4, 56)	−2.46	.017
STEP 2				
I can tell whether a person is high or low in prejudice	.28	(12, 48)	1.99	.052
Ignoring gay issues				
STEP 1				
Outness	−.33	(4, 56)	−2.65	.011
STEP 2				
Family Support	−.48	(12, 48)	−3.65	.001
Not owning up to discomfort				
STEP 2				
Family Support	−.33	(12, 48)	−2.27	.028
Focusing on the topic of homosexuality				
STEP 2				
Family Support	−.50	(12, 48)	−3.60	.001
Gay people should educate heterosexual people	−.36	(12, 48)	−3.00	.004
Stating that they do not disapprove of homosexuality				
STEP 2				
People will like me less if they know I am gay	−.29	(12, 48)	−1.97	.055
I can tell if a person is high or low in prejudice	.29	(12, 48)	2.10	.041
Use subtle prejudicial language				
STEP 2				
Heterosexuals know I am LGB by my appearance	.27	(12, 48)	2.01	.049
Treating respondent as an LGB representative				

	B	df	t	p
STEP 1				
Age	−.31	(4, 56)	−2.65	.001
Outness	−.39	(4, 56)	−3.32	.002
STEP 2				
Heterosexuals know I am LGB by my appearance	.24	(12, 48)	1.97	0.55
	B	df	t	p
Asking inappropriate or too many questions				
STEP 1				
Gender	−.28	(4, 56)	−2.35	.022
Outness	.32	(4, 56)	2.64	.011
STEP 2				
Family support	−.47	(12, 48)	−3.59	.001
Indicating that they know someone else who is gay				
STEP 1				
Age	−.25	(4, 56)	−2.00	.051
Outness	.27	(4, 56)	2.21	.031
No mistakes				
STEP 1				
Age	.27	(5, 54)	2.09	.049
STEP 1				
Age	−.25	(4, 56)	−2.00	.051
Outness	.27	(4, 56)	2.21	.031

Note: Because this is an exploratory study, results with p's of up to .06 are included in the table.

Shared reality predictors. To the extent that respondents had greater support from their families they less frequently experienced four mistakes: *Ignoring gay issues, Not owning up to discomfort, Focusing on the topic of homosexuality,* and *Asking inappropriate or too many questions.* This finding suggests that family members may be the main perpetrators of these mistakes, but that concerned family members can successfully avoid them. Likewise, to the extent that respondents believed they could tell that a person is high or low in prejudice, they less frequently experienced the mistake of well-intentioned heterosexuals' *Relying on Stereotypes,* and well-intentioned heterosexuals *Pointing out that they are not prejudiced.* This suggests that participants who are aware of heterosexuals' prejudice levels may steer clear of people who would make these mistakes. We also demonstrated several effects that we are not certain how to interpret. To the extent that respondents believed people know they are LGB by their appearance, they more frequently experienced the mistakes of well-intentioned heterosexuals (a) *Using subtle prejudicial language* and (b) *Treating the respondent as a representative of the LGB community.* Perhaps they are treated as a representative of the LGB community more because they are perceived to embrace that identity more by being more out. Finally, to the extent that respondents believed that gay people have a responsibility to educate heterosexual people, they less frequently experienced the mistake of well-intentioned heterosexuals *Focusing on the topic of homosexuality.* Perhaps they do not perceive that heterosexual people are focusing on the topic of homosexuality because they consider such behavior acceptable.

Contact hypothesis predictors. One contact hypothesis measure predicted the extent to which people had experienced mistakes: To the extent that respondents thought people would like them less if they knew they were gay, they were less likely to have experienced the mistake of *Heterosexuals pointing out that they are not prejudiced.*

Age also influenced the reports of experience with several mistakes. Older people reported experiencing the following mistakes with less frequency than younger people: *Relying on stereotypes, Treating respondent as an LGB representative, Indicating that they know someone else who is gay.* It is not clear why older people would be less likely to experience these mistakes. However, older people were more likely than younger people to agree with the statement that there are no mistakes if an individual is truly well-intentioned.

Gender predicted the extent to which respondents experienced the mistake of well-intentioned heterosexuals *Asking inappropriate or too many questions.* Women reported experiencing this mistake to a greater extent than men. People may feel more comfortable asking women personal questions. Alternatively, women may have different definitions of our terms "inappropriate questions" or "too many questions" than men do.

Outness also predicted several mistakes. Specifically, people who were more out experience the following mistakes more: *Ignoring gay issues, Asking inappropriate or too many questions,* and *Stating that they know another gay person.* Certainly it seems that people who are out would be likely to encounter any of the listed mistakes with greater frequency.

ANNOYANCE OR ANGER WITH MISTAKES

A more precise way to test the theoretical perspectives of interest to us is to examine participants' reactions to these potential mistakes (i.e., how annoying they found these mistakes to be). Therefore, a second set of regression analyses were conducted, examining the extent to which each of the mistakes angered or annoyed respondents. Because the questions concerning the respondents' level of experience with mistakes and annoyance with the mistake were highly correlated, for this set of analyses, we controlled for the extent to which respondents had experienced the mistakes by including the response to that question in the first step of the equation. Therefore, in this set of analyses demographic variables (gender, age), outness and experiences with the mistake were entered in the first step. The six predictor variables of interest were entered in the second step. The results are presented in Table 4.

Shared reality predictors. Contrary to predictions, people who believed they can tell if a person is high or low in prejudice were *more* annoyed by *Not owning up to gay issues* and *Relying on stereotypes.* Perhaps respondents who have experienced more of some types of

TABLE 4   Significant Predictors of Extent to Which Participants Are Annoyed or Angered by Mistakes in Study 2

	B	df	t	p
Using subtle prejudicial language				
STEP 1				
Experience	.68	(5, 51)	6.61	.000
STEP 2				
People will like me less if they know I am gay	.24	(13, 43)	2.01	0.50
Not owning up to discomfort				
STEP 1				
Experience	−.33	(4, 56)	−2.75	.008
STEP 2				
I can tell if a person is high or low in prejudice	−.28	(13, 47)	−2.19	.035
People will like me less if they know I am gay	−.26	(13, 47)	−1.98	.054
Relying on stereotypes				
STEP 1				
Experience	−.53	(5, 54)	−4.55	.000
STEP 2				
People will like me less if they know I am gay	−.29	(13, 47)	−2.58	.013
I can tell if a person is high or low in prejudice	−.28	(13, 47)	−2.50	.015
Ignoring gay issues				
STEP 1				
Gender	−.35	(5, 54)	−3.22	.002
Age	−.21	(5, 54)	−1.94	.058
Outness	.32	(5, 54)	2.90	.005
Experience	.55	(5, 54)	4.87	.000
Focusing on the topic of homosexuality				
STEP 1				
Experience	.37	(5, 54)	3.03	.004
Indicating they would not have known respondent is gay				
STEP 1				
Experience	.47	(5, 51)	3.97	.000
Indicating that they know someone else who is gay				
STEP 1				
Age	−.28	(5, 53)	−2.86	.006
Experience	.58	(5, 53)	5.77	.000

TABLE 4 (continued)

	B	*df*	*t*	*p*
Asking inappropriate, or too many questions				
STEP 1				
Experience	.59	(5, 53)	4.64	.000
STEP 2				
People will like me less if they know I am gay	.30	(13, 45)	2.37	.022
My work/school performance would be evaluated more harshly	−.27	(13, 45)	−1.98	0.55
Treating respondent as an LGB representative				
STEP 1				
Experience	−.58	(4, 56)	−4.52	.000
STEP 2				
Family Support	−.30	(13, 44)	−2.53	.023
Acting gay				
STEP 1				
Experience	.55	(5, 50)	4.77	.000

Note: Because this is an exploratory study, results with *p*'s of up to .06 are included in the table.

mistakes believe they are better able to discern who is high in prejudice and who is low in prejudice. Consistent with our hypotheses, people who have more supportive families were less bothered by the mistake of *Treating the respondent as an LGB representative.* Perhaps participants with more receptive families are more comfortable in that role because they spend more time helping people who are close to them understand LGB perspectives.

Contact hypothesis predictors. People who believed others will like them less if they know that they are gay were more annoyed by *Using subtle prejudicial language,* and *Asking inappropriate, or too many questions,* but less annoyed by the mistakes of *Not owning up to discomfort,* and *Relying on stereotypes.* Ironically, people who believe that their work or school performance will be evaluated more harshly are less annoyed by *Asking inappropriate or too many questions.* Therefore, our results are inconclusive with regard to the contact hypothesis predictions.

The most consistent predictor of annoyance with mistakes was the extent to which participants had experienced these mistakes. Obviously, the more often people encounter mistakes, the more likely they are to find them bothersome. Also, women found one mistake, *Ignoring gay issues,* more annoying than men did. Younger people were more annoyed than older people by heterosexual people *Ignoring gay issues,* and *Stating that they know another gay person.* Finally, people who are more out found *Ignoring gay issues* more annoying than those who were less out.

General Discussion

In these two studies, we investigated mistakes that well-intentioned heterosexuals may make when attempting to appear non-prejudiced. We approached this issue by asking gay people to describe the mistakes that they had experienced when interacting with well-meaning heterosexuals. We utilized shared reality theory and the contact hypothesis to predict the extent to which participants reported experiencing and being bothered by mistakes.

SHARED REALITY AND THE PREDICTION OF MISTAKES

We have discussed several types of shared reality that may be important in understanding LGB reactions to mistakes made by well-intentioned heterosexuals. Another dimension of shared reality concerns the closeness of the individuals involved. The supportiveness of family members may serve as a buffer for LGB people against some types of mistakes. The family support measure (which indicates both knowledge of and acceptance of LGB and individuals' LGB identity) was predictive of tolerance for at least one mistake.

People who felt that others were aware of their sexual orientation were more bothered by at least one type of mistake. The authors originally thought that people who believed others could identify their sexual orientation were being fairly intentional in their self-presentation. That is, we presumed that those who reported that others can determine their sexual orientation by their appearance were making an explicit effort to identify themselves as LGB to heterosexual people, and would be more tolerant of the mistakes of well-meaning heterosexuals. However, we found that people who believe others are aware of their sexual orientation were less receptive to heterosexuals' mistakes. The fact that these results were opposite of the original prediction suggests an alternative interpretation. Perhaps participants who reported that others were aware of their sexual orientation felt that they had no control over the extent to which others perceived them as LGB. Sexual orientation is usually viewed as a concealable stigma. However, the subjective experience of many LGB people may be that their sexual orientation is inconcealable and readily recognizable by others. This issue is worthy of future study. How does an LGB person's (lack of) ability to pass as heterosexual (if they so desire) influence their reactions to heterosexual people?

This question leads to yet another interpretation of shared reality theory as applied to LGB perceptions of heterosexual people. In some ways, the majority of heterosexual people probably share their attitudes about gay issues with LGB people who are less comfortable with their own sexual orientation. Therefore, LGB people who are less comfortable with their sexual orientation may be more accepting of heterosexuals' mistakes. This interpretation could explain the puzzling results we demonstrated concerning some of the contact hypothesis variables. For example, perhaps those who think others would like them less if they knew they were gay were more accepting of mistakes because they could empathize with other people's discomfort with sexual orientation issues.

The contact hypothesis did not have any clear effects on participants' tolerance for mistakes. Previous positive experiences with heterosexuals did not predict annoyance with any of the mistakes. In some cases, expecting negative reactions from others appeared to more likely to be annoyed by mistakes, in other cases less likely. This finding suggests that the contact hypothesis framework we have employed here is not useful for understanding LGB people's reactions to the mistakes of well-intentioned heterosexuals, perhaps because we did not pinpoint the exact types of contact that our participants had experienced with heterosexual people.

IMPLICATIONS OF THE CURRENT RESEARCH FOR INTERACTIONS BETWEEN LGB AND HETEROSEXUAL PEOPLE

We found that gay people are quite able to describe mistakes encountered by well-intentioned heterosexuals. For example, the two most common mistakes in Study 1 concerned the heterosexual person's tendency to talk about other people that they know who are gay, and their tendency to state that they are not prejudiced. Heterosexual people may not even be aware that this behavior is offensive to some LGB people. Thus, it may be useful to inform heterosexual people that such comments may be offensive to gay and lesbian people through sensitivity training workshops or other educational settings.

Many people feel ill-equipped to deal with the increasingly multicultural focus of our society. Reports have been made that college students feel uncomfortable and anxious in intergroup situations (see Stephan & Stephan, 1987, for a discussion of intergroup anxiety). It is easy to see, based on the responses of the participants in these studies, how heterosexuals may feel that they are "between a rock and a hard place" as they attempt to negotiate pleasant interactions with gay people. For example, either too much or too little attention to the topic of homosexuality can be viewed as a mistake. The right level of attention is not well-defined and is probably difficult for a well-meaning heterosexual to determine. Thus, it may be useful for LGB people to develop an understanding of the trials and tribulations of some well-meaning heterosexuals (see also Conley, Evett, & Devine, 1997).

FUTURE DIRECTIONS AND LIMITATIONS

Many interesting issues remain in the study of LGB individuals' perceptions of the mistakes made by heterosexuals. One important consideration in our sample is the possibility of selection bias. Because of the sensitive (and concealable) nature of LGB identities, it is impossible to determine if the responses of this sample accurately reflect the attitudes of the larger gay and lesbian population. We can conjecture that those who participated in this study probably are more comfortable with their sexual orientation, and more open about their sexual orientation than average, or they would not have agreed to participate in the study.

An important study in this line of research will be to address the mistakes that heterosexuals think they are making when they interact with LGB people. Understanding differences in perceptions of mistakes between these two groups may represent hope for better communication between members of different groups and smoother interactions between heterosexuals and LGB people.

References

Allport, G. W. (1954). *The Nature of Prejudice.* Reading, MA: Addison-Wesley.

Backstrom, C. H., & Hursh-Cesar, G. (1981). *Survey Research.* New York: John Wiley, Inc.

Brewer, M. B., Dull, V., & Lui, L. (1981). Perceptions of the elderly: Stereotypes as prototypes. *Journal of Personality and Social Psychology 41,* 656–670.

Conley, T. D., Devine, P. G., Rabow, J. R., & Evett, S. R. (in press). LGB people's experiences in and expectations for interacting with heterosexuals. *Journal of Homosexuality.*

Conley, T. D., Evett, S. R., & Devine, P. G. (1997). Distinguishing between hostility and discomfort in expectations for interpersonal, intergroup interactions. Presented at the 77th Annual Convention of the Western Psychological Association, Seattle, March.

Devine, P. G., Evett, S. R. & Vasquez-Suson, K. (1996). Exploring the interpersonal dynamics of intergroup contact. In R. Sorrentino & E. T. Higgins (Eds.), *Handbook of Motivation and Cognition: The Interpersonal Context, Vol. 3,* pp. 423–464. New York: The Guilford Press.

Devine, P. G., Monteith, M. J., Zuwerink, J., & Elliot, A. J. (1991). Prejudice with and without compunction. *Journal of Personality and Social Psychology, 60,* 817–830.

Hardin, C. D., & Conley, T. D. (2001). A relational approach to cognition: Shared experience and relationship affirmation in social cognition. In G. B. Moskowitz (Ed.) *Cognitive Social Psychology: The Princeton Symposium on the Legacy and Future of Social Cognition* (pp. 3–17).

Hardin, C. D. & Higgins, E. T. (1996). Shared Reality: How social verification makes the subjective objective. In R. M. Sorrentino and E. T. Higgins (Eds.) *Handbook of Motivation and Cognition: The Interpersonal Context, Vol. 3* (pp. 28–84).

Herek, G. M. (1984). Beyond "homophobia": A social psychological perspective on attitudes toward lesbians and gay men. *Journal of Homosexuality, 10,* 1–21.

Herek, G. M. (1994). Assessing attitudes toward lesbians and gay men: A review of empirical research with the ATGL scale. In B. Greene and G. M. Herek (Eds.) *Lesbian and Gay Psychology: Theory, Research and Clinical Applications* (pp. 206–228). Thousand Oaks, CA: Sage.

Herek, G. M. (1998). *Stigma and Sexual Orientation: Understanding Prejudice Against Lesbians, Gay Men, and Bisexuals.* Sage: Thousand Oaks, CA.

Herek, G. M. & Capitanio, J. P. (1996). "Some of my best friends": Intergroup contact, concealable stigma, and heterosexuals' attitudes toward gay men and lesbians. *Personality and Social Psychology Bulletin, 4,* 412–424.

Herek, G. M. & Glunt, E. K. (1993). Interpersonal contact and heterosexuals' attitudes toward gay men: Results from a national survey. *Journal of Sex Research, 30,* 239–244.

Stephan, W. G. (1987). The contact hypothesis in intergroup relations. In C. Hedrick (Ed.), *Review of Personality and Social Psychology: Vol. 9. Processes and intergroup relations* (pp. 13–40). Newbury Park, CA: Sage.

Stephan, W. G., & Stephan, C. W. (1985). Intergroup anxiety. *Journal of Social Issues, 41,* 157–175.

Fact Sheet: Lesbian, Gay, Bisexual, and Transgendered Youth Issues

14

CHAPTER

SIECUS

During adolescence, young people form their sexual identity. This SIECUS Fact Sheet reviews research on sexual orientation during adolescence and presents the available statistics on lesbian, gay, bisexual, and transgendered (LGBT) students. many of the studies are regional or local. Much of the research focuses on samples of LGBT youth who are disproportionately at risk.

Self-Concept and Identity

- Sexual self-concept is an individuals' evaluation of his or her sexual feelings and actions[1]
- Developing a sexual self-concept is a key developmental task of adolescence[2]
- During adolescence, young people tend to experience their first adult erotic feelings, experiment with sexual behaviors, and develop a strong sense of their own gender identity and sexual orientation[3]
- Gender identification includes understanding that a person is male or female as well as understanding the roles, values, duties, and responsibilities of being a man or a woman[4]

During Adolescence

These statistics are from a report written by the Safe Schools Coalition of Washington State which describes several other studies:[5]

- In Seattle, of 8,406 respondents in the ninth to twelfth grades, 4.5 percent of respondents described themselves as gay, lesbian, and bisexual (GLB). Ninety-one percent describe themselves as heterosexual. Another four percent indicated that they were "not sure" of their orientation.
- In Massachusetts, of 3,982 respondents in the ninth to twelfth grades, two percent of the students described themselves as GLB and three percent reported that they had had same-gender sexual experience.
- In Vermont, of 8,636 respondents in the ninth to twelfth grades, 5.3 percent of young men and 3.4 percent of young women reported having engaged in same-gender "sexual activity."
- In Minnesota, of 36, 254 respondents in the seventh to twelfth grades, 1.1 percent of students described themselves as "bisexual," "mostly homosexual," or "100 percent homosexual." Same-gender sexual attraction and anticipated future same-gender sexual experience was reported by 5.1 percent, and same-gender sexual fantasy was reported by 2.8 percent of respondents.
- Uncertainty about sexual orientation declined with age, from 25.9 percent of 12-year-old students to five percent of 17-year-old students.[6]
- In San Francisco, of 1,914 respondents in the ninth to twelfth grades, 0.2 percent of respondents reported same-gender sexual intercourse.
- Of 13,454 Native-American youth in the seventh to twelfth grades at reservation schools throughout the nation, 1.6 percent of students described themselves as "bisexual," "mostly homosexual," or "100 percent homosexual." Same-gender sexual experience was reported by 1.3 percent of respondents. Same-gender attraction and anticipated future same-gender sexual experience was reported by 4.4 percent and same-gender sexual fantasy by 4.4 percent of respondents.

A national survey of 1,752 college students found that:[7]

- Forty-eight percent of self-identified gay and bisexual college students became aware of their sexual preference in high school, while 26 percent found their true sexuality in college.
- Twenty percent of self-identified gay and bisexual men knew that they were gay or bisexual in junior high school, and 17 percent said they knew in grade school.
- Six percent of self-identified gay or bisexual women knew that they were gay or bisexual in junior high school, and 11 percent knew in grade school.

Sexual Behaviors

A study of 394 self-identified bisexual and homosexual adolescents in the seventh to twelfth grades who participated in the *1986–87 Minnesota Adolescent Health Survey* found that:[8]

- 35.8 percent of younger girls ("younger" was defined as 14 years of age or younger) and 14.3 percent of younger boys reported having had any kind of sexual experience with a male.
- 45.2 percent of younger boys compared to 8.2 percent of younger girls reported sexual experience with a female.
- The majority of younger girls reported fantasizing about males, and the majority of younger boys reported fantasizing about females. However, 27.1 percent of younger girls compared to 18.6 percent of younger boys reported fantasizing about both genders.
- 74.1 percent of older boys ("older" was defined as 17 years of age or older) and 26.9 percent of older girls reported sexual experience with a female.
- For older adolescents, half of the boys and girls reported fantasizing exclusively about the opposite gender, while 41.6 percent of older girls and 36.4 percent of older boys reported fantasizing about both genders.

A study of 3,816 public school students 12 to 19 years of age who participated in the *1987 Minnesota Adolescent Health Survey* found that:[9]

- Bisexual/lesbian respondents (33 percent) were as likely as their heterosexual peers (29 percent) to have ever had penile-vaginal intercourse, while those unsure of their sexual orientation (22 percent) were less likely to have engage in penile-vaginal intercourse
- Of the respondents who had ever had penile-vaginal intercourse, 62 percent of bisexual/lesbian young women said they had first done so before the age of 14, as compared with 45 percent of heterosexual respondents and 46 percent of those unsure of their sexual orientation. However, this difference was no longer statistically significant when controlled for self-reported history of sexual abuse.
- Among sexually experienced respondents, bisexual/lesbian women were significantly more likely to engage daily or several times a week in penile-vaginal intercourse (22 percent) than their heterosexual peers (15 percent) or those unsure of their sexual orientation (17 percent).

A study of ninth to twelfth grade public high school students in the *1995 Massachusetts Youth Risk Behavior Surveillance* found:[10]

- Gay, lesbian, and bisexual orientation was associated with having had sexual intercourse before 13 years of age.
- Gay, lesbian, and bisexual orientation was associated with having sexual intercourse with four or more partners both in a lifetime and in the past three months.
- Gay, lesbian, and bisexual orientation was associated with having experienced sexual contact against one's will.

Contraceptive Use

A study of 3,816 public school students 12 to 19 years of age who participated in the *1987 Minnesota Adolescent Health Survey* found that:[11]

- Among sexually experienced respondents, 44 percent of those unsure of their sexual orientation reported no use of contraception as compared with 30 percent of bisexual/lesbian respondents and 23 percent of heterosexual respondents.
- Of the respondents who used any contraceptive method, 12 percent of bisexual/lesbian respondents, 15 percent of heterosexual respondents, and nine percent of those unsure of their sexual orientation used unreliable methods (such as withdrawal or rhythm).

HIV Risk

- A study of 2,621 gay and bisexual men 15 to 25 years of age in 10 U.S. cities found that more than one fifth (22 percent) of young gay or bisexual men had never tested for HIV and over half had not tested in the six months prior to the study. This study also found that these men were more likely to test if they knew of a place where they felt "comfortable" and if they had exposure to information from a variety of prevention sources such as flyers or workshops.[12]
- A study of 3,492 gay and bisexual men, 15 to 22 years of age in seven U.S. cities found that one in six young men who had sexual intercourse with men had recently had sexual intercourse with women. In addition, nearly one fourth of these men reported recently having had unprotected sexual intercourse with both men and women. The study confirms that young bisexual men are a "bridge" for HIV transmission to women, particularly since 6.6 percent of the bisexual men in the study were HIV positive.[13]

Pregnancy

A study of 3,816 public school students 12 to 19 years of age who participate in the *1987 Minnesota Adolescent Health Survey* found that:[14]

- Bisexual/lesbian respondents reported approximately twice as great a prevalence of pregnancy (12 percent) as either unsure or heterosexual young women (five to six percent).
- Among respondents who had been pregnant, 24 percent of bisexual/lesbian respondents reported multiple pregnancies as opposed to 10 percent of heterosexual respondents and 15 percent of those unsure about their sexual orientation.

Harassment and Safety

A national survey of 496 LGBTQ students under 19 years of age who were affiliated with local youth service organizations found that:[15]

- Two out of five youth (41.7 percent) did not feel safe in their schools because they are LGBTQ.
- 86.7 percent of LGBTQ youth who felt safe in their schools still reported sometimes or frequently hearing homophobic remarks.
- Despite reporting feeling safe, 46 percent of LGBTQ youth reported verbal harassment, 36.4 percent reported sexual harassment, 12.1 percent reported physical harassment, and 6.1 percent reported physical assault in their schools.
- 91.4 percent of LGBTQ youth reported that they sometimes or frequently hear homophobic remarks in their schools (words such as "faggot," "dyke," or "queer").
- 99.4 percent of LGBTQ youth reported hearing homophobic remarks from other students (n = 481).
- Over one third (36.3 percent) of LGBTQ youth reported hearing homophobic remarks from faculty or school staff.
- Over one-third (39.2 percent, n = 184) of LGBTQ youth reported that no one ever intervened when homophobic remarks were heard. Almost half (46.5 percent) reported that someone intervened only some of the time. Other students were more often reported to intervene (82.4 percent) than were faculty (66.5 percent).
- 38.2 percent of youth did not feel comfortable speaking to school staff about LGBTQ issues.
- 47.7 percent of youth from the Midwest, 41.7 percent of youth from the Northeast, 31.6 percent of youth from the South, and 29.4 percent of youth from the West reported being uncomfortable talking to any school staff member about LGBTQ.
- 69 percent of LGBTQ youth reported experiencing some form of harassment or violence.
- 61.1 percent of LGBTQ youth reported experiences of verbal harassment, with 45.9 percent having experienced it daily, 46.5 percent reported experiences of sexual harassment; 27.6 percent reported experiences of physical harassment; and 13.7 percent reported experiences of physical assault.
- 73.7 percent of transgender youth reported hearing homophobic remarks "sometimes" or "frequently."
- 94 percent of white youth, 85.7 percent of African-American/black youth, 80.6 percent of Latino(a) youth, and 93.8 percent of Asian-Pacific Islander youth reported hearing homophobic remarks "sometimes" or "frequently."
- 98.3 percent of youth from the Midwest, 92.3 percent of youth from the South, 89.4 percent of youth from the West, and 86.4 percent of youth from the Northeast reported hearing homophobic remarks "sometimes" or "frequently."

- 40 percent of Latino(a) youth, 29.6 percent of White youth, 18.8 percent of Asian-Pacific Islander youth, and 13.4 percent of African-American/black youth reported being physically harassed at school because of their sexual orientation or gender identity.
- 40.4 percent of youth from the Midwest, 30.2 percent of youth from the West, 21.8 percent of youth from the Northeast, and 17.1 percent of youth from the South reported being physically harassed at school because of their sexual orientation and gender identity.

A study of ninth- to twelfth-grade public high school students in the *1995 Massachusetts Youth Risk Behavior Surveillance* found that:[16]

- Gay, lesbian, and bisexual youth were more than four times as likely to report being threatened with a weapon on school property.
- Gay, lesbian, and bisexual youth were almost five times as likely to report failing to attend school because of their fears about safety.
- Gay, lesbian, and bisexual youth were more likely to carry a weapon in the 30 days prior to the survey.
- Gay, lesbian, and bisexual youth were more likely to have engaged in a physical fight in the 12 months prior to the survey.

A study of 2,816 public school students 12 to 19 years of age who participated in the *1987 Minnesota Adolescent Health Survey* found:[17]

- Bisexual/lesbian respondents were more likely to report physical abuse (19 percent) than heterosexual adolescents (12 percent) and those unsure of their sexual orientation (11 percent).
- Twenty-two percent of bisexual/lesbian respondents reported a past history of sexual abuse versus 15 percent of heterosexual respondents and 13 percent of those unsure of their sexual orientation.

A study in the New York juvenile justice system estimates that anywhere from four to 10 percent of the juvenile delinquent population identify as LGBTQ.[18]

Sexual Abuse

A study of 394 self-identified bisexual and homosexual adolescents in the seventh to twelfth grades who participated in the *1986–87 Minnesota Adolescent Health Survey* found that:[19]

- The proportion of younger respondents (defined as 14 years of age or younger) with a history of sexual abuse was almost four times greater among girls (14.9 percent) than boys (4.1 percent).

- None of the younger boys and 42.1 percent of the younger girls who reported a history of sexual abuse discussed the abuse with someone.
- 30.7 percent of older girls (defined as 15 years of age or older) compared to 16.7 percent of older boys reported a history of sexual abuse.
- 54.5 percent of older boys and 45.8 percent of older girls who reported a history of sexual abuse had never discussed the abuse with anyone.

Suicide

A study of ninth- to twelfth-grade public high school students in the *1995 Massachusetts Youth Risk Behavior Surveillance* found that:[20]

- Gay, lesbian, and bisexual youth were more than three times as likely to have attempted suicide in the past 12 months.

A Massachusetts Department of Public Health study found that:[21]

- Of 4,000 Massachusetts high school students, approximately 40 percent of gay and bisexual students had attempted suicide compared with approximately 10 percent of their heterosexual peers.

Substance Abuse

A study of public high school students in the ninth to twelfth grades in the *1995 Massachusetts Youth Risk Behavior Surveillance* found that:[22]

- Gay, lesbian, and bisexual orientation was associated with an increased lifetime frequency of use of cocaine, crack, anabolic steroids, inhalants, "illegal," and injectable drugs.
- Gay, lesbian, and bisexual youth were more likely to report having used tobacco, marijuana, and cocaine before 13 years of age.

School Personnel

- In a random sample of high school health teachers, one in five surveyed said that students in their classes often used abusive language when describing homosexuals.[23]
- A national study of secondary school counselors' perceptions of adolescent homosexuals found that 25 percent perceived that teachers exhibited significant prejudice toward homosexual students and that 41 percent believed that schools were not doing enough to help gay and lesbian students adjust to their school environments.[24]

- In a random sample of high school health teachers, one third perceived the schools were not doing enough to help homosexual adolescents.[25]
- In a study gay and lesbian adolescents 14 to 21 years of age, 23 percent of females and 25 percent of males reported that they were able to talk with their school counselors about their sexual orientation.[26]

Support for LGBT Youth

A 1988 national survey of heterosexual male youths 15 to 19 years of age found that only 12 percent felt that they could have a gay person as a friend.[27] In a 14-city survey, nearly three-fourths of lesbian and gay youth first disclosed their sexual identity to friends; forty-six percent lost a friend after coming out to her or him.[28] In a study of gay and lesbian adolescents 14 to 21 years of age, fewer than one in five of the surveyed gay and lesbian adolescent students could identify someone who was very supportive of them.[29]

Student Attitudes

A national survey of 2,804 American high school students 16 to 18 years of age with an "A" or "B" grade average found that:[30]

- Nearly 40 percent say that they are prejudiced against homosexuals.
- Nearly four out of five (78 percent) feel homosexuals should be permitted to enlist in the military.
- Three out of four (74 percent) feel gays should be allowed to teach school.
- More than three out of five high-achieving teens (62 percent) believe it is okay to have a gay Girl or Boy Scout Leader.
- Two out of three (68 percent) believe gays should be able to coach youth sports.
- More than half believe gay males and lesbians should be allowed to marry (54 percent) and to join the clergy (54 percent).

Parental Support

A national survey of 1,000 American parents found that:[31]

- Seventy-six percent of parents nationwide would be comfortable talking to their children about issues related to homosexuality or gay and lesbian people.
- Sixty-seven percent of parents nationwide favor teaching children that gay people are just like other people.
- Sixty-two percent of parents nationwide would be comfortable talking to their children's teachers about issues related to homosexuality or gay and lesbian people.

- Sixty-one percent of parents nationwide said that homosexuality is "something I would discuss with my children if they asked me questions, but not something I would raise with them on my own."
- Fifty-six percent of parents nationwide favor allowing groups or clubs on school campuses to promote tolerance and prevent discrimination against gay and lesbian students.
- Fifty-five percent of parents nationwide would be comfortable if their children's teachers were gay or lesbian.
- Fifty-five percent of parents nationwide favor allowing openly gay teachers to teach in middle schools and high schools.
- Fifty-four percent of parents nationwide would be comfortable if their children's friends were gay or lesbian.
- When asked, "What is the youngest age you feel you might need to talk to your children about homosexuality?," the following responses were given:

Under five years of age—two percent
Five to six years of age—eight percent
Seven to eight years of age—eight percent
Eight to nine years of age—11 percent
Nine to 10 years of age—21 percent
11 to 12 years of age—20 percent
13 to 14 years of age—14 percent
15 to 16 years of age—four percent
17 to 18 years of age—one percent
Over 18 years of age—two percent
Do not know—10 percent

Teaching about Homosexuality

- Forty-six percent of a random sample of high school health teachers formally taught about homosexuality. Among those teachers, 48 percent spent less than one class period teaching about homosexuality.[32]
- Thirty-seven percent of high school health teachers reported that they would feel very comfortable teaching about homosexuality, while 20 percent believed that they also would be very competent at teaching the topic.[33]
- Sixty-six percent of high school health teachers identified mass media as the most commonly used source of information regarding homosexuality.[34]
- In a self-reported study, sixty-two percent of health and education professionals stated that they needed to update their knowledge or skills to discuss or teach homosexuality and bisexuality.[35]
- In one study of gay and lesbian adolescents 14 to 21 years of age, half of the students said that homosexuality had been discussed in their classes. Of those, 50 percent of females and 37 percent of males said it was handled negatively.[36]

References

1. *Facing Facts: Sexual Health for America's Adolescents* (New York: SIECUS, 1995), p. 12.
2. Ibid., pp. 10, 12.
3. Ibid., p. 10.
4. Ibid., p. 12.
5. B. Reis and E. Saewyc, *Eighty-three Thousand Youth: Selected Findings of Eight Population-based Studies as They Pertain to Anti-gay Harassment and the Safety and Well-being of Sexual Minority Students* (Seattle, WA: Safe Schools Coalition of Washington, 1999).
6. G. Remafedi, M. Resnick, R. Blum, and L. Harris, "Demography of Sexual Orientation in Adolescents," *Pediatrics,* vol. 89, no. 4 (April 1992), pp. 714–21.
7. L. Elliott and C. Brantley, *Sex on Campus: The Naked Truth About the Real Sex Lives of College Students* (New York: Random House, 1997), pp. 163–4.
8. E. M. Saewyc, L. H. Bearinger, P. A. Heinz, et al. "Gender Differences in Health and Risk Behaviors among Bisexual and Homosexual Adolescents," *Journal of Adolescent Health,* vol. 23, no. 2 (August 1998), pp. 181–8.
9. E. M. Saewyc, L. H. Bearinger, R. W. Blum, and M. D. Resnick, "Sexual Intercourse, Abuse and Pregnancy among Adolescent Women: Does Sexual Orientation Make a Difference?," *Family Planning Perspectives,* vol. 31, no. 3 (May/June 1999), pp. 127–31.
10. R. Garofalo, R. Cameron-Wolf, S. Kessel, et al., "The Association between Health Risk Behaviors and Sexual Orientation among a School-based Sample of Adolescents," *Pediatrics,* vol. 101, no. 5 (May 1998), pp. 895–902.
11. Saewyc, Bearinger, Blum, and Resnick, "Sexual Intercourse, Abuse and Pregnancy among Adolescent Women."
12. *HIV Trends in U.S. Highlight Need for Expanded Prevention* (U.S. Centers for Disease Control and Prevention press briefing at the Thirteenth International AIDS Conference, Durban, South Africa, July 10, 2000).
13. Ibid.
14. Saewyc, Bearinger, Blum, and Resnick, "Sexual Intercourse, Abuse and Pregnancy among Adolescent Women."
15. *1999 National School Climate Survey* (New York: GLSEN, 1999).
16. Garofalo, Cameron-Wolf, Kessel, et al., "The Association between Health Risk Behaviors and Sexual Orientation among a School-based Sample of Adolescents."
17. Saewyc, Bearinger, Blum, and Resnick, "Sexual Intercourse, Abuse and Pregnancy among Adolescent Women."
18. R. Feinstein, A. Greenblatt, L. Hass, et al., *Justice for All? A Report on Lesbian, Gay, Bisexual and Transgendered Youth in the New York Juvenile Justice System* (New York: Lesbian and Gay Project of the Urban Justice Center, 2001), p. 6.
19. Saewyc, Bearinger, Heinz, et al., "Gender Differences in Health and Risk Behaviors among Bisexual and Homosexual Adolescents."
20. Garofalo, Cameron-Wold, Kessel, et al., "The Association between Health Risk Behaviors and Sexual Orientation among a School-based Sample of Adolescents."
21. P. Healy, "Suicides in State Top Homicides," *Boston Globe,* (Feb. 28, 2001).
22. Garofalo, Cameron-Wold, Kessel, et al., "The Association between Health Risk Behaviors and Sexual Orientation among a School-based Sample of Adolescents."
23. S. K. Telljohann, J. H. Price, M. Poureslami and A. Easton, "Teaching about Sexual Orientation by Secondary Health Teachers," *Journal of School Health,* vol. 65, no. 1 (Jan. 1995), pp. 18–22.

24. Telljohann, Price, Poureslami, and Easton, p. 18–22; J. H. Price and S. K. Telljohann, "School Counselor's Perceptions of Adolescent Homosexuals," *Journal of School Health,* vol. 61, no. 10 (Dec. 1991), pp. 433-8.
25. Telljohann, Price, Poureslami, and Easton, p. 18–22.
26. S. K. Telljohann and J. H. Price, "A Qualitative Examination of Adolescent Homosexuals' Life Experiences: Ramifications for Secondary School Personnel," *Journal of Homosexuality,* vol. 26, no. 1 (1993), pp. 41–56.
27. W. Marsiglio, "Attitudes toward Homosexual Activity and Gays as Friends: A National Survey of Heterosexual 15- to 19-Year-Old Males," *Journal of Sex Research,* vol. 30, no. 1 (Feb. 1993), pp. 12–7.
28. C. Ryan and D. Futterman, "Lesbian and Gay Youth: Care and Counseling," *Adolescent Medicine, State of the Art Reviews,* vol. 8, no. 2 (June 1997), p. 221.
29. Telljohann and Price, pp. 41–56.
30. *Y2K Who's Who among American High School Students* (Lake Forest, IL: Educational Communications, Inc., 2000).
31. *Horizons Foundation National Survey of 1000 Parents* (San Francisco: Horizons Foundation, 2001).
32. Telljohann, Price, Poureslami, and Easton, p. 20.
33. Ibid.
34. Ibid.
35. D. L. Kerr, D. D. Allensworth, J. A. Gayle, "The ASHA National HIV Education Needs Assessment of Health and Education Professionals," *Journal of School Health,* vol. 59, no. 7 (Sept. 1989), p. 301–7.
36. Telljohann and Price, pp. 41–56.

Section

Parenting, Relationships, and Sexual Behavior

The Eight Stages of Ending a Relationship

Albert J. Angelo, M.S.Ed

CHAPTER

While many human sexuality texts examine the origins and development of love, courtship, and the building and maintaining of intimate relationships, few provide detailed information about what emotional and psychological changes occur when two people end an emotionally intimate relationship. This omission is significant, for students experiencing an ending of their relationship, often called "a breakup," frequently feel confused, depressed, isolated, and scared, and yet have limited opportunities to learn more about what they are experiencing or how to cope with their loss.

This article covers the stages one experiences when a relationship ends. I write about these stages to expand the opportunities for students to learn more about the dynamics of an ending relationship and to help them comprehend that one need not feel ashamed, confused, or isolated when a breakup occurs. As I have found men and women feel more empowered and optimistic when they understand the predictive and normative stages of an ending relationship, I hope this article is both educationally enriching and emotionally comforting to those working through their pain and loss.

The eight stages one experiences when a relationship ends are:

1. Denial
2. Anger/confusion
3. We can work it out
4. It's over: Now to grieve
5. What went wrong
6. I'm not the same person
7. No going back
8. Peace

In her book: *On Death and Dying,* Dr. Elisabeth Kubler-Ross observed that a dying person goes through five emotional stages when death is near. Her model serves as a useful tool when examining the ending of relationships as both a breakup and a death highlight one's process of coping with loss. The reader will observe that the first three stages in this article parallel Dr. Kubler-Ross' model and that her last stage of "Acceptance" shares similar components to the stage I describe and title: "Peace."

Before describing the eight stages, it is important to note that each individual experiencing an ending of a heterosexual, homosexual, or bisexual relationship will do so uniquely and with varying intensity. Factors such as the emotional significance of the relationship, one's philosophical and spiritual outlook, one's personality, and previous experiences or lack of experience with ending relationships will influence the process. Clearly, while the pattern may look similar, no two people experience a breakup exactly the same way.

The First Stage: DENIAL

The first stage on an ending relationship is "Denial." It is here where one or both partners fail to recognize and/or purposely avoid identifying serious problems within the relationship. While friends and family may see the disharmony, the person in denial remains intentionally unaware. Often, rationalization is employed as a defense against information suggesting the relationship is at risk. This process of overlooking and avoiding one's problems often frustrates others trying to help, but only when a person enters stage two will he/she be able to begin seeing the challenges that lie ahead.

The Second Stage: ANGER/CONFUSION

Feelings of anger and confusion can occur within any of the eight stages. However, in stage two one begins feeling uncharacteristically irritated and angry with his/her partner.

For the person who will end the relationship, everyday behaviors by one's partner, not bothersome in the past, like being late for dinner, or leaving dirty clothes on the floor, now provoke feelings of intense irritation and annoyance. While in this stage, this person may not understand why he/she feels these emotions and may fail to identify these reactions as a symptom of a relationship in trouble.

The person being left also goes through this stage. Feeling confused, frustrated, frightened, and powerless, a person may lash out at his/her partner. Reactions such as "Why are you so moody!" or "What's wrong with you!" can occur. Despite the anger, confusion, and frustration, or whether one will leave or be left, a person still believes his/her relationship has not yet ended.

The Third Stage: WE CAN WORK IT OUT

In this stage one or both partners realize the relationship is in serious risk of ending. Acknowledging the risk, one or both partners try to repair it back to health. Sometimes this works and sometimes it doesn't.

When both partners are in this stage, the relationship has a chance for survival. However, if only one partner is in this stage, the chances for avoiding a breakup are diminished. For example, the partner in denial may not understand the need to "fix" the relationship and the partner in the anger/confusion stage may think the problem lies within the other and not within him/herself. As a personal example, while in this stage, I recommended to my partner that we enter couples counseling. He, not being in this stage, refused my offer feeling "my" problems were not stemming from the relationship and felt no need to get involved. Predictably, when my partner entered this third stage he requested we attend therapy. His suggestion, unfortunately, came too late.

As I offer in my lectures, it does not take two people to have a relationship. It only takes one BELIEVING a relationship exists. As an example, think of one's faith in a higher power. A person can believe a spiritual relationship exists despite the lack of any physical contact or communication. Faith alone creates the relationship. This point is extremely important, for one's relationship with another never ends until the person chooses to truly believe and acknowledge that it is over. Without this acknowledgement, a person can convince him/herself the relationship lives on. This point brings to mind the fictitious story of a woman who for years every night sets a place at the dinner table for her husband lost at sea hoping he will one day return. As long as she maintains this hope, the relationship, for her, continues; the husband isn't dead, he'll be home soon and dinner will be waiting. Sadly, it also means she and others dwelling too long in this stage forfeit opportunities to be in other loving relationships. While it can feel emotionally comforting to stay in this stage hoping a lost relationship will be resurrected, it is best to know when to stay and work on difficulties and when to let go and move on.

OBSESSION

While in the "We can work it out" stage, the person being left can become completely obsessed with trying to win back his/her partner. Repeatedly telephoning, e-mailing, or visiting a partner and pleading or begging for the person to "come back" can all occur during this stage. Dr. Helen Fisher describes these obsessive behaviors in her book *Why We Love: The Nature and Chemistry of Romantic Love.* She states:

> As a person begins to realize a beloved is thinking of ending the relationship, they generally become intensely restless. Overcome by longing and nostalgia, they devote almost all of their energy, and their attention to their departing mate. Their obsession: Reunion with their lover, pp. 160–161.

Fisher states a person feeling obsessed may become so focused on their missing partner that everyday activities become reminders of one's lost love. My students have described how restaurants, neighborhoods, books, movies, and various scents and smells have acted as reminders. For me, music acted as an especially strong reminder. Love songs seemed to speak directly to my feelings of pain and loss and to my hope my relationship would somehow survive.

BARGAINING

Dr. Elizabeth Kubler-Ross describes in her book *On Death and Dying* how terminally ill patients will often "bargain" with a higher power to stay alive for a specific period of time. For example, a person with stomach cancer may pray to God to stay alive for three more months to see a daughter finish college or son get married. The process of bargaining helps patients feel they have some control in postponing their inevitable passing.

When relationships end, the process of bargaining can also occur. When attempts to work on a relationship fail, the person who doesn't want the relationship to end may seek some type of agreement, or bargain, with his/her partner. A man who asks his wife to wait and file for divorce until after their children finish high school is bargaining; he understands the relationship could end, but is hoping to delay it for a year or two. A woman who asks her partner to stay in the relationship until both are finished graduate school is also bargaining. Unfortunately, as stated, bargaining does not fix or repair the relationship; it only delays the breakup and prevents one or both partners from progressing forward.

The Fourth Stage: IT'S OVER: NOW TO GRIEVE

Once all hope of saving the relationship has disappeared and once a person acknowledges to him/herself that the relationship is over, grieving begins. Grieving is a natural and healthy process and, in my opinion, should not be avoided. It is only by working through one's grief and acknowledging one's loss that the healing process begins. This stage, though difficult, should not be rushed. In conjunction with a healthy support system such as family, friends, and/or counseling, I recommend a person take the time needed to fully grieve the relationship's passing.

The Fifth Stage: WHAT WENT WRONG

In the third stage, a person believes his/her relationship has a chance for survival and will explore ways and methods to try and keep it alive. However, when those efforts fail and the relationship does end, it is in this fifth stage and often parallel to the grieving process that one examines why the relationship couldn't last. In this analysis, one may discover that aspects of a partner's personality, lifestyle, and/or goals and ambitions were incongruent with one's own. This examination is healthy and I believe necessary for it allows one to realize that relationships often end not because a partner is bad or malicious, but because two people simply no longer find themselves in a compatible, workable situation. It also gives a person the "mental permission" to let go of the guilt for not being able to fix the relationship.

When one works through the stages of an ending relationship, two interesting reactions can occur. I term them "Regrets" and "Pleasant Surprise."

REGRETS

Within the dynamics of an ending relationship the person who initiates the breakup must live with his/her decision and actions. When this person examines why the relationship ended and begins longing for the good qualities found in his/her ex-partner, feelings of regret may develop. If a man always enjoyed the holidays with his partner and it's now Thanksgiving, he may feel a level of regret for breaking up with his partner. Feelings of regret are normal because when a relationship ends one must say goodbye to both the bad and good qualities of his/her partner.

PLEASANT SURPRISE

The person who was left and did not want the relationship to end, may have primarily concentrated on what was lost. Now, however, this person looks at what was gained from the separation. Positive feelings may develop as one realizes that the ending of the relationship equals no longer dealing with a partner's negative qualities. If a woman had a partner who liked taking vacations at the beach and she hates the beach, she may feel a sense of freedom and joy for no longer having to plan Summer vacations around sand and sea. She now has the "pleasant surprise" of realizing the freedom to travel (or not to travel) wherever she wants, whenever she wants.

The Sixth Stage: I'M NOT THE SAME PERSON

When a relationship ends, life changes. Daily routines change, interactions with others change, one's residence may change, and one's goals and outlook may change. In the sixth stage one examines as a single person how his/her life is now different or will be different. Where going camping was part of being a couple, one may now decide he/she hates camping. After being in the suburbs for twenty years, an individual may find city life more enjoyable. While it may feel scary and unsettling, this process of self-examination is important and necessary for it allows a person to understand, rediscover, and appreciate his/her individual qualities, talents, and interests. This introspection also helps one identify more clearly those attributes desired and not desired in a future partner. The process of change is often scary, but it is important to remember that only through change is one able to grow and flourish.

The Seventh Stage: NO GOING BACK

In the seventh stage, a person comprehends and accepts not only that the relationship ended but why it needed to end. This understanding can occur through the self-examination process as stated in stage six. It can also occur when one gains more insight into his/her ex-partner's personality, interests, and behavior. One student commented to me that she had a hard time "getting over" her ex-partner until she learned more about him. With additional knowledge she understood why their relationship didn't work and why it wouldn't work in the future. In this stage, any lingering questions about why the relationship ended are finally extinguished.

After progressing through the seven stages one is now ready to make peace with the ending of the relationship.

The Eighth Stage: PEACE

After working through all the previous stages, the final result is peace. I use the term "peace" because at this stage thoughts toward and/or actions from the ex-partner do not provoke strong emotional responses and one's desire to return to the relationship has vanished. Discovering an ex-partner is dating again or has fallen in love causes no anger, resentment, or hurt. In fact, there may be hope this person is happy and doing well.

This last stage does not mean all feelings toward another are gone. One can still love and care about an ex-partner. It simply means the strong emotional longing has dissipated allowing one to feel at peace with the memories and history of the past relationship. For those currently working through these stages, my wish is for you to one day find this peace in your lives so you can begin to love again, as you surely will!

References

Fisher, Helen E. (2004) *Why We Love: The Nature and Chemistry of Romantic Love.* (pp. 160–161) Henry Holt & Company.
Kubler-Ross, Elisabeth (1969) *On Death and Dying.* Simon & Schuster, Inc.

Sperm Donors Meet Their Families

Linda Villarosa

Identification of Anonymous Fathers Is More Common Now

In the early 1980s, Bob, who was a student at the time, decided to donate sperm to a sperm bank. He needed the money, but he also thought it would be nice to help a couple who wanted a child but could not conceive. He signed a waiver and was promised anonymity. He assumed that was that.

But this year, the sperm bank contacted Bob, who asked that his last name and hometown be withheld, and told him that he had a daughter who wanted to meet him. "I was bowled over, and even suspicious at first," Bob said.

But after the teenager and her mother sent letters and photographs, they decided to meet. The girl and her parents spent a weekend with Bob and his wife and young son in March, and they have exchanged phone calls and e-mail messages since.

"Seeing her was very emotional," Bob said. "The profile, the mannerisms, everything was so much like me that it was scary. We had a good time together, and I was relieved that everything went so well."

Though Bob says that there is the possibility that he has more children, this experience was so overwhelming that he is not sure that he will do it again. "If the bank comes to me and asks me to do this again, I'll probably say just release medical information but nothing other than that," he said.

Bob's experience is unusual but it is becoming more common. Though most of the 150 sperm banks in the United States offer only anonymous donors, increasing numbers are coming up with ways, sometimes highly creative, to assure that children born with donated sperm can meet the men who fathered them. Other sperm banks are considering the option.

About a dozen sperm banks offer what is called donor identification release. In these cases, when the man donates sperm, he agrees that when his offspring turn 18, they can call or write the sperm bank and get contact information. The Sperm Bank of California in Berkeley was the first to offer this option, in 1983.

The first child turned 18 in January, and she has been given the name of her donor, though she has not called him yet. This year, a total of 16 offspring from that bank will turn 18, and next year another 29 will. Several other sperm banks across the country now offer similar programs.

Sweden, Austria and the State of Victoria in Australia have mandatory donor identification release. In Canada, a bill was introduced in Parliament on May 9 calling for a mandatory sperm donor registry. It also provides for the voluntary release of donors' identities.

The increasing openness follows a similar trend in adoption. In sperm donation, it has also accelerated as more single women and lesbian couples have chosen to have children.

In the past, the consumers were overwhelmingly couples having trouble conceiving, generally because the husband was infertile or had a genetic disease. The couple would choose an anonymous sperm donor who, based on sketchy information, had physical traits similar to the husband. After the child was born, they often told no one, including the children, and the medical records were sometimes destroyed.

But now, though heterosexual couples remain the primary clients of sperm banks, improvements in assisted reproductive technology have meant they are finding ways to conceive their own biological children without the use of donor sperm.

Since being introduced in 1992, intracytoplasmic sperm injection, in which a single sperm is injected into a mature egg, has sharply increased fertility among couples with male infertility. According to the American Society for Reproductive Medicine, in 1995 the injection method resulted in 1,659 clinical pregnancies and 1,350 births. In 1998, the last year with full statistics, the numbers had jumped to 9,361 pregnancies and 7,712 births.

At that same time, growing numbers of single women and lesbian couples are choosing to conceive using donor sperm. Though no statistics can confirm it, interviews with experts in reproductive medicine and representatives of sperm banks say that lesbians and single women make up an increasing proportion of parents of the 30,000 donor offspring born each year.

"Early on, families were counseled never to disclose the fact that they had used donor insemination," said Sue Rubin, co-founder of the Ethics Practice, a service in Berkeley that provides education and consultation. She is also the chairwoman of the identity release task force at the Sperm Bank of California. "These were primarily straight couples, and the goal was to preserve the presumption of the father's identity in the family. But as more lesbians and single women became clients, the initial reason for secrecy wasn't applicable."

Francey and Laurel Liefert, a lesbian couple in Berkeley, chose an open identity donor in deciding to have children 16 years ago. In three years, when their oldest son, Marcus, turns 18, he will be able to call the agency and get information about the donor, including an address and telephone number.

"We chose a donor who was willing to be known to his offspring, because we have several friends who were adopted, and they felt frustrated by not knowing who their biological parents were," said Francey Liefert, a teacher for the visually impaired. "We didn't want our sons to have this mystery in their lives that was a mystery forever."

Some experts, though, are increasingly worried about the lack of regulations, or research, in this area. The Food and Drug Administration, which has a voluntary registry of tissue banks, will begin to regulate all banks for health and safety early next year, but has no proposed rules about contact between donors and offspring.

"Because there are no hard and fast rules about whether you should know a donor or not know a donor, it is all being played out very loosely," said Anthony Thomas, head of the male infertility section at the Cleveland Clinic Foundation and a member of the reproductive society's ethics committee. "My concern is that we don't know how all of this is going to affect the offspring. This needs to be regulated."

The Ambiguity of "Having Sex": The Subjective Experience of Virginity Loss in the United States

17

CHAPTER

Laura M. Carpenter

What do we mean when we talk about sex? At the turn of the twenty-first century in the United States, there exists no single answer to this question. Different individuals and social groups attach diverse meanings to sexual activity, variously understanding sex as an expression of intimacy, a route to physical pleasure, or a sacred part of marriage. People even disagree about which sexual acts constitute "real" sex, as became apparent during the 1998 independent council investigation of President Clinton, in which classifying certain sexual activities as sex or as foreplay was a major point of contention. In short, the meaning of the term *sex* is ambiguous in the contemporary U.S. Because sexuality comprises a central part of personal identity, what sex means matters profoundly to the women and men who must negotiate their sexual lives in an atmosphere of diverse beliefs. It is also consequential for researchers who study sexual attitudes and conduct, and for policy makers who seek to address sexuality-related issues.

The experience of virginity loss offers one vantage point from which to explore the ambiguity surrounding sex and the consequences of that ambiguity for personal identity. Societal concerns about sexuality often crystallize around virginity loss, both because it is widely perceived as one of the most significant turning points in sexual life and because of the emphasis public health and policy professionals place on first coitus and sexual initiation. In this paper, I concentrate on two subjective aspects of virginity loss. First, to what sexual experiences do women and men refer when they talk about virginity loss or the first time they had sex? Which events do they posit as producing the transition from virgin to nonvirgin identity and who do they see as eligible to make that transition? Second, how do people interpret virginity loss? How do the meanings that individuals attach to virgin and nonvirgin identity shape their expectations and choices about the transition between those identities?

In answering these questions, I address several shortcomings of the literature on early sexual experiences. First, relatively little research has explored the subjective meanings of virginity loss (di Mauro, 1995). Although first experiences with vaginal intercourse—which researchers often identify as "virginity loss"—have been staples of research on sexual behavior since the 1960s, the preponderance of literature on early sexuality has focused on its public health dimensions (Ericksen, 1999; Sprecher, Barbee, & Schwartz, 1995). Second, most studies of virginity loss have focused primarily or exclusively on the experiences of young women and on people who identify themselves as heterosexual, despite a growing body of empirical and anecdotal evidence that beliefs and behavior vary meaningfully across and within gender and sexual orientation (this evidence includes Elder, 1996; Hart, 1995; Holland, Ramazanoglu, & Thomson, 1996; Rubin, 1990; Thompson, 1995; Tolman, 1994). Third, many of the studies that are sensitive to meaning rely on data gathered more than a decade ago, before the advent of HIV/AIDS as a public problem and the full impact of the New Right backlash against liberal sexual ideology (e.g., Brumberg, 1997; Rubin, 1990; Thompson, 1995).

Theoretical Background

My analysis relies on an understanding of sexuality as profoundly shaped by social factors or *socially constructed* (Gagnon & Simon, 1973; Laws & Schwartz, 1977; Stein, 1989; Vance, 1991). Different cultural groups, both within and across societies, interpret different activities as sexual and imbue different sexual practices with specific meanings. At the same time, individuals actively interpret and reinterpret their sexual experiences over their lifetimes, thereby creating their identities as sexual beings. The patterned ways in which cultures and individuals approach sexuality can be understood as *interpretive frames,* schemas that enable people to "locate, perceive, identify, and label" occurrences within their life and the social world at large (Goffman, 1974, p. 21).

Diverse ways of framing specific aspects of sexuality, such as virginity loss, may be available in a given society at a single time. The frames that are available serve as part of the cultural "toolkit" with which individuals construct their sexual identities (Swidler, 1986). In the contemporary West, sexuality constitutes a central feature of identity; individuals are to a great degree defined by themselves and others, both socially and morally, in terms of their sexuality (Foucault, 1978; Giddens, 1992; Plummer, 1995; Weeks, 1985). Early sexual experiences, perhaps especially virginity loss, appear to be crucial steps through which individuals develop a sense of their identities as sexual beings (Gagnon & Simon, 1973; Holland et al., 1996).

In modern social life, identity (or self) comprises an ongoing project on which people expend considerable creative effort (Giddens, 1992). Sociologists typically theorize identity as a bridge linking the individual and society. One can usefully distinguish between *social identity*, the identities people attribute or impute to others, and *personal identity*, the meanings people attribute to their own selves (Snow & Anderson, 1987).[1] Social and personal identity are not necessarily congruent. For instance, a young woman may be perceived by her friends as a virgin (social identity) while knowing herself to be a nonvirgin (personal identity). Identity comprises multiple dimensions, of which sexual identity (incorporating virginity status) is only one. Various dimensions of identity are intertwined in ways that depend in part on individuals' interpretations of those dimensions. For example, people who interpret virginity as a stigma might associate virgin identity with "loser" or "geek" identity, whereas people who frame virginity as a valuable gift might link virgin identity with traditional feminine identity.

Different interpretive frames imply different evaluations of virgin and nonvirgin identity. A person may embrace or distance himself from a particular social or personal identity, depending on his and others' interpretations of it. Should he desire a different identity than the one he has, he may work to obtain a new one, either in fact (as when a virgin seeks to lose his virginity) or in appearance (as when a virgin portrays himself as a nonvirgin). Not static, identity changes over the life course, as when people adopt new social roles or statuses. Transitions from one identity to another comprise rites of passage or status passages; virginity loss, entailing the transition from virgin to nonvirgin identity, constitutes just such a passage (Glaser & Strauss, 1971; Turner, 1969; van Gennep, 1908). Although the literature on status passages typically assumes congruence between social and personal identity, transitions can presumably occur independently at either level.) Undergoing a rite of passage involves relinquishing one identity in order to replace it with another. Therefore, how people approach a status passage and how they conduct themselves afterwards depend in part on their beliefs about both the initial and new identities (as well as on the beliefs of those around them).

Definitions and interpretations of virginity loss serve as tools for constructing sexual identity at both the social and personal levels. The ways people define virginity loss determine the point at which they see themselves—and others—as moving from virgin to nonvirgin identity as well as whom they deem eligible to make that transition. Not least because they imply evaluations of the desirability of virgin and nonvirgin identity, interpretations of virginity loss influence individuals' conduct, including their decisions about when to lose virginity (i.e., when to adopt a new personal and/or social identity) and how to present themselves to others (i.e., what social identity to claim possibly distinct from

---

[1]Snow and Anderson (1987) identify a third dimension of identity, *self-concept*, which refers to a person's overarching view of herself or himself as a social, moral, and physical being and serves as a "working compromise" between social and personal identity (p. 1348).

personal identity). As we will see the ambiguity of virginity loss affords people some, if limited, discretion in constructing their sexual identities.

Changing Meanings and Definitions of Virginity Loss

Although the loss of virginity has been almost universally recognized as an important rite of passage, comprising part of the transition from childhood to adulthood, belief about the meaning of and criteria for making the transition from virginity to nonvirginity have varied considerably (Muuss, 1970; Schlegel, 1995). Within the U.S., notion about the meaning of virginity loss—rooted in a Christian tradition venerating virginity (Aries, 1985)—have changed significantly over time. In the mid- to late-nineteenth century U.S., virginity implied purity and innocence from sexual experience and desire, and was seen as a natural and necessary state for unmarried women (Nathanson, 1991; Welter, 1983). Virginity loss was framed as an irrevocable loss of innocence and, if it took place outside of marriage, as the onset of moral corruption, madness, and even death. After about 1900, new ways of framing virginity loss became ascendant, accompanied by changes in sexual conduct. At the beginning of the century, young men typically saw their own virginity as a neutral or negative attribute, whereas young women perceived theirs as a thing of value. Yet, in contrast with previous eras, the belief that virginity was valuable for women did not preclude a growing proportion of young women and men from framing virginity loss as appropriate within the context of serious premarital relationships. From about 1920 on, young people increasingly opted to lose their virginity before marriage, typically with the person they planned to marry (Brumberg, 1997; D'Emilio & Freedman, 1988; Modell, 1983; Rubin, 1990).

This pattern prevailed until the mid 1960s, when young people, especially young women, more and more came to approve of and engage in premarital sexual intercourse with partners whom they did not expect to marry (Hofferth, Kahn, & Baldwin, 1987; Jessor & Jessor, 1975; Reiss, 1960; Zelnik & Shah, 1983). Although men's virginity continued to be framed as neutral or stigmatizing, for women a new frame emerged in which virginity was neither desirable nor undesirable (Rubin, 1990). By the 1980s, some young women even adopted frames more typical of men, perceiving virginity as an embarrassment or unwanted constraint (Brumberg, 1997; Rubin, 1990; Thompson, 1995), a stance which may have grown more prevalent during the 1990s (Sprecher & Regan, 1996). Over this period, gender differences in the prevalence and timing of first coitus narrowed considerably, largely due to changes in women's conduct (King, Balswick, & Robinson, 1977; Sherwin & Corbett, 1985; though see Ehrenreich, Hess, & Jacobs, 1986).

These broad changes did not, however, entirely displace traditional notions positing virginity as a virtue in women but as a negative trait in men (Ferrell, Tolone, & Walsh, 1977; Moffatt, 1987; Sprecher & Regan, 1996; Thompson, 1990). Beginning in the mid 1980s, frames casting virginity as valuable gained renewed popularity in certain segments of society. For instance, members of the New Right promoted a new frame advocating premarital virginity for both men and women; some proponents even claimed that virginity could be regained, provided sufficient repentance and commitment to future chastity (Dobie, 1995; Ingrassia, 1994). Indeed, one study found that, between 1990 and 1995, an increasing proportion of young men expressed pride and happiness about remaining virgins (Sprecher & Regan, 1996). As a consequence of these many changes, diverse ways of framing virginity loss—and sex in general—coexist in the present-day U.S. (D'Emilio & Freedman, 1988; Seidman, 1991).

Concern with specifying exactly which sexual acts could result in virginity loss appears to be a recent phenomenon, part of a general tendency, beginning in the late nineteenth century and accelerating over the course of the twentieth, to approach human sexuality as a medical, rather than a moral, matter. Public health experts' focus on "risk behaviors" is one prominent recent expression of the medicalization of sexuality (Nathanson, 1991; Tiefer, 1995; Weeks, 1985). Before the twentieth century, virginity loss was probably understood as resulting from vaginal intercourse, but not from partnered sexual activities such as manual stimulation (van de Walle & Muhsam, 1995). Yet, the primary conceptualization of virginity loss was in moral terms—as an irreversible transition from innocence (and virtue) to experience (and corruption)—rather than in terms of the performance of specific physical acts (Nathanson, 1991). Popular literature in the highly sexually-restrictive late nineteenth century included more than one cautionary tale in which young women lost their virtue without engaging in a genital sexual act (Welter, 1983). Attempts to establish physical criteria for virginity loss could be seen as early as the 1830s, with the "invention" of petting—noncoital sexual contact intended not to compromise premarital virginity (Rothman, 1983). But it was not until the 1920s that popular understandings of virginity loss came to center on delineating the sexual activities in which virgins could engage without losing virginity. From then on, the practice of engaging in noncoital genital sexual activity with the express intent of retaining virginity became increasingly widespread. Scholars have referred to this phenomenon as *technical virginity* (Newcomer & Udry, 1985). Technical virgins almost invariably equate virginity loss with first coitus, although, as Rubin (1990) notes, the content of "everything but" coitus has changed over time, most notably to include oral sex. In every era, virginity loss appears to have been understood as possible only between a woman and a man.

In contemporary popular and academic literature, the term *virginity loss* denotes first coitus. As one advice manual for teen women explains, "Unless his penis penetrates your vagina, you're a virgin" (Solin, 1996, p. 85). Similarly, social scientists often use the terms *nonvirgin* and *virgin* as shorthand to describe people who have and have not experienced vaginal intercourse (e.g., Jessor & Jessor, 1975; Schuster, Bell, & Kanouse, 1996). Few modern scholars appear to have consciously considered the possibility that virginity loss could refer to an experience other than first coitus. Yet, despite this apparent consensus, the definition of virginity remains somewhat ambiguous. In the one study (to my knowledge) to investigate explicitly how young people define virginity loss, only four-fifths of respondents agreed that a woman would lose her virginity "if her vagina [was] fully penetrated by a penis" (Berger & Wenger, 1973, p. 669). Furthermore, anecdotal evidence suggests that young lesbians and gay men have recently begun to reframe virginity loss as including sex between same-sex partners (Elder, 1996; Hart, 1995), rather than deeming virginity loss as irrelevant to their own experiences as was common in the past (Raymond, 1994).

Definitions of sex are similarly ambiguous. On the one hand, when (heterosexual) women and men in the U.S. and Britain use the term sex, they almost always refer to vaginal-penile intercourse (Holland et al., 1996; Wight, 1994). However, Sanders and Reinisch (1999) found that many (41%) college students thought of oral-genital contact as sex and even more (81%) considered anal-genital contact sex. In light of the definitional ambiguity surrounding both sex and virginity loss, the common formula defining virginity loss as occurring the first time a person has sex appears deceptively straightforward.

Data and Research Methods

This study relies on data from in-depth case studies of 61 women and men, the majority of whom lived in the greater Philadelphia metropolitan region. Of the 33 women, 22 (67%) self-identified as heterosexual, 7 (21%) as lesbians, and 4 (12%) as bisexual. Of the 28 men, 17 (61%) described themselves as heterosexual, 9 (32%) as gay, and 2 (7%) as bisexual. Respondents came from diverse backgrounds. Almost 80% were White, 10% were African-American, 7% were Latino, and 5% were Asian-American. Two-thirds were from middle-class backgrounds, as measured by parental education and occupation, and the remaining one third were from working-class backgrounds. Fifty-five percent of respondents were both White and from middle-class backgrounds. One third (21) were raised mainline Protestant, one fourth (16) Roman Catholic, one-sixth (10) evangelical Protestant, one-eighth (8) Jewish, and one-tenth (6) nonreligious. Fifty-six of the 61 described themselves as nonvirgins at the time of the interview. Of these 56, 88% reported losing their virginity during adolescence (at age 16.4 on average).

Respondents ranged in age from 18 to 35, with an average age of about 25. Age distributions differed little by gender or by sexual orientation. My goal of situating virginity loss in the broader context of earlier and later sexual experiences prompted my decision to interview young adults (over age 17) rather than adolescents. Although I did not limit the sample to nonvirgins, in selecting respondents 18 or older, I could be assured that the vast majority would have become sexually active prior to the interview (Laumann et al., 1994). Interviewing young adults also facilitated comparison across sexual orientation. Because people who identify themselves as lesbian, gay, or bisexual seldom do so, especially publicly, before their late teens (Raymond, 1994), locating nonheterosexual adolescents to interview would have proved difficult. The upper limit of the age range, 35, was set to include people who became sexually active before as well as after HIV/AIDS became a prominent public health issue, but to exclude those who became teenagers before the so-called Sexual Revolution was well established (in the early 1970s).

To locate study participants, I used the purposive snowball sampling method. Initial respondents were recommended by professional contacts and special-interest organizations; I then asked every person I interviewed to introduce me to others who might agree to take part in the study. Snowball sampling offered several advantages crucial to achieving my research aims. Recruiting study participants through their own social networks may have helped overcome reluctance to participate in research on a topic typically perceived as very private (Sterk-Elifson, 1994; Thompson, 1995). (Although large-scale sexuality surveys have successfully employed random samples—e.g., Laumann, Gagnon, Michael & Michaels, 1994—such methods may not be appropriate for gathering in-depth subjective accounts of sexual experiences.) Snowball sampling moreover enabled me to identify gay and bisexual women and men, who are not numerically common, readily "visible," or evenly distributed throughout the U.S. population (Biernacki & Waldorf, 1981).

Drawbacks of snowball samples include their nonrandom, nonrepresentative nature, which prevents the researcher from directly generalizing findings to a broader population. Additionally, because social networks tend to be relatively homogeneous, the members of each snowball are likely to hold similar beliefs.[2] To counter this potential source of bias and to increase sample diversity, I started several snowballs in each of the four main gender-sexual orientation categories and limited each snowball to five members.[3] The typically small size of snowball samples also hinders the ability to generalize. Yet, a small, nonrandom sample may be sufficient for researchers who are concerned primarily with discovering the range of ideas or behaviors available in a given culture, rather than their prevalence in a population. Indeed, one of the most striking aspects of the 61 interviews I conducted is the frequency with which different respondents raised the same general themes. Glaser and Strauss (1967) refer to this phenomenon as saturation. Given the focus of my research, then, the advantages of the snowball sampling method outweighed the drawbacks.

INTERVIEW METHODS

To gather data for this project, I relied on in-depth, semi-structured interviews. Most questions were open ended so that participants could speak freely and at length about

---

[2]Focusing on an event that typically preceded the interview by several years may help mitigate this type of selection bias. While adult friends probably hold similar views on sexuality, shared beliefs about virginity per se may be less salient in adult than teen friendships (on teen peers, see Billy & Udry, 1985; Kinsman, Romer, Furstenberg, & Schwartz, 1998; Thompson, 1990). None of the clusters of friends I interviewed included people who had known one another at the time of their own virginity loss.

[3]People who are willing to participate in sexuality research may be unusually comfortable talking about sexuality or may perceive their own conduct and attitudes as consonant with social norms. Nonetheless, my sample included several very conservative and several radical respondents. Regrettably, I have no way to ascertain how many people were not included among potential participants because acquaintances declined to recommend them.

what they perceived as the salient aspects of virginity loss, thereby enabling me to collect a wealth of detailed data on subjective interpretations and experiences. Yet every interview asked about the same categories of information—the definition and meaning of virginity loss, learning about virginity loss, personal sexual history, and virginity-related social interactions—facilitating comparisons among respondents. In-depth interviews provide respondents with the opportunity, often lacking in traditional social science surveys, to explain experiences that defy simple categorization. They also enhance participants' ability to ascertain the trustworthiness of the interviewer, and thus may promote more extensive, detailed, or truthful accounts. Conversely, closed-ended questions presume a priori knowledge of the possible range of understandings that people bring to phenomena like virginity loss. Exploratory studies such as mine provide a necessary foundation for surveys seeking to illuminate the subjective aspects of virginity loss.

Interviews lasted from 1 to 3 hours and took place at a location chosen by the respondent (typically the respondent's home or office, or my office). Participants were informed that their identities would remain confidential and anonymous and that they could stop the interview at any time; they were not compensated for taking part in the study. The Human Subjects Committee of the Institutional Review Board of the University of Pennsylvania approved the study design, interview protocol, and consent form.

I conducted every interview in person between April 1997 and October 1998. This period overlapped with the independent council investigation of the relationship between President Bill Clinton and Monica Lewinsky, which arguably prompted a national consciousness raising about the definitional ambiguity of sex. Twenty-five interviews took place in or after late January 1998, when allegations that Lewinsky had performed fellatio on Clinton were first widely publicized. Five of these 25 respondents mentioned the Clinton-Lewinsky controversy during our interviews; 6 of the 25 self-identified as heterosexual. People seldom question the commonsense equation of sex with vaginal-penile intercourse, unless they have personally experienced (and recognized) desire for same-sex partners. (The seeming "naturalness" of heterosexuality is a key component of the phenomenon Rick, 1980, named *compulsory heterosexuality*.) Therefore, although I expected that gay and bisexual respondents would have interrogated the sex-coitus equation during the process of coming out (and thus well before the interviews), I was concerned that the extraordinary circumstances of the Clinton-Lewinsky investigation might have prompted heterosexual respondents to revise their definitions of virginity loss, thus biasing later interviews. Fortunately, the timing of the interviews appeared not to affect their content. Regardless of when I spoke with them, most heterosexual respondents initially defined virginity loss with a simple statement such as "[Virginity loss is] the first time having sex" (Lavinia, 30, heterosexual), by which they meant vaginal intercourse.[4] In contrast, virtually every lesbian, gay, or bisexual participant responded

---

[4]To preserve confidentiality, all respondents are identified by pseudonyms.

by raising the issues of sex between same-sex partners, often referring more generally to the existence of different ways of defining sex.

METHODS OF ANALYSIS

To code and analyze interview data, I relied primarily on the systematic procedures referred to as *grounded theory* (Glaser & Strauss, 1967). Developed to optimize analysis of qualitative data, the grounded theory approach stresses the inductive development of the analytic categories guiding the researchers's inquiries. This strategy helps the researcher focus on the meaning of experiences to study participants. My analysis thus seeks to represent faithfully the means through which real people make sense of their social world. To uncover patterns in respondents' talk about virginity loss, I read transcripts of each interview several times, allowing salient themes to emerge from them. For example, I did not ask study participants whether they saw virginity as a gift or as a stigma; that respondents thought about virginity in these metaphorical terms emerged during the course of the interviews and analysis. Using these emergent themes, along with key topics as cited in the relevant literature, I developed a guide for coding the interviews, which I then reread, identifying these themes and topics as they appeared.

Findings

DEFINING VIRGINITY LOSS

Participants in my study were in complete agreement about a few aspects of the definition of virginity loss. In particular, every respondent believed that vaginal-penile intercourse would constitute virginity loss, if it were the first partnered sexual activity in which a woman or man had engaged. Furthermore, every respondent stipulated that a person could not lose her or his virginity without the involvement of a human partner and the stimulation—by more than manual means alone—of at least one partner's genitalia. Less agreement existed regarding other sexual acts that could take place between a woman and a man.[5] About one fourth (17) of respondents believed that a woman or a man who engaged in oral sex with an opposite-sex partner would lose her or his virginity. For example, Marty (26, heterosexual) said of oral sex, "That's fooling around, in my terminology." More respondents—56%—thought that anal intercourse between a man and a woman could constitute virginity loss.[6]

---

[5] I did not ask separate questions about fellatio and cunnilingus, nor did I inquire specifically about perceptions of giving versus receiving oral sex. Respondents' remarks at various junctures indicated disagreement as to whether performing oral sex would be sufficient to cause virginity loss.

[6] Qualitative researchers typically favor terms such as *many, seldom,* and *often* over percentage statistics for fear that readers will misinterpret the latter as representing the distribution of beliefs and behaviors among a broader population. Yet, words like "many" can be vague and imprecise. For the sake of precision in meaning, I use both percentage statistics and qualitative expressions. In no case should the reader assume that these percentages can be directly generalized to young adults in the U.S. overall.

The prevalence of anti-gay sentiment in the U.S. notwithstanding, a majority of study participants claimed that it was possible to lose one's virginity with a same-sex partner. Four fifths of respondents (49) believed that both men and women could lose their virginity with a same-sex partner. Another 10% believed that men could lose their virginity with same-sex partners, but that women could not. Only 4 respondents argued that virginity loss could take place only through coitus. Respondents who saw same-sex virginity loss as possible took two different perspective regarding the sex, or sexual orientation, of the virgin and her/his partner. About half of participants (29) posited different standards of virginity loss for sex between same- and opposite-sex partners. For example, Meghan (22, heterosexual) said: "I guess virginity has to be defined within each type of relationship, like woman-woman, man-man, heterosexual . . . If that is their way of making love . . . I think probably no, they wouldn't be a virgin." Another one third (20) believed that anal sex, oral sex, and coitus were equally capable of resulting in virginity loss, regardless of the sex of the partners involved. For example, Seth (19, gay) explained: "I think of oral sex as sex, and I think of anal sex as sex, and I think of vaginal sex as sex. Those are kind of like the three things that I think of as sex." (On the tendency to create hierarchies among sexual acts, see Rubin, 1984.)

Definitions of virginity loss varied by sexual orientation, in ways that correspond to the particular concerns of people who are heterosexual and people who are not. For example, all but one of the nonheterosexual respondents contended that both women and men could lose their virginity with partners of either sex, compared with just under three fourths of heterosexual participants. Lesbians, gay men, and bisexuals were also considerably more likely than heterosexual women and men to say that vaginal, oral, and anal sex would all result in virginity loss, regardless of the sex of the actors (59% and 18%, respectively). Several respondents suggested that people who support such a single-standard definition of virginity may do so out of a desire to establish equal status or acceptance for gay sex, an issue arguably of greater concern to gay and bisexual women and men than to their heterosexual counterparts.

There was little agreement about nonconsensual sex experiences. Just under half of the respondents (26) believed that rape would constitute virginity loss. For example, Karen (21, heterosexual) said: "[Rape] would definitely be intercourse, so I wouldn't consider them a virgin. Unfortunately." About one third (22) felt that a person absolutely could not lose their virginity as a result of rape. According to Matt (24, heterosexual):

> I guess losing your virginity is at least partially defined by the experience you gained about sex and relationships. And I think that there's so much that's strange about [rape and molestation] that they may not really fall into that category.

The remaining 13 participants fell somewhere in between these two extremes, arguing that although a person who was raped was technically (i.e., physiologically) no longer a virgin, in many ways they still were. For instance, Carrie (20, heterosexual) said:

> I see virginity as definitely something that you can choose into, and people . . . don't get to choose into rape . . . If their only sexual experience has been something like a rape, I would call them a virgin even though technically, um, something did happen.

In short, respondents disagreed as to whether nonconsensual sex should be categorized as a form of sex, albeit an undesirable one, or whether it was, in some sense, not really sex at all. They also disagreed as to whether virginity loss could or should occur only on a voluntary basis.

Beliefs about virginity loss and nonconsensual sex were patterned by gender, consistent with the distinctive concerns women and men have regarding sexuality. Nearly two thirds of women in the study said that rape could never or could only technically constitute virginity loss, compared with only half of men. This gender difference appears to stem from a variety of social factors, especially women's greater susceptibility to rape and the greater likelihood that women respondents had themselves experienced a nonconsensual sexual encounter. (For national data, see Laumann et al., 1994.) One fourth (8) of the women in the study had bene victims of forced sex, compared with only one man. None of these nine respondents believed that virginity could be lost through coerced sex.

Another dimension of social identity along which definitions of virginity loss were patterned was age. Younger respondents (25 and under) were more likely than their older counterparts to view same-sex virginity loss as possible (91% and 67% of younger and older respondents, respectively) and to believe that nonconsensual sex could not or could only technically result in virginity loss (55% and 15% of younger and older respondents, respectively). The extent to which younger participants thought it possible to lose virginity with a same-sex partner suggests a growing legitimization of gay and lesbian sexuality in the U.S. over time. Similarly, the greater tendency of younger respondents to exclude rape from their definitions of virginity loss may indicate partial incorporation of feminist ideas about rape into mainstream understandings of sexuality. It is noteworthy that younger respondents appear to be redefining virginity loss rather than choosing to abandon the concept of virginity altogether. Their decisions stand as testimony to the continuing social significance of the categories of virgin and nonvirgin in the face of a changing sexual landscape.

IDENTIFYING PERSONAL VIRGINITY-LOSS EXPERIENCES

Another way to evaluate what people mean when they talk about virginity loss is to look at which experiences they identify as the point at which they lost their own virginity. Of the 56 respondents who were not virgins at the time of the interview, four fifths said that they had lost their virginity the first time they engaged in coitus. Eight participants reported losing their virginity the first time they gave or received oral sex and 2 identified the first time they had anal sex as the point at which they lost their virginity. (Five of the respondents who identified a first same-sex encounter as the point at which they lost their virginity did so only in retrospect; at the time of the encounter, they had not yet questioned the common definition of virginity loss as a person's first experience with coitus.)

Which experiences respondents identified as resulting in their own loss of virginity varied by sexual orientation. All 37 nonvirgin heterosexual respondents and 4 of 5 nonvirgin bisexual respondents reported losing their virginity the first time they engaged in coitus. In contrast, only one third of gay and lesbian respondents said that they lost their virginity via coitus. Lesbians were quite a bit more likely than gay men to have lost their virginity through coitus: 4 of 6 nonvirgin lesbian respondents had done so, compared with only 1 of 8 non-virgin gay men. Only one respondent, a gay man named Seth, reported losing his virginity with an opposite-sex partner by engaging in some act other than coitus (reciprocal oral sex). Of the 48 respondents who had ever engaged in coitus, 2 did not currently identify their first experience of coitus as the point at which they lost their virginity. Sarah (33, lesbian) said she lost her virginity the first time she performed oral sex on another woman; she engaged in one act of coitus 2 years later. As an adult, Geoff (30, gay) pinpointed his loss of virginity as the first time he exchanged oral sex with another boy (at age 5); but as a teen, he had thought of himself as losing his virginity the first time he engaged in coitus (at age 12).

INTERPRETING VIRGINITY LOSS

Over the course of their lives, the women and men who participated in my study drew primarily on three distinctive metaphors to make sense of virginity and the experience of virginity loss. About half (30) of them at some point likened virginity to a gift and virginity loss to gift-giving. For instance, Kelly (24, heterosexual) said that virginity is:

> . . . supposed to be something special and cherished and wonderful and something to keep and you give to someone who is. . . . I don't know if lose is the right word. . . . I'll say you give to someone, whenever you find the right person.

Just over half (34) of respondents compared virginity and virginity loss to stages in a broader process or rite of passage. According to Emma (24, heterosexual):

> I see everything in life as kind of a process and, losing your virginity is kind of the start of a process. . . . In general . . . the first time with anything tends to be a little awkward at best, you know. And so . . . it's just kind of the start of something that progresses.

Finally, just over one third (23) of participants at some point turned to the metaphor of virginity as a stigma to understand their experiences. As Kendall (28, gay) recalled:

> I think almost every teen-like movie . . . was about getting laid or not getting laid, and what an idiot you were for not getting laid. And then girls, you now, hemming and haw-ing, "Should I put out? Should I not put out?" Growing up it's always been a stigma, it's always been a bad thing . . . to be a virgin. I'm sure I knew a lot more virgins than let on. But, couldn't be a virgin in public.

As described here, the three primary interpretive frames are best understood as ideal types (see Weber, 1946). In practice, the boundaries between the frames, and the experiences of those who employed them, were somewhat indistinct. Moreover, about one third of respondents reported that their perspectives on virginity had changed over time, often in response to new experiences.

These metaphorical interpretive frames profoundly shaped respondents' expectations, experiences, and retrospective evaluations of virginity loss. When people think metaphorically, they compare two phenomena and expect those phenomena to resemble one another (Lakoff & Johnson, 1980). Thus, respondents who spoke of virginity as a gift anticipated the experience of "giving" their virginity to resemble giving a gift more generically. Perceiving virginity as a very valuable gift, not least because of its nonrenewable nature, these women and men were concerned primarily with finding partners who would appreciate the worth of their gift and, more important, reciprocate it with a gift of similar value (typically the recipient's own virginity or increased commitment to the relationship). The norm of reciprocity stipulates that every gift must be returned; therefore, a single gift can set in motion an endless series of exchanges, each of which strengthens the bond between the givers. Yet, while a giver can increase the odds of reciprocity by selecting a recipient who seems likely to return her gift, she cannot compel reciprocation. Givers are, therefore, always somewhat subject to the whims of recipients (at least in societies like the contemporary U.S., where social controls are relatively weak). (For more details, see Mauss, 1925; Schwartz, 1967.)

In a similar manner, participants who interpreted virginity as part of a process expected the experience of virginity loss to resemble other familiar processes, such as education or marriage, which entail a transition from one social status to another. These men and women believed that virginity loss, like social transitions in general, would increase their knowledge (about sexuality or themselves) and leave them feeling transformed. Adherents to the process frame saw virginity loss as both an inevitable and a desirable transition, but disagreed as to whether it was rapid and dramatic or gradual and incremental. (On the sociological aspects of status passages, see Glaser & Strauss, 1971; Turner, 1969; van Gennep, 1908.)

Finally, respondents who viewed virginity as a stigma were eager to discard that stigma as soon as practically possible. They typically emphasized the importance of not incurring additional stigmas, such as a reputation for sexual ineptitude, during the campaign to lose virginity. Cognizant of the ever-present possibility that their stigma could be discovered, exposed, and derived by others, many in this group sought to conceal their virginity so long as it existed. These concerns are characteristic of people who bear a temporary stigma. (For a classic statement on stigma, see Goffman, 1963.)

PATTERNS BY GENDER AND SEXUAL ORIENTATION

Study participants drew on different interpretive frames to understand virginity depending in part on their gender. Women and men were equally likely to have ever seen virginity loss as part of a larger process, as we see in Table 1. However, almost twice as many women as men had thought about virginity as a gift (61% of women, compared with 36% of men). Conversely, men were nearly three times more likely than women to have ever viewed

TABLE 1   Interpretation of Virginity Ever by Gender and Sexual Orientation

	Gift	Stigma	Process	Other[a]	Total[b]
Women	61% (20)	21% (7)	52% (17)	9% (3)	54% (33)
Men	36% (10)	57% (16)	61% (17)	11% (3)	46% (28)
Heterosexual	54% (21)	38% (15)	46% (18)	5% (2)	143% (39)
Lesbian/gay	31% (5)	38% (6)	73% (12)	25% (4)	167% (16)
Bisexual	67% (4)	33% (2)	67% (4)	0% (0)	167% (6)
Total	49% (30)	38% (23)	56% (34)	10% (6)	153% (61)

[a]Four respondents (three gay men and one lesbian) at some point interpreted virginity as irrelevant to their own experience; two respondents (both heterosexual women from evangelical Protestant backgrounds) described maintaining virginity as a way to honor one's commitment to God.
[b]Percentages total more than 100 because some respondents reinterpreted virginity over time.

virginity as a stigma (57% of men and 21% of women). This pattern is consistent with the resilient, if evolving, sexual double standard (Ferrell, et al., 1977; Moffatt, 1987; Rubin, 1990). Notably, gender differences were more pronounced among older respondents (26 and over), suggesting a possible weakening of the double standard over time.

Interpretations of virginity were also patterned by sexual orientation. As shown in Table 1, the propensity ever to interpret virginity as a stigma varied little by sexual orientation. However, many more lesbians and gay men adhered to the process frame than did their heterosexual counterparts (73% and 46%, respectively). Conversely, heterosexual respondents were more likely to have ever thought of virginity as a gift than were their gay and lesbian counterparts (54% compared with 31%). Bisexual respondents fell somewhere in between, with two thirds interpreting virginity as a gift and two thirds viewing it as a stage in a process. Gay and bisexual respondents were especially likely to have seen virginity loss as part of a process, in part because, for them, virginity loss was closely intertwined with the process of coming out.

INTERPRETATIONS, EXPECTATIONS, AND CONDUCT

These interpretive frames are of particular interest because each was associated with a fairly distinctive constellation of sexual beliefs and conduct, including sexual behavior and presentation of self before and after virginity loss, relationships with virginity-loss partners, contraceptive use during virginity loss, and satisfaction with the experience of virginity loss overall. Here, I briefly discuss the ways that interpretive approaches to virginity loss shaped respondents' decisions about how to present themselves to others, especially their virginity-loss partners. In presenting themselves as virgins or nonvirgins, participants claimed particular social identities, sometimes based on and sometimes despite their personal identities (see Table 2).

Before losing their virginity, respondents who viewed virginity as a gift typically spoke openly about their virginity status with people they knew. In fact, they were often quite

TABLE 2 Selected Aspects of Virginity-loss (VL) Experiences by Interpretation of Virginity Loss

Aspect of experience	Interpretation of Virginity Loss		
	Gift	Stigma	Process
Presentation of self before/after VL.	Most likely to be proud of virginity; most likely to be ashamed of virginity loss.	Most likely to conceal virginity; most likely to brag about virginity loss (when possible).	Typically open about virginity status before and after VL, but neither proud nor ashamed.
Communication with VL partner.	Invariably admitted own virginity to VL partner. Failure to discuss reciprocity concerns could lead to dissatisfaction.	Least likely to admit virginity to VL partner. Concealed virginity often undetected (esp. among younger virgins), but discovery could be devastating.	Typically told partners about own virginity. Able to overcome physically or emotionally unpleasant experiences by talking with partner.
Relationship to VL partner.	Most likely to lose virginity in a serious dating relationship, when in love, or with a "soulmate."	Most likely to lose virginity with a stranger or "temporary" partner (e.g., a friend).	If hetero- or bisexual, typically dating VL partner. If lesbian or gay, VL often with friend (VL part of coming out process).
Contraceptive use at VL (for those whose VL was coitus).	Most likely to use contraceptives (79%); most likely to use the Pill (36% of users), often in combination with condoms.	Least likely to use contraceptives (59%); often unwilling to discuss contraception with VL partner, for fear of appearing inexperienced.	Second-most likely to use contraceptives (67%); non-users often planned to use, but didn't because VL encounter unplanned.
Overall satisfaction with VL experience.	Most dependent for satisfaction on the conduct of VL partners (due to emphasis on reciprocation).	Typically satisfied merely by losing virginity, but devastated if ridiculed by VL partner.	Pleasurable experiences common. Where VL not pleasurable, generally satisfied with VL as a "learning experience."

proud of being virgins. These men and women invariably discussed their virginity with their sexual partners, in part to ensure that their partners realized what a special gift they were about to receive. Such self-disclosure also served as a way to encourage reciprocity. Bryan (18, heterosexual), who had made a point of discussing his virginity with his girlfriend before they had sex, explained, "If you feel as though you're not loved as much as . . . you love this other person, and you actually decide to have sex with this person, I think you kind of feel slighted." Communication about virginity status may have been facilitated by the nature of the relationship adherents to the gift frame had with their virginity-loss partners: They were the group most likely to lose their virginity in serious dating relationships and to be in love with their partners or to describe them as "soulmates." Respondents who interpreted virginity as a gift were the most likely to use contraceptives when they lost their virginity (79% did), a tendency apparently related to both willingness to communicate and the relationship between partners. (Data are for respondents who lost their virginity by engaging in coitus.) On the downside, however, the five respondents (all women) whose partners failed to reciprocate described their virginity-loss experiences as emotionally devastating and as diminishing their value as persons. The norm of reciprocity effectively empowers recipients at the expense of givers; therefore, participants who saw virginity as a gift were particularly vulnerable to distressing virginity-loss experiences precisely because they framed virginity as a gift.

From a policy perspective, encouraging young people to interpret virginity as a gift—a stance consistent with many abstinence-only sex education programs—is a double-edged sword, protecting against one negative potential consequence of sexual activity (pregnancy and/or STD transmission) but increasing the likelihood of another deleterious consequence (emotional distress due to partner's nonreciprocation). In contrast, even adherents to the stigma frame whose partners ridiculed them experienced virginity loss as positive on balance, inasmuch as they lost their stigma. Participants who saw virginity loss as a process achieved the goal of gaining knowledge merely through losing their virginity, thus their partners could in practice wield little power over them. I discuss the relationship among interpretive frames, gender, and sexual agency in more detail elsewhere (Carpenter, 2000).

In contrast, participants who saw virginity as a stigma were extremely reluctant to admit their virginity to anyone they knew. Many worked to disguise their virginity, either actively—by falsifying their sexual histories—or passively—by allowing or encouraging others to assume that they were no longer virgins. Not surprisingly, people who interpreted virginity as a stigma were the most likely to conceal their virginity from their virginity-loss partners. For instance, Bill (31, heterosexual) decided not to tell his partner that he was a virgin because "It was so obvious to me that she wasn't [a virgin], that I felt demeaned by, if I had [told her]." Indeed, many respondents in this group lost their virginity with relative strangers, from whom they might more easily conceal their sexual status. Most clandestine virgins avoided detection by their partners; however, the three respondents whose partners either ridiculed them as virgins or as sexually incompetent were profoundly dissatisfied with the manner in which they lost their virginity (albeit relieved to have expunged their stigma). Men were far less successful than women at concealing their virginity and sexual inexperience, perhaps due to popular stereotypes of men as sexually active and women as sexually passive. Respondents who lost their virginity at relatively advanced ages were also less successful at concealment, apparently because their similarly-aged partners were already sexually experienced. The desire of adherents to the stigma frame to avoid being stigmatized as virgins also affected their use of contraceptives. The group least likely to employ a form of contraception (59% did), a number of these respondents declined to discuss contraception—or to insist on practicing safer sex— precisely in order to avoid appearing inexperienced or foolish to their partners. Bill recalled:

> I was so nervous, it was my first time and . . . I didn't want to look foolish, so I ended up having sex with her without any protection. And she said that she was okay, she had that taken care of. And I didn't go into any great details, I was just so nervous.

Finally, women and men who thought of virginity loss as a step in a process were typically frank about their virginity status, seeing it as cause for neither pride nor shame. Almost all of these respondents told their virginity-loss partners that they were virgins, which may have facilitated later discussions of awkward or unpleasant aspects of virginity loss. In fact, people who interpreted virginity as part of a process proved to be the best-equipped to work through physically or emotionally negative experiences by talking with their partners, generally in ways that helped ensure more positive sexual experiences later on. For example, Jennifer (25, heterosexual) expected virginity loss with her boyfriend of three months to be physically and emotionally enjoyable. Instead, she found sexual intercourse to be so unpleasant and tedious that she had no desire to have sex again. She had, however, enjoyed losing her virginity on an emotional level; this, plus her boyfriend's support and encouragement were crucial in convincing her that the physical aspects of sex would improve over time. She said:

> I didn't even enjoy it. . . . It just made me think it was a waste of my time [laughs]. . . . I told him, "That's it?" He's like, "Isn't that enough?" [laughs]. And I said, "No" [laughs]. He had lost his virginity with a girl he had been with before. And so I think going through it with her . . . he kind of knew that it wasn't that pretty the first time.

Respondents who saw virginity as a stage in a process were almost as likely as adherents to the gift frame to use contraceptives when they lost their virginity (67% did), probably for much the same reasons: open communication and close relationships with partners. Interestingly, of the four adherents to the process frame who lost their virginity without using contraceptives, three had at some point discussed contraception with their partners and had planned to use condoms. However, consistent with their understanding of virginity loss as stemming naturally out of a series of experiences, these young people lost their virginity when "one thing led to another" in circumstances where contraceptives were unavailable.

Discussion

These findings demonstrate that considerable ambiguity surrounds the definition and interpretation of virginity loss. This ambiguity provides young women and men with a degree of flexibility: Within constraints, they may choose which specific definitions and interpretations of virginity and nonvirginity they will use in constructing their sexual identities. In recent decades at least, virginity loss has by and large ben defined with reference to physiological rather than to moral criteria, and has been specifically equated with first coitus. Indeed, participants in my study defined virginity loss almost exclusively in physiological terms, with scarcely any mention of virtue or sin. Not one respondent disputed the common belief that otherwise sexually inexperienced individuals would lose their virginity the first time they engaged in coitus. However, a majority contended that, with same-sex partners, people could also lose their virginity without engaging in vaginal intercourse. Moreover, about half believed that nonconsensual coitus could not truly result in virginity loss. Given the popular equation of virginity loss with "first sex," new definitions of virginity loss suggest new understandings of sex in general. Defining virginity loss to include same-sex encounters implies an understanding of "real" sex that challenges heterosexist norms. Likewise, defining virginity loss to exclude rape implies that coercive sexual acts are not "really" sex. My study thus corroborates previous findings of disagreement over the definition of virginity loss (Berger & Wenger, 1973) and sex (Sanders & Reinisch, 1999). It also advances the literature by revealing definitional ambiguities related to sex with same-sex partners and to coercive sex (both previously unexamined).

Definitions of virginity loss constitute claims about identity, for how people define virginity loss determines how and when they believe the transition between virgin and nonvirgin identity occurs. To the extent that virginity loss forms an important part of the passage from childhood to adulthood, different definitions of virginity loss render people differentially eligible for achieving status as sexual adults. For example, the traditional equation of virginity loss with first coitus effectively denies nonvirgin identity and sexual adulthood to people who do not wish to engage in vaginal intercourse. Conversely, defining virginity loss as possible through oral or anal sex with same-sex partners extends the status passage of virginity loss to gay, bisexual, and heterosexual people alike. By a similar token, to exclude coercive sex from the definition of virginity loss is to claim that the transition from virgin to nonvirgin identity cannot be imposed by another but rather must be chosen by the person making the transition.

Given their implications for identity, it is not surprising that definitions of virginity loss were patterned by group membership, reflecting group concerns. Lesbian, gay, and bisexual respondents, whose sexual repertoires depended less on coitus than did those of their heterosexual counterparts, were considerably more likely to argue that oral and anal sex could result in virginity loss, especially between same-sex partners. These men and women thereby proposed assigning virgin and nonvirgin social identity in ways consistent with their understanding of themselves as sexual adults for whom coitus is not the central sexual act. These criteria moreover correspond with many of these respondents' own experiences of adopting nonvirgin personal identity without engaging in vaginal intercourse. Likewise, women respondents, far more likely than men to experience coercive sex, were disproportionately likely to argue that virginity loss could not occur without the virgin's consent. They therefore asserted that virgin and nonvirgin identity are to some extent voluntary.

By challenging traditional definitions of virginity loss, individuals and social groups can help alter prevailing criteria for assigning social identity and possibly also promote greater social equity. The definitional ambiguity of virginity loss allows people some discretion in choosing the point at which they adopt personal identity as nonvirgins, as when a self-identified lesbian rejects heteronormative definitions to locate her own loss of virginity at her first sexual encounter with another woman. A person whose own definition of virginity loss diverges considerably from prevailing understandings may find that others assign her a social identity that differs from her personal identity. Yet, as more individuals adopt nontraditional definitions of virginity loss, new criteria for assigning social identity may emerge and supplant older approaches. Younger respondents were more likely than their older counterparts to offer nontraditional definitions, suggesting that such changes may be underway.

Previously, scholars have established that diverse interpretations of virginity loss and sex are available in the contemporary U.S. (D'Emilio & Freedman, 1988; Seidman, 1991; Thompson, 1995). Participants in my study framed virginity loss in ways corresponding roughly to previously described understandings of virginity as valuable, stigmatized, and relatively neutral. However, my research presents a more subtle and useful picture of diverse perspectives on virginity loss. Because metaphorical ways of thinking posit similarities between two phenomena—in this case, between virginity loss and gift-giving, stigma, and learning processes—it is possible to illuminate virginity loss by drawing on sociological knowledge about the phenomena with which people compare it. The metaphorical frames for virginity loss that emerged as respondents recalled their experiences may therefore offer a particularly promising framework for future research on early sexual experiences.

My findings further extend previous studies by demonstrating the continuing evolution of interpretations of virginity loss. Like researchers before me, I found that women and men tended to interpret virginity loss differently, with women more apt to view virginity as a valuable gift and men more likely to see virginity as a stigma. Also as in earlier studies, a handful of women and men in my project embraced gender atypical views of virginity; younger participants were considerably more likely to cross this gender boundary. Yet, my interviews revealed a third way of interpreting virginity loss—as a step in a longer process—which largely transcended gender; such an interpretation has seldom been mentioned in previous research (Rubin, 1990, notes a value-neutral stance toward virginity among women but not among men). These findings suggest an ongoing trend whereby the meanings attributed to virginity loss are increasingly dissociated from gender.

Like definitions, interpretations of virginity loss serve as tools for the construction of sexual identity. When a person decides to lose her virginity, she is effectively electing to adopt a new personal identity and potentially a new social identity, should she (or another) choose to disclose her new status. Respondents based their choices about virginity loss (and related phenomena like self-presentation and contraception) on their interpretations of virginity and on what those interpretations imply about virginity and nonvirginity as identities. Adherents to the gift frame viewed virginity as a worthy personal and social identity which they were proud to claim. They strove to maintain their identity as virgins (at both levels) until they were able to make the transition to an equally respectable nonvirgin identity—one which signaled the deepening of a committed relationship with a loving, reciprocating partner. In contrast, respondents who saw virginity as a stigma endeavored to conceal their personal identity when they were virgins, to project a nonvirgin social identity (even when discrepant with personal identity), and to achieve the nonvirgin personal identity they desired under almost any circumstance. People who drew on the process frame perceived both virginity and nonvirginity as acceptable social and personal identities, depending on individual circumstances, and typically adopted a social identity congruent with their personal identity both before and after virginity loss. They spoke of deciding to undergo the transition to nonvirgin personal identity when the time felt "right." The interpretive ambiguity of virginity loss allowed respondents to select from among different approaches to virginity loss, each associated with different stances toward virgin and nonvirgin identity. These diverse interpretations guided people's choices about virginity loss—the adoption of nonvirgin identity—along different paths with distinctive consequences.

Conclusion

In this paper, I have explored ambiguities int he definition and interpretation of virginity loss as a specific case of the ambiguities of "sex." I have also shown how individuals use definitions and interpretations of virginity loss as tools for constructing sexual identity at both the social and personal levels. Definitions of virginity loss and sex are ambiguous; with the exception of coitus, people disagree about which sexual activities can result in virginity loss and thus, by extension, about which activities are "really" sex. A similar ambiguity pertains to interpretations of virginity loss and sex, for different people ascribe diverse meanings to all manner of sexual experiences. Different definitions of virginity loss enable people to construct personal identity in different ways, by allowing them to choose, within constraints, the point at which they move from virgin to nonvirgin identity. Diverse interpretations of virginity loss likewise guide people's choices about losing virginity—and adopting a new identity—along different paths, based in part on what specific interpretive frames imply about virgin and nonvirgin identity. Having changed dramatically in the past, definitions and interpretations of virginity loss and sex continue to evolve, often apparently in response to social movements like feminism and gay rights.

Taken together, my findings challenge researchers to broaden their understandings of virginity loss and sex. Scholars need to realize that women and men in the contemporary U.S. do not simply equate virginity loss and sex with coitus. Although a few studies have adopted relatively inclusive definitions of sex (e.g., Laumann et al., 1994), more need to follow suit. In addition, researchers must bear in mind the coexistence of diverse approaches to virginity loss and sex, which may not directly correspond with gender or other aspects of social identity. Recognizing that definitions and interpretations of virginity loss vary is an important step toward developing a thorough understanding of adolescent sexuality. Such knowledge is important for its own sake as well as for the success of future research, sex education curricula, and public policy initiatives. For example, given diverse perspectives on virginity loss, survey participants may approach the same questions from different interpretive standpoints. Likewise, sex education programs that assume homogeneity in beliefs may fail to affect their audiences as intended.

The research reported here can be usefully extended in several ways. In light of previous studies suggesting distinctive patterns by racial-ethnic background (Aneshensel, Fielder, & Becerra, 1989; Horowitz, 1983; Schuster et al., 1996; Smith & Udry, 1985), and given the relative racial and ethnic homogeneity of my sample, future research should evaluate the ambiguities of virginity loss and sex among a more diverse group. Especially crucial from a public policy perspective, future investigations should also seek to establish the prevalence of these patterns in a large probability sample. Finally, research on the depiction of virginity loss in mass media would expand scholars' knowledge about the cultural resources young people possess when they approach early sexual experiences. Young people construct their identity as sexual beings in part through virginity loss, but in the contemporary U.S. the meaning of virginity loss is ambiguous, as is the meaning of sex. Better understanding of the many potential meanings of virginity loss thus constitutes a crucial step in developing the comprehensive picture of adolescent sexuality on which sex education, research, and adolescents themselves depend.

References

Aneshensel, C. S., Fielder, E. P., & Becerra, R. M. (1989). Fertility and fertility-related behavior among Mexican-American and non-Hispanic white female adolescents. *Journal of Health and Social Behavior, 30,* 56–76.

Aries, P. (1985). St. Paul and the flesh. In P. Aries & A. Bejin (Eds.), *Western sexuality: Practice and precept in past and present times* (pp. 36–39). Oxford, England: Blackwell.

Berger, D. G., & Wenger, M. G. (1973). The ideology of virginity. *Journal of Marriage and the Family, 35,* 666–676.

Biernacki, P., & Waldorf, D. (1981) Snowball sampling: Problems and techniques of chain referral sampling. *Sociological Methods and Research, 10,* 141–163.

Billy, J. O. G., & Udry, J. R. (1985). Influence of male and female best friends on adolescent sexual behavior. *Adolescence, 0,* 21–32.

Brumberg, J. J. (1997). *The body project.* New York: Random House.

Carpenter, L. M. (2000, August). Gender and the meaning and experience of virginity loss in the contemporary United States. Paper presented at the Annual meeting of the American Sociological Association, Washington, DC.

D'Emilio, J., & Freedman, E. B. (1988). *Intimate matters: A history of sexuality in America.* New York: Harper & Row.

di Mauro, D. (1995). *Sexuality research in the Untied States: An assessment of the social and behavioral sciences.* New York: The Social Science Research Council.

Dobie, K. (1995, January/February). Hellbent on redemption. *Mother Jones, 20,* 50–54.

Ehrenreich, B., Hess, E., & Jacobs, G. (1986). *Re-making love: The feminization of sex.* New York: Doubleday.

Elder, L. (1996). *Early embraces.* Los Angeles: Alyson Publications.

Ericksen, J. A. (1999). *Kiss and tell: Surveying sex in the twentieth century.* Cambridge: Harvard University Press.

Ferrell, M. Z., Tolone, W. L., & Walsh, R. H. (1977). Maturational and societal changes in the sexual double-standard: A panel analysis (1967–1971; 1970–1974). *Journal of Marriage and the Family, 39,* 255–271.

Foucault, M. (1978). *The history of sexuality.* New York: Vintage.

Gagnon, J. H., & Simon, W. (1973). *Sexual conduct: The social sources of human sexuality.* Chicago: Aldine.

Giddens, A. (1992). *The transformation of intimacy.* Stanford, CA: Stanford University Press.

Glaser, B. G., & Strauss, A. L. (1967). *The discovery of grounded theory: Strategies for qualitative research.* Chicago; Aldine.

Glaser, B. G., & Strauss, A. L. (1971). *Status passage.* Chicago: Aldine-Atherton.

Goffman, E. (1963). *Stigma: Notes on the management of spoiled identity.* New York: Simon and Schuster.

Goffman, E. (1974). *Frame analysis: An essay on the organization of experience.* Cambridge, MA: Harvard University Press.

Hart, J. (1995). *My first time.* Los Angeles: Alyson Publications.

Hofferth, S. L., Kahn, J. R., & Baldwin, W. (1987). Premarital sexual activity among U.S. teenage women over the past three decades. *Family Planning Perspectives, 19,* 49.

Holland, J., Ramazanoglu, C., & Thomson, R. (1996). In the same boat? The gendered (in)experience of first heterosex. In D. Richardson (Ed.), *Theorising heterosexuality* (pp. 143–160). Bristol, PA: Open University Press.

Horowitz, R. (1983). *Honor and the American dream: Culture and identity in a Chicano community.* New Brunswick, NJ: Rutgers University Press.

Ingrassia, M. (1994, October 17). Virgin cool. *Newsweek, 124,* 58–69.

Jessor, S. L., & Jessor, R. (1975). Transition from virginity to nonvirginity among youth: A social-psychological study over time. *Developmental Psychology, 11,* 473–484.

King, K., Balswick, J. O., & Robinson, I. E. (1977). The continuing premarital sexual revolution among college females. *Journal of Marriage and the Family, 39,* 455–459.

Kinsman, S. B., Romer, D., Furstenberg, F. F., Jr., & Schwartz, D. F. (1998). Early sexual initiation: The role of peer norms. *Pediatrics, 102,* 1185–1193.

Lakoff, G., & Johnson, M. (1980). *Metaphors we live by.* Chicago: University of Chicago Press.

Laumann, E. O., Gagnon, J. H., Michael, R. T., & Michaels, S. (1994). *The social organization of sexuality: Sexual practices in the United States.* Chicago: University of Chicago Press.

Laws, J. L., & Schwartz, P. (1977). *Sexual scripts: The social construction of female sexuality.* Hinsdale, IL: Dryden Press.

Mauss, M. (1925). *The gift.* New York: Norton.

Modell, J. (1983). Dating becomes the way of American youth. In L. P. Moch & G. D. Stark (Eds.), *Essays on the family and historical change* (pp. 91–126). College Station, TX: Texas A & M University Press.

Moffatt, M. (1987). *Coming of age in New Jersey.* New Brunswick, NJ: Rutgers University Press.

Muuss, R. E. (1970). Puberty rites in primitive and modern societies. *Adolescence, 1970,* 109–128.

Nathanson, C. A. (1991). *Dangerous passage: The social control of sexuality in women's adolescence.* Philadelphia: Temple University Press.

Newcomer, S. F., & Udry, J. R. (1985). Oral sex in an adolescent population. *Archives of Sexual Behavior, 14,* 41–46.

Plummer, K. (1995). *Telling sexual stories.* London: Routledge.

Raymond, D. (1994). Homophobia, identity, and the meanings of desire: Reflections on the cultural construction of gay and lesbian adolescent sexuality. In J. M. Irvine (Ed.), *Sexual cultures and the construction of adolescent identities* (pp. 115–150). Philadelphia: Temple University Press.

Reiss, I. L. (1960). *Premarital sexual standards in America.* Glencoe, IL: Free Press.

Rich, A. (1980). Compulsory heterosexuality and lesbian existence. In A. Snitow, C. Stansell, & S. Thompson (Eds.), *Powers of desire: The politics of sexuality* (pp. 177–205). New York: Monthly Review Press.

Rothman, E. K. (1983). Sex and self-control: Middle-class courtship in America, 1770–1870. In M. Gordon (Ed.), *The American family in socio-historical perspective* (pp. 393–410). New York: St. Martin's Press.

Rubin, G. (1984). Thinking sex: Notes for a radical theory of the politics of sexuality. In C. S. Vance (Ed.), *Pleasure and danger: Exploring female sexuality* (pp. 267–319). Boston: Routledge.

Rubin, L. (1990). *Erotic wars: What happened to the sexual revolution?* New York: Farrar, Strauss & Giroux.

Sanders, S., & Reinisch, J. M. (1999). Would you say you "had sex" if. . . ? *Journal of the American Medical Association, 281,* 275–277.

Schlegel, A. (1995). The cultural management of adolescent sexuality. In P. R. Abramson & S. D. Pinkerton (Eds.), *Sexual nature, sexual culture* (pp. 177–194). Chicago: University of Chicago Press.

Schuster, M. A., Bell, R. M., & Kanouse, D. E. (1996). The sexual practices of adolescent virgins: Genital sexual activities of high school students who have never had vaginal intercourse. *American Journal of Public Health, 86,* 1570–1576.

Schwartz, B. (1967). The social psychology of the gift. *American Journal of Sociology, 73,* 1–11.

Seidman, S. (1991). *Romantic longings: Love in America, 1830–1980.* New York: Routledge.

Sherwin, R., & Corbett, S. (1985). Campus sexual norms and dating relationships: A trend analysis. *The Journal of Sex Research, 21,* 258–274.

Smith, E. A., & Udry, J. R. (1985). Coital and non-coital sexual behaviors of white and black adolescents. *American Journal of Public Health, 75,* 1200–1203.

Snow, D. A., & Anderson, L. (1987). Identity work among the homeless: The verbal construction and avowal of personal identities. *American Journal of Sociology, 92*, 1336–1371.

Solin, S. (1996). *The* Seventeen *guide to sex and your body*. New York: Simon and Schuster.

Sprecher, S., Barbee, A., & Schwartz, P. (1995). "Was it good for you, too?" Gender differences in first sexual intercourse experiences. *The Journal of Sex Research, 32*, 3–15.

Sprecher, S., & Regan, P. C. (1996). College virgins: How men and women perceive their sexual status. *The Journal of Sex Research, 33*, 3–15.

Stein, A. (1989). Three models of sexuality. *Sociological Theory, 7*, 1–13.

Sterk-Elifson, C. (1994). Sexuality among African-American women. In A. S. Rossi (Ed.), *Sexuality across the life course* (pp. 99–126). Chicago: University of Chicago Press.

Swidler, A. (1986). Culture in action: Symbols and strategies. *American Sociological Review, 51*, 273–286.

Thompson, S. (1990). Putting a big thing into a little hole: Teenage girls' accounts of sexual initiation. *The Journal of Sex Research, 27*, 341–361.

Thompson, S. (1995). *Going all the way: Teenage girls' tales of sex, romance, and pregnancy*. New York: Hill and Wang.

Tiefer, L. (1995). *Sex is not a natural act and other essays*. Boulder, CO: Westview.

Tolman, D. L. (1994). Doing desire: Adolescent girls' struggles for/with sexuality. *Gender and Society, 8*, 324–342.

Turner, V. (1969). *The ritual process*. Ithaca, NY: Cornell University Press.

van de Walle, E., & Muhsam, H. V. (1995). Fatal secrets and the French fertility transition. *Population and Development Review, 21*, 261–279.

van Gennep, A. (1908). *The rites of passage*. Chicago: University of Chicago Press.

Vance, C. S. (1991). Anthropology rediscovers sexuality: A theoretical comment. *Social Science and Medicine, 33*, 875–884.

Weber, M. (1946). The social psychology of world religions. In H. H. Gerth & C. W. Mills (Eds.), *From Max Weber: Essays in sociology* (pp. 267–301). Oxford, England: Oxford University Pres.

Weeks, J. (1985). *Sexuality and its discontents*. London: Routledge.

Welter, B. (1983). The cult of true womanhood: 1820–1860. In M. Gordon (Ed.), *The American family in socio-historical perspective* (pp. 372–392). New York: St. Martin's Press.

Wight, D. (1994). Boys' thoughts and talk about sex in a working class locality of Glasgow. *The Sociological Review, 42*, 703–738.

Zelnik, M., & Shah, F. K. (1983). First intercourse among young Americans. *Family Planning Perspectives, 15*, 64–70.

Manuscript accepted February 28, 2001

Conceptual Models of Sexual Activity

CHAPTER 18

Al Vernacchio, M.S.Ed.

We've all heard the lines before. We may have even used them ourselves. "Did you score?" "I got to second base last night." "Watch out. I hear he plays for the other team." Baseball metaphors are used to talk about sexual activity from playgrounds in Middle School to dorm rooms in colleges, to break rooms in corporate offices. Even when the actual baseball-related terms are no longer used, because we think they are too juvenile, many people nevertheless still use baseball as a conceptual model to organize their thinking about sexual activity. Far from being harmless word play, the expectations about sexual activity that result from using baseball as a conceptual model lead to unfulfilling, restrictive and inequitable sexual experiences and relationships. We need a new conceptual model for sexual activity, one that sets up expectations for satisfying, healthy, diverse, and equitable expressions of that activity. This article will examine the unhealthy expectations set up by using the baseball model and then offer an alternative model for consideration which may lead to more healthy expectations for sexual activity.

Writing in the early 1990s, Deborah Roffman, in her article "The Power of Language: Baseball as a Sexual Metaphor in American Culture", (1991) points out how ". . . insidiously powerful, singularly effective, and very efficient this [baseball] metaphor is as a vehicle for transmitting and transferring to successive generations of young people all that is wrong and unhealthy about American sexual attitudes" (Roffman, 1991, p. 2). Over a decade later, in my work with students at both the high school and graduate school levels, I continue to find this to be true. Both groups of students can easily generate a list of baseball language that relate to sexual activity, and while both groups say they rarely use this terminology in their day-to-day conversations, they readily agree that the framework provided by these metaphors informs how they think about sexual activity and, often, how they behave with it comes to sexual activity. The baseball model has staying power in our culture, especially because it goes unexamined. Since our culture is so negatively affected by this model, unless we challenge its assumption we will continue to be led blindly around the bases.

The first step in challenging the baseball model is to examine some of the common terminology it presents. I gathered the list below simply by asking my students for base-ball-related terms they've heard regarding sexual activity. They were instructed not to invent new terms, just to repeat ones they had heard. In short order they came up with this list. Think about what terms you might be able to add.

- "pitcher" = the active (insertive) partner in sexual activity
- "catcher" = the passive (receptive) partner in sexual activity
- "first base" = kissing or "making out"
- "second base" = "touching above the waist" / "feeling up the shirt" / fondling the breasts
- "third base" = "touching below the waist" / "petting" / fondling the genitals
- "sloppy second base" = breast stimulation with the mouth
- "sloppy third based" = oral sex
- "score" or "hit a home run" = to have vaginal intercourse
- "strike out" = fail to get as far in sexual activity as one hoped
- "bench warmer" = someone who isn't involved in sexual activity (with the implication that they are not "good enough" to do so) / can also be a term for a virgin (whether by choice or inexperience)
- "bat" = penis
- "nappy dugout" = a vagina
- "a glove or catcher's mitt" = condom
- "if there's grass on the field, play ball" = if a woman has pubic hair she's old enough for sexual activity
- "switch-hitter" = a bisexual person
- "plays for the other team" = a gay/lesbian person

In different communities what constitutes each "base" may be different. At a recent gathering of sexuality educators, a colleague who works with the mentally challenged reported that one of her clients named her first base as holding hands, second based as a kiss on the cheek, third base as a kiss on the lips and a home run as marriage. While the meaning of the bases may change, the fact remains that each community has bases that they can reference when using this model. Another thing revealed by these terms, and noted by Roffman in her article, is their inherent sexism. When "second base" is defined as touching above the waist, it seems only to apply to fondling female breasts. No one gets to second by touching a man's breasts. These terms assume that the male is the active party in the sexual activities. No doubt some young women own this language, being proud of their ability to "round the bases" as well as any young man, but many see only males "playing the game" and women as the field upon which the game is played. "Bat" describes a man's penis as a powerful tool to be used, while "nappy dugout" suggests a vagina is a place of waiting or a place for the team (of men, of course) to gather. Beyond the sexism inherent in these terms, note also the homophobia and biphobia present. Baseball as a conceptual model for sexual activity speaks only to heterosexuals and defines sexual activity as a male-female dynamic. Those who are not heterosexual are placed on the outside. "Switch hitters" may be versatile, but they are also seen as a bit odd. "Playing for the other team" places gay, lesbian, bisexual, and transgender people not on the "home team" but rather in the place of the "other". Simply thinking about the assumptions conveyed by these terms is enough to see how this model sets up inequitable relationships. This terminology, as damaging as it is, results from an even more damaging overall conception of sexual activity as tied to baseball. If we examine not terminology, but rather the game of baseball itself, we can begin to see how this conceptual model sets up sexual activity to be competitive, goal-directed, and restrictive.

Baseball is such a part of the American consciousness that it can be difficult to tease out its elements so that they can be examined. Ask someone to talk with you about baseball and you are likely in for game highlights, player statistics, declarations of team-based loyalty, or even comments about the business of baseball. To get to the heart of baseball as a conceptual model for sexual activity requires stripping down the game to its essential elements and rules. To do that, imagine aliens have come to Earth from another planet and want to know about baseball. They have no prior knowledge at all, so they need the basic concepts around which the game is built. Stripped down to its essential concepts, baseball might look something like this:

1. Baseball requires two opposing teams: The nature of baseball is competitive. Two opposing teams play against (and never along with) each other.
2. Baseball involves a series of offensive and defensive maneuvers: Each team alternates playing offense and defense. Offensive players try to get into the field and then return home. Defensive players try to keep the offensive players off the field or limit their penetration into the field.
3. Baseball has a strict order of play: The bases can only be rounded in a specified order (to do otherwise is to commit an error). Each defensive player has a set position which focuses on a limited part of the field. Offensive players approach the plate in a strict batting order. Other rules designate the number of players per team, number of strikes and balls allowed for each batter, etc. Baseball is a rule-bound game, and playing it well requires strict observance of those rules. In fact, umpires are employed to make sure that players follow the rules and maintain the integrity of the game. It is the game itself and not the players that are of primary importance in baseball.
4. Baseball has a specific goal to be achieved within a designated length of time: Baseball is a goal-directed activity. The aim is to score more runs than the opposing team in the allotted nine innings and therefore win the game. It's an all-or-nothing proposition; no credit is given for moving part of the way around the bases, and

only one team gets to win. In fact, "real" baseball is rarely played without keeping score or just for the fun of it. The time frame of a baseball game may be lengthened or shortened, but only in the service of achieving the all-important goal of winning the game.

5. Baseball requires specified equipment and a specified skill set: A host of equipment is needed to play a game of baseball. While some improvisation is possible, it is difficult to play the game without the equipment (indeed, in some cases the game ceases to be baseball and becomes "stick ball" or simply "catch"). More importantly, baseball requires a specific skill set. The ability to hit and throw the ball, run the bases, catch, and a whole host of physical and mental attributes are essential for being a "good" player. While people without this skill set can certainly play the game, they might feel inferior on a team with more skilled players, and would certainly not find themselves highly valued. In a competitive game of baseball, unskilled players might find themselves in the position of "bench warmers" who simply sit on the sidelines and never get to play at all.

6. Baseball is a team sport: It is difficult, if not impossible to play by yourself.

7. Baseball is seasonal: "Real" baseball (the games that count) is played during a specific season. Baseball can be played out of season, but it is not an activity that can easily take place all year round.

With baseball as our conceptual model for sexual activity, we can begin to see how these concepts translate into messages about that activity. When these messages influence, or in more extreme cases control, our approach to sexual activity, the following messages result:

1. Sexual activity is a competitive, oppositional activity: That is, the participants are playing against each other rather than on the same team.

2. Sexual activity involves a series of offensive and defensive maneuvers: It is made up of a series of moves where one person aggressively tries to move the activity forward (the offensive player/team) while the other person resists or tries to slow the forward motion (the defensive player/team).

3. Sexual activity has a strict order: This is perhaps the most damaging message of the baseball construct. The restriction to round the bases only in a particular order corresponds to a scripted and often stagnating repertoire for sexual activity where kissing precedes fondling which precedes oral sex which precedes vaginal intercourse. This also sets up a hierarchy of behavior where vaginal intercourse has the highest importance and all other sexual activity is somehow less than it. Stopping sexual activity before engaging in intercourse is tantamount to leaving the game unfinished. This strict, rule-bound order also sets up a system where each player has a specified role that must not be violated. This is seen most obviously when strict gender roles are overlaid on sexual behavior. We have already seen how the terminology implies that the man must be the "pitcher" while the woman is the

"catcher." It is the man's responsibility to try to move around the bases and the woman's job to control how far he can go. Other myths such as: men are always ready for sex, women are more concerned with relationships than pleasure, all physical contact between men and women is a precursor to sexual activity, and many others can be viewed in light of the baseball model as playing one's designated position. Just as a center fielder should not wander into the infield, males and females should play their own designated positions and not cross into each other's territory.

4. Sexual activity is goal-directed, with a specific endpoint to be achieved in a specified amount of time: Achieving orgasm through vaginal intercourse ("getting to home plate") is the goal of sexual activity. Again the primacy of vaginal intercourse is emphasized at the expense of other activities (even ones that might bring more sexual, emotional, or physical satisfaction). While the length of time for sexual activity certainly varies from encounter to encounter, each encounter is nevertheless held to a specific endpoint involving one (at least the offensive player, but hopefully the defensive player as well) achieving orgasm, ideally through vaginal intercourse. This point also encourages the elusive goal of the simultaneous orgasm so that the game can end at the same time for both teams.

5. Sexual activity is a team sport: It is not a solo activity, thus masturbation is not considered "real" sexual activity and self-exploration as a form of sexual activity doesn't put one "in the game". Another aspect of the team sport concept, especially for males, is that sharing stories of one's prowess on the field with other team members is part of the game. Thus, men get to brag about how well they performed, offering a play-by-play for their "fans" and fellow teammates. Women certainly have done this as well, although when considered to be the field upon which the game is played, this may be more difficult. In either case, when sexual activity becomes a spectator sport intimacy, privacy, and a special bond between the partners may be lost.

6. Sexual activity requires specified equipment and a specified skill set: The message of having proper equipment may be a positive one in this age of safer sex (i.e. having condoms or other barrier methods to prevent sexually transmitted infections or methods to prevent unwanted pregnancy). However, more often this message has negative connotations. The equipment message is often related to body size and shape (especially penis size as men brag about who has a bigger, more powerful bat). This may lead to body shame and insecurity about one's ability to satisfy their partner if they think their equipment doesn't measure up. Note again the inherent sexism in this, as vaginal size does not enter into the discussion. Women are certainly not immune to the equipment message, however, as we see in the explosion of cosmetic procedures used to alter a body so that its equipment might be seen as more desirable. Believing that a specified skill set is necessary for "proper"

sexual activity can lead to further insecurity as people wonder whether they know the "right" way to pleasure their partner. The huge industry of sexual self-help books, videos, and seminars speaks to our collective insecurity around our performance in sexual activity. Another way to see this message is that once one's skill set or equipment is past its peak one should "get out of the game". Our society's denial of and lack of comfort with sexual activity among seniors, the disabled, those with chronic diseases or anyone who is not at the top of their game brings an elitism into the realm of sexual activity. It ceases to be something for all of us and becomes something for only a specific sub-set, those "in shape" enough to play the game well.

7. Sexual activity must have a specified time and place: While some may argue that this is not a bad message, it does restrict sexual activity, making it not for all times and seasons.

If baseball really does serve as our conceptual model for sexual activity, then we are set up for inequitable, scripted, and in many cases unfulfilling sexual experiences. In looking at these messages, is it any wonder our society is so unhealthy in its approach to sexual activity? When faced with the prospect of not playing the game properly, winding up on a "losing team", or being a "bench warmer", sexual activity becomes a completely goal-driven activity. Only methods that enhance the pursuit of the all-important orgasm through vaginal intercourse, and only achieved through the "proper" series of events, are valued. In trying to discover whether one is affected by the baseball model of sexual activity, consider some of the following questions:

1. Do I see sexual activity as goal-directed? Is it all about getting to vaginal intercourse and/or orgasm?
2. Do I prioritize sexual behavior into a hierarchy where vaginal intercourse is more prized than other expressions of sexual activity?
3. Is sexual activity oppositional? Is one party playing offense while the other plays defense? Is it someone's job to push things further? Is someone else charged with slowing the pace?
4. Do I worry about the equipment I bring to "the game"? Do I worry whether I have performed at a certain level of proficiency?

If we find our concept of sexual activity, or our actual behavior, burdened by these expectations, perhaps it is because our conceptual model has set us up for a negative sexual experience rather than a positive one. What would be helpful in this case is an alternative conceptual model. In searching for one, we need to find something that is as universally understood in our culture and as accessible (or even more accessible) as baseball. It must be a model based upon something that people usually associate with a positive and satisfying experience. It must also be a model that sets up a series of expectations about sexual activity that lead to a more equitable, less goal-oriented, and more satisfying experience than the baseball model. At the risk of sounding absurd, I believe we can find all of these aspects in a new conceptual model centered on pizza.

While certainly there are some people who do not like pizza, it is a common part of most Americans' diet. Pizza can be part of a celebration, a social gathering, a romantic evening just for two, or a solitary pleasure. It can be an event unto itself or it can be a part of a larger event. It is something we are familiar with and feel competent discussing; everyone can be well versed in pizza without ever having to memorize a box score. Again, the first step in working with pizza as a conceptual model for sexual activity is to draw out its essential elements. If we try to explain pizza to aliens who have no concept of it, we might find ourselves making the following points:

1. Pizza is a food used to satisfy hunger; it is readily available and not bound by any season: Ideally, we have pizza because we *want* to have pizza. We experience a hunger, a craving, sometimes even a need for it. While pizza may be a default option to the eternal question "What's for dinner?" at its best it is chosen because pizza is the best thing to satisfy our present hunger. And since there is no "season" when pizza becomes available, it can be enjoyed anytime. No matter what the time of year, or what meal, people can have pizza. It is enjoyed for lunch, dinner, snacks, and even breakfast! It fits most every situation, and is always available to satisfy our cravings when they occur.

2. Pizza offers many choices, so discussion or dialogue is important before ordering: Bring people together to have pizza and a conversation begins. Sometimes it may be very simple, "Should we get our usual?" Other times debate or negotiation is necessary. "Do you like mushrooms?" "I'd rather have pepperoni." "No anchovies, please—yuck!" One of the best things about pizza is that it can be ordered to suit perfectly the needs and wants of those ordering it, provided those involved have enough discussion to ensure everyone involved will be satisfied.

3. Pizza comes in a variety of shapes, sizes, and styles and may be eaten in a variety of ways: While some styles and varieties of pizza may be more popular than others, there is no established hierarchy. A square pizza is just as acceptable as a round one. Pineapple may not be your thing, but it isn't "wrong" to put it on a pizza. Crusts may be thin and crispy or thick and chewy, all based on individual preference. Once the pizza arrives, how one eats it is again up to individual preferences. Use a knife and fork, fold the slice in half, eat the crust first—it's all based upon what works best for you, and all methods are equally valid ones, even though we may have a strong preference for one over another. Unlike baseball, there is no specific equipment or skill set needed to enjoy pizza.

4. At its best, pizza arrives appealing to the senses: The anticipation of enjoying a freshly made pizza is enhanced by its appeal to our senses. The sight of the steam

rising off of the pizza, the smell of fresh ingredients, the warmth of the crust, and the taste of the first bite all contribute to the enjoyment of eating pizza. The senses are engaged, stimulated, and ultimately satisfied.

5. If there is any "goal" to eating pizza, it is simply satisfaction: We eat and enjoy it until we feel satiated. For some, one piece is more than enough; others can finish a whole pizza at a sitting. There are no rules that dictate how much one has to eat. In fact, overindulging leads to us feeling bloated rather than satisfied. Each person involved sets their own limit for when they are finished.

6. Eating pizza can be a solo, shared, or group activity: Unlike baseball, it's easy and quite acceptable to eat pizza by yourself. It's also OK to share it with others. Pizza also removes the spectator aspect of the baseball model. There is no need to brag about one's ability to eat pizza. It is an experience shared by those participating in it; it doesn't need to involve anyone else.

As we did with the baseball model, translating these ideas about pizza into ideas about sexual activity provide a very different set of expectations for what that activity can be:

1. Sexual activity should spring from desire and not be bound by a set season: The impetus for sexual activity should be desire—ideally for connection, for intimacy, for relationship, and for pleasure. It should not be something entered into out of obligation, or worse coercion. What determines when and how sexual activity takes place is an individual decision based on individual wants, needs, and values. Its occurrence should not be ruled by set seasons, schedules, or times of day. No event or situation (the date, the prom, or even the wedding night) can dictate when sexual activity should take place. Rather, sexual activity may be included or excluded in every situation based on the desire of the participants.

2. Sexual activity requires communication and negotiation before any activity takes place: I have always believed that couples who can't talk about their sexual activity together shouldn't be engaging in that activity with each other. Couples who are able to set parameters, negotiate behavior, and discuss their sexual activity before the activity takes place will experience greater intimacy, enhanced communication in their relationship and more enjoyable sexual activity together. They will also limit the chance of negative consequences such as sexually transmitted infections, unwanted pregnancy, or emotional upset that results from different expectations about what sexual activity might mean. Communication and negotiation removes the oppositional component that is so significant in the baseball model. The people involved in the sexual activity negotiate to make it the best experience for the parties involved; it is not a negotiation to see who will ultimately "win", but a way to ensure that everyone's needs are met.

3. Sexual activity contains a wide range of options, all of which are acceptable and equally valid: One of the greatest benefits of the pizza model is the eradication of a

hierarchical system of behaviors in sexual activity. Couples select activity based on their individual preferences and goals. Removing the primacy of vaginal intercourse and orgasm gives couples access to many more options for pleasure. It also makes sexual contact valid no matter what the gender or sexual orientation of the participants. Thus, the pizza model is inclusive of lesbian, gay, and bisexual relationships. Further, with no required equipment or skill set, sexual activity becomes truly egalitarian and open to all, regardless of age, ability, body types, or any other factor.

4. At its best, sexual activity should be appealing, enticing, and pleasing to the senses: Sexual activity is a whole body experience. All of the senses should be engaged; sights, smells, touches, tastes, and sounds all contribute to a satisfying sexual experience. Again there is no hierarchy of senses to be found here and also no primacy given to the genitals. All senses and all parts of the body should be engaged. The more senses that are appealed to, and the more the whole body is involved, the better the experience.

5. Sexual activity is not a goal directed activity; its main objective should be satisfaction not the achievement of some artificial standard of completion: With pleasure and satisfaction as the main foci, couples are free to create sexual activity that involves as many or as few sexual behaviors as they wish. With the measuring stick of mandatory vaginal intercourse and orgasm (and especially the simultaneous orgasm) gone, couples may define for themselves what amount of pleasure makes them feel satisfied and what is considered their own appropriate ending point. This model also allows the couple to have fluctuating end points depending on the situation. Some may choose an encounter that culminates in vaginal intercourse with orgasm at one time and at other times find satisfaction in kissing and fondling each other whether that results in orgasm or not. Sexual activity becomes directed not by a set of external rules but rather by the needs, desires, and decisions of the people engaged in it.

6. Sexual activity can be a solitary or shared experience: Bringing masturbation and sexual self-exploration into the definition of sexual activity allows those for whom partnered sexual activity is unwanted or unavailable to be included. We are sexual beings from our birth to our death. Our sexuality does not depend on being in a relationship with another person. No one is forced to be a "bench warmer" in the pizza model.

The pizza model frees the concept of sexual activity from the restrictions and external rules imposed by the baseball model. It establishes the primacy of individual desire and the decisions of the participants as the controlling factors in sexual activity. It opens the participants to a wider range of behaviors that can be expressed and allows them to define the parameters of their own sexual activity. It sets up more equitable, flexible, and hopefully fulfilling sexual activity.

Conceptual models are very powerful tools for setting expectations, defining behaviors, and bringing values to light. If we find some set of behaviors in our life to be uncomfortable or unsatisfying, it would do us well to attempt to examine the conceptual model that drives those behaviors for, as our model is so shall our behavior be. Attempts at behavior change without addressing the conceptual model behind that behavior has little chance of succeeding. However, if we can critically examine and alter the conceptual model, behavior change can flow more easily from that point.

American society is awash in unhealthy sexuality. We have soaring rates of teenage pregnancy and sexually transmitted diseases. Sexual assault, sexual harassment, and sexual coercion seem to be epidemic. A huge number of marriages end in divorce, not uncommonly driven by the couple's dissatisfaction with their sex life. While the source of these problems cannot all be attributed to the baseball model of sexual activity, it is true that such a model leads us to beliefs about sexual activity and behaviors that contribute to our nation's state of unhealthy sexuality.

Sexuality and sexual activity are forces that can bring out the best in us. Sexual activity can help us to create intimate, constructive, and fulfilling interactions and relationships. In order for sexual activity to do this, it must be based upon a model that is open, equitable, and respectful of differences. In examining our own sexual lives, we should strive to bring them closer to this goal. An examination of the conceptual model that drives our idea of sexual activity can be an important first step in this process.

Reference

Roffman, Deborah M. (1991). The Power of Language: Baseball as a Sexual Metaphor in American Culture. *SIECUS Report, 19*(5), 1–6.

Section VI

Sexual Health, Aging, Sexual Victimization, and Disabilities

Facts in Brief: Sexual and Reproductive Health: Women and Men

CHAPTER 19

Alan Guttmacher Institute

Men and women experience similar sexual and reproductive events, but with some important differences.

Sexual Activity

- Men experience first intercourse at age 16.9, on average, and women at age 17.4. Men spend slightly longer being sexually active before getting married: nearly 10 years, on average, compared with just under 8 years for women.
- By their late teenage years, at least 3/4 of all men and women have had intercourse, and more than 2/3 of all sexually experienced teens have had 2 or more partners.
- Among sexually experienced people in their 20s, 31% of men and 20% of women had more than one sexual partner in the past year.
- In their 30s and 40s, when the great majority of men and women are married, most have only one sexual partner in a given year.

Contraceptive Use

- In their first experience with intercourse as adolescents, more than 2/3 of men and women rely on the condom.
- Condom use declines among both men and women as they grow older. Only 16% of men and women 35–39 used condoms in the past month, either alone or with another method.

The Alan Guttmacher Institute (AGI), *Sexual and Reproductive Health: Women and Men, Facts in Brief*, New York: AGI, 2002, http://alanguttmacher.org

- As they grow older, both men and women are more likely to rely on female methods of contraception, whether they are married, cohabiting or single. By their late 20s, 45% of men and 44% of women use only female methods.
- By their late 30s, 15–20% of men and women rely on vasectomy for contraception. However, female methods continue to provide the greater part of overall protection: 24% of men and 31% of women in this age-group rely on female sterilization, and 21% of men and 14% of women on other female methods.

Sexually Transmitted Infections

- At all ages, women are more likely than men to contract genital herpes, chlamydia or gonorrhea.
- Adolescents and youth in their 20s are much more likely than older men and women to contract chlamydia and gonorrhea.
- During 2001, adolescent and adult women represented 26% of new AIDS cases, compared to only 11% in 1990 and 6% in 1982. 13% of men who received AIDS diagnoses in 1999 were exposed to HIV solely through heterosexual activity, a proportion that has grown substantially in recent years.

Abortion

- Pregnancies that result in abortion are almost twice as likely to involve teenage women as they are to involve teenage men (22% as opposed to 13%).
- The majority of abortions involve men and women aged 20–29: 53% of abortions involve men in their 20s, and 55% involve women in their 20s.
- 34% of abortions involve men 30 or over, and 24% involve women 30 or over.

Pregnancy, Childbearing and Parenting

- Teenage women are more than twice as likely as teenage men to be involved in a pregnancy, and nearly three times as likely to become parents.
- Approximately 1/2 of all births involve men and women in their 20s, and the percentage of men and women involved in pregnancies each year is roughly equal at this stage in life (14% for men and 15% for women). However, women begin childbearing slightly earlier than men, with half of women having a child by age 26 and half of men by age 28.5.
- In their 30s, women are more likely than men to have had children: 82% of women, compared with only 67% of men. By their 40s, this disparity virtually disappears: 85% of men and 87% of women have children.

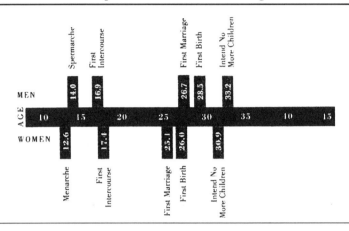

chart a
Sexual and Reproductive Timeline

*Men and women experience important sexual
and reproductive events at similar ages.*

Source: AGI, *In Their Own Right,* page 8.

- By their 40s, 13% of women have one child, 35% have 2 children, and 39% have 3 or more. Among men in their 30s, 16% have one child, 38% have 2 children and 31% have 3 or more. 13% of women and 15% of men in their 40s have no children.
- In 1998, married women with children younger than 18 spent one and a half times as much time with them as fathers did. Between 1965 and 1995, however, the average amount of time father spent with their children increased by an hour per day.
- Most births, and most abortions, involve people in their 20s and early 30s.

Marriage

- By their early 20s, slightly over 1/4 of all women, but fewer than 1/5 of men, are married. As men approach their late 20s, their rate of marriage sharply increases; by their late 20s, 42% of men and 48% of women are married.
- In their 30s, approximately 2/3 of men and women are married. However, women's likelihood of being divorced, separated or widowed sharply increases, reaching 16%, almost twice that of men.

TABLE I Distributions of Births and Abortions

Most births, and most abortions, involve people in their 20s and early 30s.

Age at conception	% distribution			
	Births		Abortions	
	Men	Women	Men	Women
15–17	2	8	5	10
18–19	5	8	8	12
20–24	21	26	29	33
25–29	28	27	24	22
30–34	25	22	15	14
35–39	14	8	11	8
40–44	5	1	8	2

*Source:*Darroch JE, Landry DJ and Oslak S, Pregnancy rates among U.S. women and their partners in 1994, *Family Planning Perspectives,* 1999, 31(3):122–126 & 136; and Deardorff KE, Hollmann FW and Montgomery P, *U.S. Population Estimates, by Age, Sex, Race and Hispanic Origin: 1990 to 1994,* Washington, DC: U.S. Bureau of the Census.

- By their 40s, a larger proportion of men than of women are married (78% and 69%, respectively). Women's likelihood of being divorced, separated or widowed in their 40s remains substantially higher than that of men.

Disadvantage

- On nearly every indicator—including early parenthood, divorce rates, rates of sexually transmitted infection and health insurance coverage—poor women and men fare worse than those who are better-off, and minority women and men fare worse than whites.
- As adolescents, approximately 1/5 of men and women lack health insurance coverage.
- Both men and women are more likely to lack insurance coverage in their 20s than at any other period during the reproductive years (ages 15–49). Nearly 40% of men and nearly 30% of women 20–24 have no health insurance.
- As adults, men are more likely than women to lack health insurance; levels of private (employer-based) insurance coverage are similar, but women are more likely than men to be covered by Medicaid.

Services

- Many federally and state funded reproductive health programs are designed to serve women but not men, and do not offer male services.
- Most women begin seeing a doctor for routine reproductive health care services after they become sexually active, and women who have children become linked to the health system when they are pregnant and giving birth. Men do not have a similar routine channel for obtaining sexual and reproductive health services.
- An appropriate sexual and reproductive health "service set" for both men and women should include counseling and education, as well as purely medical services.

Sources of Data

Sources include research conducted by The Alan Guttmacher Institute (AGI) and published in *In Their Own Right: Addressing the Sexual and Reproductive Health Needs of American Men* and the peer-reviewed journal *Family Planning Perspectives,* and unpublished AGI tabulations of the 1988–1994 National Health and Nutrition Examination Survey,s the 1991 National Survey of Men, the 1992 National Health and Social Life Survey, the 1992–1994 National Survey of Families and Households, the 1995 National Survey of Adolescent Men, the 1995 National Survey of Family Growth and the 1999 Current Population Survey. Additional sources include the Centers for Disease Control and Prevention and the Bureau of the Census.

This fact sheet was prepared, in part, with support from The Bill and Melinda Gates Foundation.

The Young Men's Clinic: Addressing Men's Reproductive Health and Responsibilities

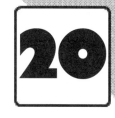

CHAPTER

Bruce Armstrong

Interest in men's health, including their sexual and reproductive health, has been growing over the past two decades. The 1994 International Conference on Population and Development in Cairo and the 1995 Fourth World Conference on Women in Beijing both recognized the effect of men's behavior on women's health, highlighted the importance of shared responsibility and sparked interest in developing interventions to increase male involvement in reproductive health programs.[1] A 2002 report by The Alan Guttmacher Institute emphasized that the sexual and reproductive health concerns of men are important in their own right, not only because males play important roles as fathers and sexual partners.[2] The National Survey of Adolescent Males, the Youth Risk Behavior Survey, and studies and reports sponsored or produced by other organizations have significantly contributed to the growing body of knowledge about men's sexual and reproductive health concerns, beliefs, attitudes and behaviors.[3]

Since 1997, the Office of Family Planning in the Office of Population Affairs at the Department of Health and Human Services has funded diverse community-based programs to learn how to engage with and provide reproductive health services to males.[4] This special report describes sexual and reproductive health services and how they have evolved at one of those programs—the Young Men's Clinic, an ambulatory clinic for adolescent and young adult males in New York City.

Armstrong, B. The Young Men's Clinic: Addressing men's reproductive health and responsibilities, *Perspectives on Sexual and Reproductive Health*, 35(5), 220–225.

The Young Men's Clinic

The clinic is a component of a reproductive health program jointly operated by the Center for Community Health and Education at Columbia University's Mailman School of Public Health and New York-Presbyterian Hospital. It is located in the upper Manhattan community of Washington Heights, which has the highest concentration of Hispanic residents in New York City.[5] Created in 1987, the Young Men's Clinic is the only facility in the city specifically tailored to address the sexual and reproductive health needs of adolescent and young adult men, and has been recognized for many years as an important model of the delivery of community-based health care services to young males.[6]

The Young Men's Clinic provides medical, social work, mental health and health education services at two clinic sessions each week. Services are provided in the clinical space used by the Center for Community Health and Education's reproductive health program, which serves adolescent and adult women at more than 25,000 visits each year. Between 28 and 35 men are served at each session. Use of the clinic has almost tripled since 1998: Some 1,452 men made 2,522 visits in 2002, compared with 506 men who made 908 visits in 1998.

The target age range for the clientele of the Young Men's Clinic is 13–30. Seventy-five percent of patients are 20–29, and 46% are 20–24 (the male age-group with the highest rates of gonorrhea and chlamydia[7]). Ninety-five percent are Hispanic (the majority of whom identify themselves as Dominican); 3% are black. Approximately half of the men are employed either full- or part-time. Only 25% of patients receive Medicaid benefits, and 3% have some form of private insurance.

HISTORY

The Young Men's Clinic evolved out of the adolescent family planning program that has been operated by the Center for Population and Family Health (now the Heilbrunn Department of Population and Family Health) since 1976. Both the scope and the use of services have shifted with fluctuations in funding and with increased knowledge about the needs of young men.

Use of reproductive health services by males was generally low during the 1970s (few of the male involvement demonstration projects sponsored by the Office of Population Affairs during that period attracted many males.) However, the emergence of HIV and AIDS, concerns about rising teenage pregnancy rates, and increases in the proportion of teenage births that were nonmarital prompted renewed interest in developing strategies to reach young men during the early 1980s.

Knowledge of young men's sexual and reproductive health needs and behaviors was limited during the mid-1980s, and the available information was typically obtained from women. To increase knowledge of factors that female and male Hispanic adolescents perceived as barriers to using contraceptives and family planning clinics, researchers from the

Center for Population and Family Health conducted and videotaped focus groups with youth from the community.[9] Several of the male participants said they were reluctant to visit a clinic close to their homes because they did not want to be identified as sexually active ("What if my aunt sees me!"). Participants also believed that family planning clinics are for women only, and that talking about birth control is not "manly" ("Men are supposed to know these things"; "Women expect you to take charge"). Embedding sexual and reproductive health care within a broader menu of services was endorsed as one way of reducing men's embarrassment over being seen at the clinic ("If I could limp in like I hurt my ankle playing basketball, I'd tell the doctor I had a drip").

The focus groups triggered a substantial (and unexpected) level of interest among the young men. Several returned to the hospital to watch the videotaped sessions (which were followed by discussions about HIV and condoms), and suggested other recreational activities that could be taped and used to connect men to services. Videotaping was extended to include break dancing in the streets, performances at school talent shows and basketball games in local parks. These activities attracted young male performers and athletes to the hospital clinic, and most young men enthusiastically participated in discussions about HIV and sexually transmitted diseases (STDs) after viewing their videotape.

These young men also functioned as gatekeepers, linking faculty at the Center for Population and Family Health to adults at community-based organizations. As common missions, interests and needs were identified, partnerships were forged between the burgeoning "men's program" and agencies that were deeply rooted in the community. For example, leaders of community-based organizations accompanied young men from their programs to the health discussions. In return, faculty and students at the Center for Population and Family Health chaperoned dances and cosponsored basketball tournaments (purchasing T-shirts, and refereeing and videotaping games). Training in cardiopulmonary resuscitation was arranged at the hospital for a local scout troop, and the scouts reciprocated by distributing flyers about the new program throughout the community.

Building on the connections established by the focus group youth and partner organizations in the community, faculty conducted in-depth interviews with high school football coaches, Little League baseball coaches, clergy and other adult "key informants" to hear what sexual and reproductive health services young men needed and how services should be designed. The consistent message that emerged from these interviews was that young men in Washington Heights had little access to routine physical examinations that were needed for participation in school, sports and work.

Informed by these responses and encouraged by the success of the videotaping outreach initiative, the Center for Population and Family Health applied to the Office of Population Affairs in 1987 for a "special initiatives" grant and received $20,000 to expand services for young men at the family planning clinic. This supplemental funding was used to develop a Monday evening clinic session exclusively for males. Pediatrics residents provided services under the supervision of an attending physician, and faculty from the

Center for Population and Family Health trained first-year medical students to provide health education. With the advent of the new evening sessions, the Young Men's Clinic shifted forma street outreach and health education program to a clinical model that was complemented by occasional outreach activities.

CURRENT SERVICE MODEL

The Young Men's Clinic currently provides a limited package of such health care services as physical examinations for school and work and treatment of sports injuries, acne and other conditions. The clinic's main focus is addressing the sexual and reproductive health needs of young men—e.g., screening and treatment of STDs, confidential HIV counseling and testing, and condom education and distribution. An attending physician, a nurse practitioner and a master's-level social worker make up the core clinical team. Family medicine resident physicians augment the medical staff during six months of the year. Medical and public health students from Columbia University provide health education services under the supervision of public health faculty. Although the majority of patients at the Young Men's Clinic speak English, 90% of the salaried clinical and support staff speak both Spanish and English.

Medical students complete psychosocial histories and provide health education at initial and annual visits. Sessions are tailored to each individuals' concerns and developmental level. "Teachable moments" are maximized so that men have opportunities to discuss how to use condoms, communicate with their partner about contraception, perform testicular self-examinations and maintain a regular schedule of visits to the clinic (e.g., for regular STD screening). Young men with significant psychosocial needs (e.g., referrals for mental health or employment services) are referred to the social worker.

Public health students design health education activities that they conduct in the waiting room. Discussions focus on STDs and other health issues that concern men (e.g., hernias and stress management), as well as beliefs related to the outcomes of and widespread acceptance of such preventive health behaviors as limiting the number of sexual partners and supporting a partner's use of a contraceptive method.

To create a male-friendly environment, clinic staff show sports and entertainment videos when group activities are not being conducted, and distribute magazines such as *Sports Illustrated* and *Men's Health.* Paintings of men engaged in health-promoting behaviors (e.g., holding a baby) are placed in strategic locations throughout the clinic, and photographs of distinguished men of color (e.g., Secretary of State Colin Powell and former Surgeon General David Satcher) are displayed on the clinic's Wall of Fame.

The social worker provides mental health and social services during clinic sessions and short-term case management services throughout the week. Some of these services do not require young men to revisit the clinic. For example, the social worker provided more than 800 telephone consultations in 2002. Consultations typically are brief (10 minutes or less) and focus on health education (e.g., symptoms of herpes), decision-making (e.g., how to help a girlfriend decide on a contraceptive method), interpersonal skills (e.g., how to talk to a partner about getting tested for STDs) and finding necessary services at other agencies (e.g., support groups for gay adolescents). Even though telephone counseling is not a reimbursable service, logs capture the full range and volume of this important activity, and summary statistics are reported to funders.

Outreach

The increasing number of clients visiting the Young Men's Clinic challenges the notion that men are hard to reach and demonstrates that young men will engage in programs that are accessible, affordable, culturally sensitive, rooted in the community and tailored to their needs. The following outreach interventions were designed to ensure that the clinic has high visibility in the community:

- A social marketing cartoon series that portrays men as competent, caring and involved in health-promoting activities has been developed. Cartoons are printed in English and Spanish on brightly colored cards and distributed through several channels. Story lines address emergency contraception, urine-based chlamydia screening, male support for female contraceptive use, hernia, and referral services at the Young Men's Clinic. A cartoon about dual protection against pregnancy and STDs is being developed. Information about the clinic (location, days and hours of operation, and telephone number) is embedded in each script.
- Medical and public health students are sent to community events such as evening basketball games. Wearing colorful clinic T-shirts, students distribute cartoons and engage men in "life space interviews" about clinic services.
- The results of formative research at the clinic in 2001 suggested that young men delay seeking health care because they fear hearing bad news. In addition, concerns were frequently expressed about the confidentiality of test results and about pain associated with laboratory tests (especially penile probes). A seven-minute digital video about urine-based screening was produced to address these concerns. In the video, satisfied patients give "testimonials" about the clinic and describe the benefits of being tested ("I sleep better at night knowing everything is all right"). The clinic's attractive facility is shown while merengue music plays in the background. Copies of the video are distributed to community-based organizations and downloaded onto computers at school-based clinics run by the Center for Community Health and Education.
- The social worker leads discussions in the family planning clinic to help women link their partners to the Young Men's Clinic. Cartoons are distributed and discussed, and women are encouraged to make appointments for their partners. After these groups were instituted, the proportion of new male patients who were referred by family planning patients increased sharply, from 25% in 1999 to 53% in 2001.

- Although most residents of Washington Heights have limited financial resources, close family and friendship networks provide invaluable support. These networks also create entry points for introducing information about men's sexual and reproductive health services. A standard talking point during waiting room groups, for example, focuses on what men can do to take care of their sexual and reproductive health, their partner's health and the health of their children. Telling friends about the clinic is proposed as one possible action. Tapping into these networks appears to be an effective strategy: Some 25% of the men who came to the Young Men's Clinic for the first time in 2001 said they had heard about the clinic from another patient; in addition, almost two-thirds of the men who made revisits in 2000 and 2001 reported that they had told another man about the clinic since their last visit.

FUNDING

The Young Men's Clinic has been supported over the years by a patchwork of funding that has included in-kind institutional contributions (e.g., the clinic facility, volunteer students and Columbia faculty), private foundation and state grants, patient fees and third-party Medicaid reimbursement. The clinic has never received funds from either New York-Presbyterian Hospital or Columbia University.

Administrators from the Center for Community Health and Education strongly believe that to prevent transmission of STDs in women and reduce the incidence of unintended pregnancy, men must be included in reproductive health services. Since 1987, when medical services for young men were introduced, some funds from the family planning operating budget have been committed to cover medical, social work and support staff at the Young Men's Clinic.

Title X funding specifically designated for men's services was first received in 1998, when the clinic was designated as an Office of Population Affairs male demonstration project. The Young Men's Clinic received funding from the New York Community Trust that same year. These additional funds enabled the clinic to hire a part-time medical directory and a full-time social worker, and to expand to two sessions each week. But although these funds provided a more secure financial base, they did not cover the total cost of operating the clinic.

The total annual operating expenses for the Young Men's Clinic are approximately $311,000, excluding administrative overhead and indirect expenses, such as rent for the clinic facility. Of that amount, $150,000 comes from the Office of Population Affairs through the New York State Department of Health, and approximately $88,000 from Medicaid billing and out-of-pocket patient fees. Other grants and funding sources provide $73,000. Uninsured patients who are 19 or older pay a nominal fee based on income, pursuant to Title X guidelines. A new Medicaid entitlement benefit that covers family planning and reproductive health care services for men and women with incomes less than 200% of the federal poverty level (Family Planning Benefit Program) has been in place in New York State since October 2002.

Organizing Concepts

EMPOWERING

The Young Men's Clinic attempts to empower men to adopt and sustain behaviors that improve their health and the health of their partners. This is challenging because many of the clinic's patients, like other low-income young men of color, experience environmental and structural barriers to meeting their most basic needs on a daily basis. Many are recent immigrants, and few have jobs that provide a living wage or employer-sponsored health insurance. Shifting eligibility requirements for Medicaid coverage since the institution of welfare reform in 1996 have left many confused, fearful and distrustful of medical and other service providers.[10]

To improve staff members' ability to increase young men's self-efficacy and engage them as partners in their own health care, the clinic trains them to help young men identify and use personal and environmental resources to make changes in their lives (e.g., initiating condom use); avoid responding to patients in a manner that sounds blaming, threatening or minimizing and that diminishes men's motivation to take action; and communicate confidence that men can change their behavior and affect their environment. For example, when completing a psychosocial history with an adult who has never finished high school, staff are trained to ask "How did you decide to leave school before you graduated?" rather than "Why did you drop out?" When providing health education about genital warts, staff help young men save face by telling them "It's okay; many men haven't heard about viruses like this one" instead of "You should know about this by now; it's a common infection."

TEACHABLE MOMENTS

Parents, teachers and health care providers regularly miss opportunities to talk with young men about sexual health concerns and fail to provide them with the knowledge and skills they need to protect themselves.[11] As a result, many young men are uninformed about sexual and reproductive health, unfamiliar with the health care system, uncomfortable talking with physicians and reluctant to seek help even when they have symptoms.[12] A visit to the Young Men's Clinic may present one of the few opportunities men have to discuss sexual and reproductive health.

The clinic maximizes teachable moments so that young men have multiple opportunities to ask questions, obtain information, learn skills and think about their behaviors. Graduate students leading group activities in the waiting room focus conversations on factors that are associated with using condoms and with partner communication (e.g., concerns that condoms will affect sexual pleasure). Students inject these issues into discussions so they can be explicitly explored (e.g., asking whether women *always* feel insulted if a man wants to use a condom).

Downtime in the waiting room is also used to inform men about cancers of the male reproductive tract, describe how the testicles are examined during a comprehensive physical, demonstrate testicular self-examinations and provide guidance about what to do if symptoms are observed (i.e., call the clinic). Encouraging men to perform testicular self-examinations and to use the Young Men's Clinic as their medical home raises men's awareness of their reproductive health, establishes a baseline of what is normal and creates opportunities for expressing concerns that may warrant attention (e.g., symptoms of herpes or genital warts).

COLLABORATION

Healthy People 2010 states that developing community partnerships is one of the most effective ways to improve the health of communities.[13] The Young Men's Clinic collaborates with several governmental, nonprofit and community-based organizations to leverage resources and create a comprehensive package of services. A linkage with the New York City Department of Health, for example, allows the clinic to offer urine-based screening for chlamydia and gonorrhea to every patient at no cost to the clinic. (The prevalence of chlamydia among clinic clients was about 11% in 2002. All of the men who tested positive were successfully treated with a single dose of azythromycin.)

EngenderHealth, an organization that provides technical assistance related to reproductive health throughout the world, funded the clinic's social marketing cartoons. Family medicine residents have increased the number of in-kind medical providers and facilitated referrals to the family medicine outpatient clinic when diabetes and other chronic conditions are diagnosed. A Harlem Health Promotion Center health educator is assigned to the Young Men's Clinic and provides smoking cessation services during clinic sessions.

Challenges and Responses

Although the substantial increase in clinic use since 1998 is encouraging and provides evidence that men are willing to participate in sexual and reproductive health care, the success of the Young Men's Clinic has created some of its most vexing problems. marketing activities and informal word-of-mouth outreach by satisfied male and female users of the family planning and reproductive health programs run by the Center for Community Health and Education have dramatically increased the clinic's visibility, but the growing demand for services is outpacing the clinic's capacity. Some 5–10 nonemergency walk-in patients have to be turned away and rescheduled at every clinic session. Although the clinic has adapted by collaborating with government and community-based agencies, enlisting graduate students to provide health education services, maximizing recovery of reimbursable revenue and seeking additional sources of funding, the financial challenges facing the clinic are formidable.

The Young Men's Clinic serves men who are the least likely to be insured and the most likely to be disconnected from health care. Men in their 20s are too old for the State Children's Health Insurance Program (SCHIP) and are rarely eligible for Medicaid. moreover, many of the clinical, counseling and health education services men need are not reimbursable.[14]

The clinic also serves a large number of immigrants, both legal and undocumented. New York State court decisions have restored full Medicaid eligibility to legal immigrants who were eligible for Medicaid before the state implemented federal welfare reforms, but undocumented adults still do not qualify for coverage except for prenatal and emergency services.[15] The policy at programs of the Center for Community Health and Education, including the Young Men's Clinic, is that no one is denied services because of inability to pay. This includes undocumented immigrants. The clinic administration and staff believe that any other position would be unethical. Moreover, health care costs would ultimately be driven up if men had to be treated at emergency rooms and their partners had to be hospitalized with pelvic inflammatory disease and other complications of untreated chlamydial infections.

As at most male involvement programs in the Untied States, especially those serving low-income, uninsured, minority communities, securing adequate and stable funding to provide and (given the high level of interest and need) expand services has been the most pressing dilemma. Few funding sources target men's sexual and reproductive health.[16] The decision to allocate scarce resources to men's services is difficult for managers of Title X-funded programs because of the rising costs of providing services and inadequate Medicaid reimbursement rates. Moreover, despite Title X's extraordinary success in helping to prevent millions of unintended pregnancies over the last 30 years, funding for the program has not kept pace with inflation. The growing federal budget deficit and pressures on states to balance budgets have created even greater financial uncertainties.[17]

Limited funding in the face of the high demand for services has constrained the capacity of the Young Men's Clinic to implement several important activities, including the expansion of health education services at community venues. During the summer of 2003, however, the clinic applied for funding to launch a community-based health education and condom distribution intervention at 14 community-based organizations in Washington Heights and neighboring Harlem, and for an additional medical provider to serve newly recruited patients. If this intervention is funded, a health educator will deliver a three-session group curriculum that uses the social marketing cartoons and digital video. A slide program that walks men through a typical clinic visit by showing digital photos of staff (e.g., receptionists), space (e.g., the lab) and activities (e.g., taking blood pressure) will also be used. Men will be encouraged to visit the clinic for STD screening. Building on the success of the In Your Face school-based intervention, developed by the Center for Community Health and Education,[18] the health educator will escort each young man who visits the Young Men's Clinic through his initial visit.

Although formative evaluations have informed the development of culturally sensitive outreach interventions such as the video and cartoons, and process evaluations (e.g., patient flow analyses, chart reviews and patient satisfaction surveys) have identified service delivery problems so that corrective action could be taken, funding constraints have limited the clinic's ability to conduct rigorous outcome evaluations. The clinic is currently seeking funding to support systematic evaluations of clinic interventions (e.g., the effectiveness of waiting room group activities on knowledge, beliefs and behaviors), as well as outcome studies that measure changes in condom use and partner communication among clinic users.

Conclusions

The sexual behavior of adolescent males has changed for the better in recent years.[19] Nevertheless, more progress is needed to achieve not only the Healthy People 2010 goal of eliminating health disparities, but also increased condom use among adolescents who are sexually active, and lower rates of pregnancy and chlamydial infection.[20] It is particularly important to increase primary and secondary prevention efforts that target men in their early 20s, who are more likely than younger males to engage in risky sexual behaviors and to have adverse reproductive health outcomes.[21] Achieving reductions in sexual risk-taking among men in their early 20s similar to those observed among adolescent males could contribute to further declines in unintended pregnancy and STD rates among young women.

The Young Men's Clinic is successfully engaging young men of color who are poorly served by the U.S. health care system. To improve young men's access to comprehensive and integrated sexual and reproductive health care throughout the country, health organizations and community-based agencies will increasingly need to pool resources, strengthen linkages and craft strategies for incorporating sexual and reproductive health into services. Most important, public and private funding specifically earmarked for men's services must be increased.

References

1. United Nations (UN), International Conference on Population and Development, Programme of Action, <www.iisd.ca/linkages/Cairo/program/p04009.html>, accessed Apr. 15, 2003, and UN, Fourth World Conference on Women, Beijing Declaration and Platform for Action, <www.un.org/womenwatch/daw/beijing/platform>, accessed Apr. 15, 2003.

2. The Alan Guttmacher Institute (AGI), *In Their Own Right: Addressing the Sexual and Reproductive Health Needs of American Men,* New York: AGI, 2002.
3. Sonenstein FL et al., Changes in sexual behavior and condom use among teenaged males: 1988 to 1995, *American Journal of Public Health,* 1998, 88(6):956–959; Grunbaum JA et al., Youth risk behavior surveillance—United States, 2001, *Morbidity and Mortality Weekly Report Surveillance Summary,* 2002, Vol. 51, No. SS-04, Rich JA and Ro M, *A Poor Man's Plight: Uncovering the Disparity in Men's Health,* Community Voices Publication Series, Battle Creek, MI: W.K. Kellogg Foundation, 2002, No. 476; Sonenstein FL, ed., *Young Men's Sexual and Reproductive Health: Toward a National Strategy,* Washington, DC: Urban Institute, 2000; and Sandman D, Simantov E and An C, *Out of Touch: American men and the Health Care System, Commonwealth Fund Men's and Women's Health Survey Findings,* 2000, <http://www.cmwf.org/programs/women/sandman_men'ssurvey2000_374.asp>, accessed Apr. 1, 2003.
4. Male Advocacy Network, *Components That Work in Male Reproductive Health and Education Programs,* Washington, DC: Male Advocacy Network, 2002.
5. Citizens' Committee for Children of New York (CCC), *Keeping Track of New York City's Children,* New York: CCC, 2002.
6. Armstrong B et al., Involving men in reproductive health: the Young-Men's Clinic, *American Journal of Public Health,* 1999, 89(6):902–905; Steinhauer J. At a clinic, young men talk of sex, *New York Times,* Sept. 6, 1995, pp. B6–7; Stolberg SG, Men's reproductive health care gets new emphasis, New York Times, Mar. 19; 2002, p. B6; Sonenstein FL et al., *Involving Males in Preventing Teen Pregnancy: A Guide for Program Planners,* Washington, DC: Urban Institute, 1997; AVSC International, Selected U.S. reproductive health clinics serving men: three case studies, New York: AVSC International, 1997; and Hanson M, ed., *Maternal and Child Health Program Design and Development: From the Ground Up: Collaboration and Partnership: A Casebook,* New York: Columbia University School of Social Work, 1997.
7. Centers for Disease Control and Prevention (CDC), *Sexually Transmitted Disease Surveillance,* 2001, Atlanta: CDC, 2002.
8. Schulte MM and Sonenstein FL, Men at family planning clinics: the new patients? *Family Planning Perspectives,* 1995, 27(5):212–216 & 225.
9. Darabi KF, Barriers to contraceptive use and clinic utilization among Hispanic teenagers in New York City, New York: William T. Grant Foundation, 1985.
10. Adams A and Armstrong B, Connecting the disconnected: involving male minority youth in reproductive health, unpublished document, Columbia University, Mailman School of Public Health, New York, 1999.
11. Porter LE and Ku L, Use of reproductive health services among young men, 1995, *Journal of Adolescent Health,* 200, 27(3):186–194; Kaiser Family Foundation and *Glamour, Survey of Men and Women on Sexually Transmitted Diseases,* Menlo Park, CA: Kaiser Family Foundation, 1998; Lindberg LD, Ku L and Sonenstein FL, Adolescents' reports of receipt of reproductive health education, 1988–1995, *Family Planning Perspectives,* 2000, 32(5):220–226; and Holtzman D and Rubinson R, Parent and peer communication effects on AIDS-related behavior among U.S. high school students, *Family Planning Perspectives,* 1995, 27(6):235–240 & 268.
12. Sandman D. Simantov E and An C, 2000, op. cit. (see reference 3).
13. U.S. Department of Health and Human Services (DHHS), *Healthy People 2010: Understanding and Improving Health,* second ed., Washington, DC: U.S. Government Printing Office, 2000.

14. Sonenstein Fl, 2000, op. cit. (see reference 3).
15. Bachrach D and Lipson K. *Health Coverage for Immigrants in New York: An Update on Policy Developments and Next Steps.* New York Commonwealth Fund, 2002.
16. Sonenstein FL, 2000, op. cit. (see reference 3)
17. Gold RB, Nowhere but up: rising costs for Title X clinics, *Guttmacher Report on Public Policy,* 2002, 5(5):6–9; Dailard C, Title X family planning clinics confront escalating costs, increasing needs, *Guttmacher Report on Public Policy,* 1999, 2(2):1–3; Gold RB, Title X: three decades of accomplishment, *Guttmacher Report on Public Policy,* 2001, 4(1):5–8; and Dailard C., Challenges facing family planning clinics and Title X, *Guttmacher Report on Public Policy,* 2001, 4(2):8–11.
18. Tiezzi L et al., Pregnancy prevention among urban adolescents younger than 15: results of the "In Your Face" program, *Family Planning Perspectives,* 1997, 29(4):173–176 & 197.
19. Sonenstein FL et al., 1998, op. cit. (see reference 3); and Grunbaum IA et al., 2002, op. cit. (see reference 3).
20. DHHS, 2000, op. cit. (see reference 13).
21. Ku L et al., Risk behaviors, medical care, and chlamydial infection among young men in the United States, *American Journal of Public Health,* 2002, 92(7):1140–1143; Bradner CH, Ku L and Lindberg LD, Older, but not wiser: how men get information about AIDS and sexually transmitted diseases after high school, *Family Planning Perspectives,* 2000, 32(1):33–38; Ku L, Sonenstein FL and Pleck JH, Young men's risk behaviors for HIV infection and sexually transmitted diseases, 1988 through 1991, *American Journal of Public Health,* 1993, 83(11):1609–1615; and Ku L, Sonenstein FL and Pleck JH, The dynamics of young men's condom use during and across relationships, *Family Planning Perspectives,* 1994, 26(6):246–251.

HIV/AIDS Diagnosis

National Women's Health Resource Center

21

CHAPTER

The first tests for HIV antibodies were introduced in 1985 to screen donated blood. Since then, their use has been expanded to include evaluating persons at risk of HIV infection. The three standard HIV tests are the Enzyme Immunosorbent Assay (EIA), the Western Blot (WB) and the Immunofluorescence Assay (IFA). Persons are informed that they are positive only when they test positive repeatedly by EIA the results are confirmed by the more specific Western Blot or Immunofluorescence Assay.

The EIA detects antibodies produced in response to HIV infection. Even though some people refer to this initial reaction as a positive result, it should not be considered positive until confirmed by a second, supplemental test on the same blood sample. If two or more blood tests are "reactive" on EIA, then the results are confirmed using a second, more specific antibody test such as the Western blot or an Immunofluorescence assay. This more specific second test can differentiate between HIV antibodies and other antibodies that react to the EIA, causing positive results even when the person is not actually infected with HIV. Although false-positive EIA results are uncommon, they can occur when the test mistakes other antibodies that the body has made for HIV antibodies.

If your HIV antibody test is negative, you are either uninfected or in the early stages of infection before the production of HIV antibodies. This early period before development of HIV antibodies, which would not be detectable on a test, is called the seroconversion time or period. Some have referred to this time as the "window period" since this is the window of opportunity for persons to unknowingly infect others. It can take up to three months for the body to produce detectable amounts of HIV antibodies. In some cases a test result is indeterminate or equivocal, meaning HIV antibodies have not yet fully developed or your blood has produced something not HIV-related to cause a test reaction.

Reprinted with permission of the National Women's Health Resource Center, Inc. www.healthywomen.org. 1-877-986-9472 (toll free).

If an indeterminate reading continues for six months or longer, you are considered uninfected.

Rapid antibody tests that produce results within a half hour have been developed. In late 2002, the FDA approved the Oraquick rapid test, a blood test that can be read in 20 minutes. Like other HIV tests, the results should be confirmed with other tests. The other rapid HIV test licensed for use in the U.S. is the Single Use Diagnostic System for HIV-1 (SUDS). The SUDS test requires serum or plasma as opposed to fingerstick whole blood for analysis, requires more steps, takes longer to run, and requires refrigeration.

An effective alternative to blood testing is an oral fluids test called OraSure, an HIV antibody testing system that uses a cotton pad placed in the mouth to collect oral secretions. Specimens are sent to a laboratory for analysis. The test, which is available only in clinics or health care professionals' offices, is as accurate as a blood test and costs about the same as a blood test. As with both rapid tests, positive OraSure tests should be confirmed with standard HIV testing.

An over-the-counter HIV test that you can perform in your home also is available. Although there are several home tests advertised, only one, Home Access Express HIV-1 Test System, is approved in the U.S. The Home Access test uses a simple finger prick process for collecting blood. The specimen is placed on special paper and mailed to a laboratory. Each test comes with a confidential or anonymous personal identification number. You receive test results by making a toll-free call. If this type of test is of interest to you, ask your health care professional for more information about where to purchase it and how to use it correctly. Once you are diagnosed with HIV, you should search for an HIV specialist or a health care professional who has experience treating HIV patients. The HIV field changes so fast that most general practice physicians cannot keep up with the latest treatment advances. Being HIV-positive, you may also face unique psychological and social challenges. Whom to notify, how to handle your feelings, when to start treatment and where to find financial assistance are some of the major issues that you face after diagnosis.

An HIV specialist also will be informed about the unique ways that HIV infection impacts a woman's health. For example, HIV-infected women are more likely to experience certain gynecological disorders than HIV-negative women, and are much more likely to have abnormal Pap smears. Consequently, screening every six months is advised for women with symptomatic HIV infection, prior abnormal Pap smears or signs of human papillomavirus infection (HPV), a sexually transmitted disease that also causes genital warts and lesions.

A Genuine Feel-Good Story: Sex May Help Prevent Prostate Cancer

CHAPTER

Carl T. Hall

Not too many studies these days conclude that a little sex is good, and even more sex is better.

But in one of the first major attempts to gauge the cancer risk of male sexual activity, researchers at the prestigious National Cancer Institute discovered to their great surprise that a lot of orgasms do a guy no harm—and may even do him some good.

It matters not if they happen during sexual intercourse with a man or a woman, or if they occur spontaneously during sleep. Even masturbation, scientifically speaking, is good for you.

"As epidemiology studies go, this is about as good as it gets," said John Witte, a genetic epidemiologist at UCSF, who was not one of the study's authors but was familiar with the results. "In this day and age, when most of the health warnings are negative—'don't do this, don't do that'—this is kind of a fun one. So ejaculation is something people don't have to feel bad about."

The study, which appears in the latest Journal of the American Medical Association, is by far the most ambitious attempt yet to clear away some of the confusion surrounding male sexual function and one of mankind's deadliest cancers.

This year, an estimated 230,000 men in the United States will be diagnosed with prostate cancer, and nearly 30,000 will die, making it second only to lung cancer on the list of the leading causes of male cancer deaths.

The research was done as part of the well-regarded Health Professionals Follow-up Study, a comprehensive look at the health and habits of nearly 52,000 predominantly white middle-aged men, launched in 1986. Experts said they had no reason to suspect the results would have been substantially different if a broader population mix were included.

The prostate study includes results for 29,342 men. The health professionals filled out detailed survey forms every two years from 1992 to 2000, estimating how many ejaculations they had had per month on average during their 20s, their 40s and the past year. Sexual climaxes during intercourse and masturbation, as well as nocturnal emissions, all counted the same.

Nearly all the previous studies suggested a link between sexual activity and elevated risk of prostate cancer, possibly because of high testosterone levels or exposure to infectious agents among men engaging in frequent sex. A small study in Australia last year suggested the opposite might be true, but those results were largely dismissed.

The new study is the first careful attempt to track a large group of men for a number of years, using statistical tools to take into account differences in diet, exercise and other disease factors that might influence prostate cancer rates. All the men were cancer-free when the study began.

The questionnaires were used to divide the men into categories of sexual activity, ranging from those estimating an average four to seven orgasms a month to those reporting at least 21 per month. Only a handful of men admitted to having fewer than one orgasm a week—not enough to make up their own category. So those few unfortunates were lumped in with the four-to-seven orgasms a month group.

Results were striking: Men having the most orgasms reduced their prostate cancer risk by a full third compared with those men reporting the fewest orgasms. The same pattern held true for those who landed in between the extremes, including an 11 percent reduced cancer risk for those estimating eight to 12 monthly ejaculations and a 14 percent decrease for those in the 13–to-20 ejaculation group.

In their formal account of their findings, the authors seemed to play down the apparent protective effects of male orgasm, in part because there is no agreement as to what might account for the protection.

"The really good news," said Dr. Michael Leitzmann, an investigator at the National Cancer Institute in Bethesda, Md., and one of the study's lead authors, is "that a high frequency of ejaculations does not increase your risk" of contracting a potentially fatal cancer as you age.

One possible explanation, said Leitzmann and other scientists, may be that the prostate accumulates carcinogens, which are perhaps cleared out during the male sex act. The walnut-size prostate gland produces fluids that are contained in semen.

Australian epidemiologist Graham Giles at the nonprofit Cancer Council in Melbourne said one of the big remaining questions was the effect of frequent orgasms during one's teenage years. Like early childbirth in women, a lot of orgasms early in a man's life span may be "like running an engine," he said, prompting youthful cells in the critical region to "fully develop into a whole lot of nice prostate cells."

But the epidemiologists said they had no intention of launching a new pro-masturbation public-health campaign aimed at teenage boys. No need for that, they said.

Whatever Happened to June Cleaver? The Fifties Mom Turns Eighty

23

CHAPTER

Laura Katz Olson

Abstract

June Broson Cleaver represents the quintessential American woman of the 1950s. Because of social pressures, women were encouraged to stay at home and make marriage and motherhood their primary career. These were reinforced by institutional barriers, legal restrictions and business practices that limited women's employment options considerably. Thus women were expected to be dependent on their husbands financially. Those who did work were relegated to low-paid jobs that offered few—or no—benefits. At the same time, the vast majority of African American females had to work to support themselves and their family; they were among the lowest paid employees, barely earning a subsistence wage. This article shows how women of the 1950s, who followed the "prescribed rules", fared during their retirement years. Because of their labor force situation as well as the structure of the Social Security System, based on female dependency and male workforce and retirement patterns, a significant percentage of single older women—especially minorities—end up living in poverty or near-poverty conditions.

Keywords

nineteen fifties, domesticity, marriage and motherhood, female employment, African American women, Social Security, older women.

June Broson Cleaver, the quintessential American mother and wife of the 1950s television series "Leave It To Beaver," is probably approaching 80 years old today. As depicted by her television persona, her fulfillment as a woman accrued from cooking, shopping, attending church meetings, crocheting, making curtains, and, most importantly, tending to the needs of her two children, Wally and Beaver, and husband Ward. Similarly to other wives on family sitcoms at the time, such as Margaret Anderson ("Father Knows Best"),

Donna Stone ("The Donna Reed Show"), and Harriet Nelson ("Ozzie and Harriet"), the kitchen was the center of June's life. In contrast to her husband, we know little of her past life except that she attended a state university and did volunteer work at the USO during World War II. Thus, the college educated June Broson's real life begins, as so many women of the times were told it should, with marriage and motherhood.

In fact, the 1950s were a unique time for women and their families, one that rested on a sharp demarcation of gender roles. For one, after World War II, the United States experienced a period of great fear along with rising expectations. The nation became hysterical about the menaces of communism, both internally and externally, and its presumed threat to the American way of life. The nuclear family came to symbolize the ideal social unit in a free-enterprise system, and even democracy itself: "Marriage and family, it was insisted, were the bedrock of our society, the foundation of capitalism" (Ford, 1999). And full-time mothers were needed to inculcate democratic values and appropriate morals in their children (Kaledin, 1984).

The cold war in a nuclear age, with its risk of annihilation, was a constant source of anxiety and stress, as well. The domestic realm would offer "a secure private nest removed from the dangers of the outside world" (May, 1988). In order to secure fully their safety and protection, middle-class young women were advised to choose solid, reliable husbands as breadwinners (Harvey, 1993).

At the same time, it was an era of unprecedented economic prosperity, consumerism, and materialism. The United States was in a privileged financial position world wide, in terms both of its manufacturing potential and the ascendancy of the dollar. Pent-up desires along with enhanced purchasing power among the population fueled the production of consumer goods; during the military conflict, Americans had accumulated more savings than in any equivalent period of time (May, 1988). Young married couples bought cars, televisions, washing machines, dishwashers, vacuum cleaners, and other assorted modern appliances and household furnishings. From 1945 to 1960, the GNP increased by approximately 250 percent, and per capita income rose by 35 percent, further stimulating the economy (Coontz, 1992).

Second, the middle-class nuclear family, ensconced in a suburban ranch house, became the mark of success, the achievement of the American dream. Aided by government-supported low-interest mortgages and federal subsidies for highways, by 1960 sixty-two percent of American families owned their own homes, up from forty-three percent in 1940; eighty-five percent of the new construction was in the suburbs (Coontz, 1992). The primary beneficiaries were white middle- and working-class families.

Third, married women, including those with young children, had been encouraged—indeed actively recruited—to enter the labor force during the war. A significant number had obtained well-paid jobs in heavy industry, such as in automobile and steel plants, previously reserved for men. By 1945, nearly 25 percent of all married females were working (May, 1988). Although most of these women indicated an interest in retaining their positions, they were either summarily fired or pressured into leaving, through a variety of forces, to make room for returning veterans.

Domesticity was promoted relentlessly by political leaders, educators, psychologists, the popular media, and other social commentators, and women's choices narrowed appreciably during the period (Ford, 1999). Brett Harvey (1993) observes:

> . . . in the fifties as in no other decade, the current of the mainstream was so strong that you only had to step off the bank and float downstream into marriage and motherhood.

Women's and girl's magazines, including *The Ladies Home Journal, Saturday Review, Fortune, McCall's, Redbook, Life,* and *Seventeen,* which exalted housework and glorified motherhood, urged women to return to the home. Working women were castigated for neglecting their children.

Television emerged as the major form of entertainment, and by 1960 nearly 90 percent of all Americans owned at least one set. Dramas and sit-coms depicted the model female as achieving her primary identity and ultimate fulfillment through motherhood and the domestic life. Harvey (1993) notes that the 1950s was actually a "decade-long celebration of maternity," as womanhood became equated with motherhood.

Advertisers, which financed the shows, unabashedly fostered images of wife and mother that would promote the newly booming market in household and children's products. And, as Eugenia Kaledin (1984) suggests, television "catered to advertisers' dreams of what the ideal woman consumer should be." These images were brought straight in the living rooms of Americans across the nation.

A wide variety of other commercial interests joined in. Even a wedding industry emerged, complete with etiquette guides, bridal registries, showers, and special magazines, encouraging consumerism and glamorizing marriage (Ford, 1999).

In fact, many psychologists and popular writers of the era insisted that personal happiness could not be achieved without marriage and children. They claimed that since a woman's nature and genetic makeup render her best suited for home management and child rearing, these roles should be her primary occupation. Not only must husband and children come first in her life, but she also must subordinate her own needs to theirs.

Moreover, in the late 1940s, Alfred Kinsey had documented a high incidence of premarital sex among young adults. In an effort to control this practice, psychologists, social workers, public officials, and others promulgated the message that health and satisfying sexual expression could only take place between husband and wife; they urged early marriages (May, 1988). Importantly, abortion was illegal in every state, and therapeutic abortions were increasingly restricted during the 1950s. Since single-parenthood was not socially acceptable, marriage and motherhood constituted the only viable option for white, middle-class single women who did engage in sex and become pregnant.

Educators, including those at the college level, began launching programs and curricula aimed at making women better wives and mothers. Courses in home economics, child development, interior decorating, gardening, and other domestic programs proliferated, especially at women's colleges (Chafe, 1972). Marriage also often meant the end of higher education for middle class females. Though larger numbers of women began college in the 1950s than in previous decades, only 37 percent actually graduated (Kaledin, 1984; Harvey, 1993).

Those who did not succumb to an exclusively domestic role through social pressures faced institutional barriers, legal restrictions, and business practices that limited their options considerably. Kaledin (1984) tells us that the work world "openly discriminated against women."

As suggested earlier, many economic opportunities were closed off to women after the war. For one, Congress had passed the Selective Service Act, which, in practice, granted veterans the right to displace women workers who had been hired during the war. In some jobs throughout the 1950s, including that of airline stewardess, the employee had to quit when she married; at age 35 she was forced to retire. William Chafe (1972) found that some large firms, such as Detroit Edison, Thompson Aircraft, and IBM, imposed regulations against hiring married women. In the vast majority of occupations, pregnant women were expected to quit; those who did not do so voluntarily were fired when their condition became noticeable. Lack of publicly-supported child care also kept many women out of the labor force. In fact, by early 1946 Congress had closed the limited number of nurseries that had been set up for working women during the war (May, 1988).

For the most part, except for nursing, teaching or social work, women's professional choices were severely limited. Institutional policies, including ceilings on the percentage of women admitted into professional schools, restricted their opportunities. For example, medical schools enforced a five percent quota on female admissions, most hospitals denied women residencies, and many medical associations refused them membership (Chafe, 1972; Kaledin, 1984). Professional women, who were disparaged as unfeminine and neurotic, often were forced to choose between family and career. Consequently, a decreasing percentage of women even aspired to professional occupations or pursued graduate study (Mintz & Kellogg, 1988). Barbara Deckard (1983) shows that the percentage of female college professors, scientists, mathematicians, and the like actually declined during the fifties.

The mix of social pressures, public policies, and institutional barriers produced impressive results:

> For the first time in more than 100 years, the age for motherhood and marriage fell, fertility increased, divorce rates declined and women's degree of educational parity with men dropped sharply (Coontz, 1992).

According to Steven Mintz and Susan Kellogg (1988), these patterns differed substantially from those both historically and in the years that followed. By 1959, nearly half of all brides had married before reaching nineteen years of age, and only 21 percent of women were single, compared to 31 percent in 1940 (Harvey, 1993). For every 1000 women between ages 15 and 24, there were 123 births (Kaledin, 1984). The birth rate for a third child doubled and for a fourth one tripled between 1940 and 1960 (Chafe, 1972). Moreover, children were born sooner after marriage and were closer in age than in prior years (May, 1988).

Harvey (1993) concludes, "women were expected to seek—and find—everything in marriage and family: love, identity, excitement, challenge, and fulfillment." Those who did not adhere to these social norms were labeled "unnatural," maladjusted, immature, deviant, and/or emotionally disturbed (Coontz, 1992). Like June Cleaver and other television moms of her ilk, wives were expected to be submissive and dependent on their husbands both emotionally and financially. Women could not borrow money in their own name, purchase a home, secure insurance or even sign a contract on their own. Self-supporting women were viewed suspiciously (May, 1988).

Yet, despite these constraints, female employment climbed through the 1950s, and there was a growing split between the image of the ideal middle-class household and the reality of women's lives (Mintz & Kellogg, 1988). By the end of the decade, women comprised approximately 35 percent of the labor force; forty percent of all women over sixteen had jobs (Chafe, 1972; Rowbotham, 1997). Significantly, a third of all wives were working, up from only 15 percent in 1940 (Kaledin, 1984).

Many women who had been fired or forced out of their war jobs either remained in or soon returned to the labor force, shifting into lower paid positions. As Harvey (1993) puts it: "Rosie the Riveter didn't necessarily leave the work force; she just moved—or was moved—over into clerical and sales jobs . . ." Most of these workers were married women over age 35 who had already fulfilled their role as mother—a significant minority was middle-class (Chafe, 1972). The number of females in the labor market over age 35 increased from 8.5 million to over 13 million from 1947 to 1956 (Kaledin, 1984).

Most single, middle-class women also worked, but it was viewed as a holding pattern until "Mr. Right" came along, presumably someone like Ward Cleaver. A large number of wives helped put their husbands through college and/or graduate or professional school. Many young married women stayed in the labor force until they became pregnant with their first child.

However, the traditional middle-class household of the 1950s was short-lived as these couples entered middle- and later, old age. In her study of 1950s suburban housewives, Harvey (1993)found that nearly all of the women experienced substantial changes in their lives during the two decades after the 1950s: some finished college; others went to work. As their children entered school, growing numbers of suburban moms began to move back into the paid labor force (Ford, 1999). Since most women had completed their families in their late twenties, they were not needed for full-time child care by the time they reached their mid-thirties (May, 1988). At the end of the 1950s, 39 percent of women with children aged 6 to 17 held jobs (May, 1988; Kaledin, 1984).

As Sheila Rowbotham (1997) explains:

> . . . the gap between assumption and actuality was being experienced by more and more white middle-class women . . . They were compelled to adapt to a cultural schizophrenia in which economic pressures pulled one way and prevailing attitudes the other. An uneasy compromise was struck: women's work was seen as helping out, a secondary income rather than a career.

Instead of challenging the cultural imperatives of the times, these women contended that they sought employment to improve their family's standard of living, pay off mortgages, send children to college, save for a vacation, or afford luxuries (Mintz & Kellogg, 1988). They did so while maintaining prevailing domestic power relationships, their main identity as homemakers and mothers, and their husband's role as primary breadwinner (Coontz, 1992; Rowbotham, 1997).

The labor market became strikingly gendered, as well (Deckard, 1983). The postwar boom had generated an ongoing demand for clerical and sales jobs, secretaries, and bank tellers, pink-collar work that was advertised in sex-segregated newspaper advertisements. Whether working for "extras" or out of economic need, women were relegated to these poorly paid positions, most of which offered few benefits or opportunities for advancement (Harvey, 1993). Within large firms, the percentage of women allowed to participate in company-run training programs, one of the primary routes for upward mobility, was often severely restricted (Kaledin, 1984).

Consequently, the Women's Bureau found that the median wage of working women in 1959 was 61 percent that of men (Deckard, 1983). And, according to "Womenpower in Today's World," a study by the National Manpower Council, women performing identical work as men earned one-third less (Kaledin, 1984).

Not all middle-class women, of course, joined the labor force full-time. May (1988) writes:

> As they moved into the expanding suburbs and settled in with their growing families, they put their best efforts into living out the post-war version of the American Dream.

By the end of the 1950s, about 70 percent of white American households looked similar to the Cleavers: a breadwinner, housewife, and two or more children (Mintz & Kellogg, 1988). Many suburban mothers worked intermittently and/or obtained part-time positions. Others pursued volunteer work in their community while their children were at school. A substantial percentage of women viewed being a housewife as their life work, and found immense satisfaction in rearing their children, serving as their husband's help mate, and participating in a wide variety of community and charity activities (Mintz & Kellogg, 1988; May, 1988). Coontz (1992) found evidence that the actual amount of time spent on child care and house work actually increased during the 1950s. The husband's income was viewed as the family wage; there was never any serious thought given to paying wives directly for their domestic work.

RACE AND THE 1950S EXPERIENCE

There was, of course, an underside to the 1950s culture, "The Other America," as described by Michael Harrington (1962) and others. Suburbia was not part of the African American experiences—few residents in these areas were single adults, elderly or members of any minority group (May, 1988; Mintz & Kellogg, 1988). While June Cleaver lived in an indistinct suburban neighborhood, her African American counterpart resided in an equally indistinct urban ghetto, a commuter ride away.

Beginning in the 1940s and accelerating in the 1950s, millions of African Americans had migrated from the south into urban areas, where they faced multiple problems such as overcrowding, crime, drugs, and oppressive discrimination. Legally sanctioned segregation in the south, as well as redlining, restrictive covenants and other forms of institutional racism in the north, prevented minorities from moving into the suburbs (Coontz, 1992). By 1960, a majority of African Americans resided in cities, mostly ghettos, as compared to three-quarters who lived in southern agricultural districts before the war.

Moreover, though the expansion of the economy in the 1950s generated growing real wages, by 1959, fifty-five percent of African American families lived in poverty compared to seventeen percent of whites (U.S. Census Bureau, 1998a). At the same time, there was a massive immigration of Puerto Ricans, most of whom found themselves in a similar plight.

Cultural expectations differed markedly: whether single or married, African American women, like their mothers and grandmothers, expected to work in order to support themselves and their family. Since employed African American men averaged about half the wages of white men in 1960, husbands rarely earned a family wage. In 1970, the labor force rate for married African American women was 70 percent compared to 49 percent for white wives (Daily, 1998). As Coontz (1992) reports: "The June Cleaver . . . homemaker role was not available to the more than 40 percent of black women with small children who worked outside the home." Nearly 25 percent of African American women headed their own households.

For the most part, however, African American women were the lowest paid employees in the country, barely earning subsistence wages; despite the fact that some were finding pink- and white-collar jobs for the first time, the vast majority worked as domestic servants or other subordinate sectors of the labor market (Rowbotham, 1997). In 1950, their income remained less than half that of white women (Kaledin, 1984). Both African American men and women also suffered steadily rising unemployment and periodic layoffs, contributing substantially to their dire economic situation.

On the other hand, according to May (1988), the popular imperative for motherhood was so pervasive during the 1950s that minorities and various ethnic groups had trends in fertility similar to those of middle-class whites living in suburbia. In addition, choices for poor, pregnant, unmarried African American women were even more limited than those for whites since they had less access to safe abortions (Harvey, 1993). Overall, African

American women experienced greater poverty, single parenthood and divorce, and a lower rate of re-marriage than their white counterparts (Coontz, 1993).

June Cleaver Reaches Eighty: Social Security and Older Women

The Social Security system, while initially structured in 1935, was shaped by the same middle-class, white values and household composition prominent in the 1950s: "traditional" families consisting of a primary male breadwinner and an unpaid female housewife/caregiver who is economically dependent on her husband; any income earned by the wive is not considered essential to the family unit. The design of the program measures work and productivity by male standards and stages throughout the life cycle. As Nancy Dailey (1998) suggests, retirement has been viewed, through the ideological lens of white men, as a single event. Yet women's pattern of employment differs—they tend to move in and out of the labor force, raising children and caring for their elders.

The system actually penalizes those who do unpaid caring work. Benefit levels are based both on wage levels and on continuous thirty-five year participation in the labor force; unwaged domestic responsibilities are calculated as zero earnings, thereby lowering any pensions earned by women in their own right. Consequently, only 20 percent of women, compared to sixty percent of men, have the minimum 35 years of covered earnings (GAO, 1997).

Because they experience lower average earnings as well as interrupted work histories, many women forego Social Security benefits based on their own record. In 1998, although two-thirds of female beneficiaries earned benefits as workers, half of them—who were dually entitled—received the higher spousal amounts (SSCA, 1999a,b).

As a result most married women, regardless of whether they participated in the labor force, collect auxiliary pensions based on their husbands' wage records. When they become widowed or divorced, the vast majority depend on these pensions for nearly all of their financial support. And there is no minimum benefit that meets their basic needs. Consequently, older women are more likely than older men to live in absolute as well as relative poverty. Nearly twenty-five percent of all single elderly females have incomes below the official poverty level—$7,800 in 1998 (U.S. Census Bureau, 1998b); they comprise 73 percent of the aged poverty population.

So whatever happened to June Cleaver? Her life might have taken one of several paths as she aged, relegating her to a number of divergent economic circumstances. As did many of her white middle-class contemporaries, June could have remained a housewife throughout the decades, retiring with her husband, when he reached age 65, to a warm climate.

Today, they would be economically comfortable, presumably with some savings and an annuity from his private pension. In fact, forty-one percent of older white couples receive revenue from a private pension, and 78 percent from their assets (SSA, 1999a). Their income from Social Security alone, consisting of Ward's primary benefit and June's fifty percent dependent's allowance, would be about $15,712 in 1998, the median for white couples (SSA, 1999b); this amount would be actuarially reduced if Ward retired at age 62, the average age for men (Dailey, 1998). Given their potential access to such diverse sources of support, only 5 percent of all older married white women are poor (SSCA, 1999b).

Even if June had entered the labor force, either full or part-time, after her children went to school, as suggested earlier it most likely would have been in low-wage clerical, sales or service work. It is doubtful she would qualify for a private pension, and she would receive very little even if she did. Moreover, though she would have contributed thousands of dollars into the Social Security System, her benefit would be exactly the same amount as if she had not worked at all. As one observer reports, Social Security imposes some of the heaviest marginal tax rates on working women (SSCA, 1999a).

Most probably, however, at age 80 June is widowed, living alone, and struggling to support herself on Social Security. Women, whose average longevity is greater than men, tend to outlive their husbands. At birth, the life expectancy for white men and women is 74 and 80, respectively. For whites reaching age 65, men can expect to live another 16 years compared to 20 years for women (GAO, 1996).

Significantly, forty percent of single women depend on Social Security for 90 percent of their total income; for twenty-five percent, the program is their only source of support (SSCA, 1996; GAO, 1997). If Ward had died after retirement, the odds are that June's benefit would be reduced to approximately $8,824, the median income for nonmarried white beneficiaries (SSA, 1999b). His death at a much earlier age would result in measurably lower amounts.

It is questionable whether she is relying on Ward's private pension for significant support, even if he had one; if the annuity was not terminated upon hies death, it would be providing her, as a surviving spouse, only about half of the original amount, averaging around $3,468 (SSCA, 1999a; SSA, 1999c). And these pensions are vulnerable to inflation since they generally are not indexed to the rising cost of living. Moreover, as with many widows, she may have been forced to slowly spend down any assets she and Ward had accumulated (SSCA, 1999a).

Currently there are 1.4 million aged widows, approximately 18 percent of the total, who live below the poverty level (SSCA, 1999b). As Colette Browne (1998) points out, more than half of the widows living in poverty were not poor before the death of their husband.

Suppose, however, that after thirty or more years together, June and Ward had dissolved their marriage. Underneath "the image of domestic tranquility celebrated in the popular media" were many unhappy couples (Mintz & Kellogg, 1988). Fearing social ostracism and/or maladjusted children, few individuals viewed splitting up as a viable option during the early years of their marriage. However, according to several analysts, from twenty-five to thirty-three percent of marriages forged in the 1950s eventually did end in divorce (Coontz, 1992; Mintz & Kellogg, 1988).

In her fifties, having spent her years promoting Ward's career, caring for the family, volunteering for charities, and/or working at low-paid jobs, June would have had limited earning ability. At age 60, she would become eligible for half of her ex-husband's Social Security benefit when he decided to retire, and his widow's pension if he died. On average, divorced women received about $4,365 from the program in 1998 (SSA, 1999d). She might secure a portion of whatever assets the couple had accumulated together, and perhaps a piece of his private pension if she is successful in court. About 22 percent of divorced aged women experience an impoverished old age SSCA, 1999b).

As Mintz and Kellogg (1988) indicate:

> The fifties ideal of a marital partnership was based on the assumption of a wife's role as hostess and consort. This was essential for the smooth running of the household and for the promotion of her husband's career.

Many men were able to rise in the business and professional worlds partly because of their wives' social functions (Kessler-Harris, 1981). Ward would be well-situated by his fifties for a decent retirement income.

Regardless of her current status, the odds are that June had some responsibilities for elder care during her middle-age years or later, further disadvantaging her position in the labor force and any future Social Security benefits in her own right. More than one in four families, primarily women, are involved in caring for an older relative (Gould, 1999); many now spend more years tending aging parents than they do raising children (Abel, 1991; Gannon, 1999).

In a few years, she will need help herself; approximately half of the elderly over age eighty-five require assistance with at least some activities of daily living (Baines, Evans, & Neysmith, 1995). Frail older men generally receive hands-on aid from their wives. Despite a lifetime of providing care to others, women are more at risk than men of lacking any assistance for themselves (Hooyman, 1999). At the more advanced ages, elderly women tend to live alone, and consequently when they become chronically ill and dependent have difficulty remaining in their own homes. If June's income is typical of widowed or divorced older women, she will not have the resources for purchasing sufficient help privately, and if she does, will deplete her assets in a few years.

Nor will she be entitled to publicly supported home and community care. Medicaid, the major financial source for government long-term care, pays primarily for nursing homes, and only after residents exhaust any of their accumulated assets. Unless single women can rely on their adult children—for the most part daughters—to attend to their needs, they often end up in institutions. June must depend on the assistance of her two sons, or more likely that of her daughters-in-law, if she is to avoid institutionalization. Nearly one-quarter of people age eighty-five and over, mostly unmarried females, reside in a nursing home (Birenbaum, 1995).

And June Cleaver's African American female counterpart? It is questionable whether she reached age eighty: her life expectancy at birth was 74 years. However, if she attained age 65, she could have expected to live, on average, another 18 years. (African American men have a life expectancy of 64 and average only 14 more years at age 65, GAO, 1996).

Most likely, prior to retirement she was a single head of household who had worked for forth years or more at low wages. Because of the regressive nature of the Social Security payroll tax, she had paid more in payroll taxes during this period than in income taxes. At age 80, there is a good chance that she is unmarried—fifty-four percent of all older African Americans are single females—and dependent on her own worker's Social Security benefit, an amount that is probably less than that of a widow of a high earner, such as June Cleaver. In 1998, single African American women averaged $6,813 annually from Social Security while married African American couples obtained $12,700 (SSA, 1999b). Nearly 7.8 million older women, mostly immigrants of color, receive no Social Security benefits at all due to their work as domestics (Browne, 1998).

Only a small number of widowed, divorced or never married female African Americans have income from assets or private pensions 19 percent and 13 percent, respectively (SSA, 1999a). Overall, they experience a poverty rate of over 30 percent (SSCA 1999a).

Conclusion

Political leaders in the twenty-first century are focusing on strengthening the financial integrity of the Social Security program. Most recommendations maintain its current design but tinker with the benefit formula. However, by solving the economic problems faced by the system, certain changes potentially could worsen the financial situation of vulnerable groups.

Raising the normal and/or early retirement age, for example, translates into a benefit cut for those in poor health, limited job prospects, and an already inadequate retirement income, particularly older minorities (GAO, 1996). Increasing the period of time for calculating benefits means more zero years, and therefore lower benefits for women who take time out for child care, and increasingly to assist their elderly parents. Lowering cost-of-living adjustments, or other across-the-board reductions, burdens women, minorities and other low-income elderly the most, especially those who are hovering at the poverty level. Any cuts in dependent benefits, of course, would disadvantage females.

Raising payroll taxes is another strategy that seeks to restore the long-term solvency of the system while maintaining its traditional structure. This solution would increase the regressive aspect of our federal taxes even further, burdening those with the lowest wages.

Other public officials and analysts concentrate on restructuring the system, urging some form of privatization. Individual accounts, for instance, would move the program away from its current emphasis on defined benefits toward a defined contribution system, advantaging high-income earners (GAO, 1999). Such an approach stresses individual equity over income adequacy; while there is greater potential for higher rates of return (and risk), it would be difficult to maintain the progressive benefit formula that helps working women, especially women of color. Individual accounts also do not protect against inflation, again harming women disproportionately since they tend to live longer than men (SSCA, 1999a). Adequate support for dependents and survivors could be in jeopardy as well, especially if the breadwinner has had more than one wife (SSCA, 1999b).

Despite public debate on the subject, there appears to be only limited concern over the adverse impact of various reform proposals on single older women and minorities. There is even less interest in improving their economic situation; none o the recent Social Security reform packages strives to better meet the financial needs of disadvantaged sectors of our population. Such proposals could include a wage-indexed, adequate minimum benefit to keep older women out of poverty (SSCA, 1999a), an increase in the allowable years for caregiving, earnings sharing between couples, and exempting a portion of wages from Social Security taxes. Moreover, some solutions that could measurably improve the solvency of the program without affecting low-income wage earners are rarely considered (i.e., expanding the tax base to include assets and other sources of individual wealth). If we ensure the system's stability without enhancing features to protect single women, African Americans and other economically deprived groups, June Cleaver's granddaughter could find herself and her African American friends in similarly adverse financial circumstances.

Bibliography

Abel, E. K. (1991). *Who cares for the elderly?: Public policy and the experiences of adult daughters.* Philadelphia: Temple University Press.

Baines, C., Evans, P., & Neysmith, S. (1998). Women's caring: Work expanding, state contracting. In C. Baines, P. Evans, & S. Neysmith (Eds.), *Women's caring: feminist perspectives on social welfare,*pp. 3–22. New York: Oxford University Press.

Birenbaum, A. (1995). *Putting health care on the national agenda.* Westport, CT: Praeger.

Brody, E. (1995). Prospects for family caregiving: Response to change, continuity and diversity. In R. Kane & J. Penrod (Eds.), *Family caregiving in an aging society.* Thousand Oaks, CA: Sage.

Browne, C. V. (1998). *Women, feminism and aging.* New York: Springer.

Chafe, W. (1972). *The American woman: Her changing social, economic and political roles 1920–1970.* New York: Oxford University Press.

Coontz, S. (1992). *The way we never were: American families and the nostalgia trap.* New York: Basic Books.

Dailey, N. (1998). *When baby boom women retire.* Westport, CT: Greenwood.

Deckard, B. S. (1983). *The women's movement.* New York: Harper & Row.

Ford, C. B. (1999). *The girls: Jewish women of Brownsville, Brooklyn 1940–1995.* Albany: State University of New York Press.

Gannon, L. G. (1999). *Women and aging: Transcending the myths.* New York: Routledge.

Gould, J. Ed. (1999). *Dutiful daughters: Caring for our parents as they grow old.* Seattle: Seal.

Harrington, M. (1962). *The other America: Poverty in the United States.* Baltimore: Penguin.

Harvey, B. (1993). *The fifties: A woman's oral history.* New York: Harper Collins.

Hooyman, N. R. (1999). Research on older women: Where is feminism. *The Gerontologist,* 39:115–18.

Kaledin, E. (1984). *American women in the 1950s: Mothers and more.* New York: G. K. Hall.

Kessler-Harris, A. (1981). *Women have always worked.* Old Westbury, NY: The Feminist Press.

May, E. T. (1988). *Homeward bound: American families in the cold war era.* New York: Basic Books.

Mintz, S. & Kellogg, S. (1988). *Domestic revolutions: A social history of American family life.* New York: Free Press.

Rowbotham, S. (1997). *A century of women.* New York: Penguin.

Social Security Administration (SSA). (1999a). Income sources by age, sex, and marital status: Percent of aged units 55 or older with money income from specific sources 1998. *Social Security Bulletin,* Annual Statistical Supplement, Washington: Government Printing Office.

Social Security Administration (SSA). (1999b). Income from social security benefits by sex, marital status, race, and hispanic origin: percent of aged units 65 or older 1998. *Social Security Bulletin,* Annual Statistical Supplement. Washington: Government Printing Office.

Social Security Administration (SSA). (1999c). Income from private pensions or annuities by sex and marital status: Percentage distribution of persons aged 65 or older 1998. *Social Security Bulletin,* Annual Statistical Supplement, Washington: Government Printing Office.

Social Security Administration (SSA). (1999d). Table 6.D3, Number and average monthly benefit for wives and husbands, by age and sex 1998. *Social Security Bulletin,* Annual Statistical Supplement. Washington: Government Printing Office.

U.S. Census Bureau. (1998a). Current population survey, Table 2. Poverty status of people by family relationship, race, and Hispanic origin 1959–1990. Washington: Government Printing Office.

U.S. Census Bureau. (1998ab. Current population survey, Table 3.E1. Weighted average poverty thresholds for nonfarm families of specified size 1959–1998. Washington: Government Printing Office.

U.S. General Accounting Office (GAO). [1999]. *Social security: Criteria for evaluating social security reform proposals.* Testimony before the subcommittee on social security, committee on ways and means (March). Washington: Government Printing Office.

U.S. General Accounting Office (GAO). [1997]. *Social security reform: implications for the financial well being of women.* Statement by Jane L. Ross (April). Washington: Government Printing Office.

U.S. General Accounting Office (GAO). [1996]. *Social security: Issues involving benefit equity for working women* (April). Washington: Government Printing Office.

U.S. Senate. (1999a). Hearings before the special committee on aging (SSCA), (February). *Women and social security reform: Are individual accounts the answer?* 106th Cong. 1st sess., Washington: Government Printing Office.

U.S. Senate. (1999b). Hearings before the special committee on Aging (SSCA), (June). *The impact of social security reform on women* 106th Cong. 1st sess., Washington: Government Printing Office.

Sex Offenders: Myths and Facts

24

CHAPTER

Catherine Piliero-Surbeck, Ph.D.

Myths

There are many myths in our society about sexual offenders and the crimes they commit. Lack of accurate information, stereotypes of sex offenders and victims, and media portrayal of sex crimes contribute to these myths. Some commonly held misperceptions about sex offenses are that:

- they occur as a result of an uncontrollable sexual urge, or due to severe mental disorders;
- sex offenders can be recognized by the way they look. For example, they are men in trenchcoats who loiter in public bathrooms and schoolyards, or they are men considered too unattractive to find a consenting sexual partner;
- gay men pose a special risk to children because they are prone to molesting boys;
- most sex offenses occur in dark, isolated places against women walking alone;
- men with "mental deficiencies," such as mental retardation, are more prone to sexual aggression than "normal" men;
- sex offenders are men and their victims are women or girls; and
- rape is not an act of sex but of violence.

Contrary to these beliefs, sex offenders are not usually "crazed" or psychotic attackers who are driven by uncontrollable sexual urges. Nor are individuals with mental retardation or "mental deficiencies" more prone to commit sex offenses than those without mental handicaps. In fact, these groups, the mentally retarded and mentally ill, are more likely to be *victims* of sexual abuse, rather than perpetrators. Regarding gender, more sex offenders are male than female, but women do commit acts of sexual aggression, and are increasingly being recognized in the courts as sex offenders. This writer has worked with

Reprinted by permission of Catherine Piliero-Surbeck.

women who have molested children, raped adolescents and committed incest. In terms of the gender of victims, it is important to recognize that both males and females are sexually abused. The sexual abuse of males is not uncommon, and males are most at risk for sexual abuse during their late childhood and early adolescent years. Some experts in the field of sexual abuse consider boys to be at almost equal risk as girls. In a 1994 study of sex offenders conducted by this writer, it was found that almost half (47%) of the victims abused by the offenders in the study were male. This is consistent with a recent survey conducted by this writer of the victim gender patterns of child molesters. This survey found nearly equal rates of sexual abuse against male and female children.

Facts

Sex offenders can be persons of either gender. They can come from lower, middle or upper social classes. They can have advanced education and work in elite, respected professions, or they can be poorly educated and work in blue-collar jobs. They are not more likely to be homosexual than heterosexual. A homosexual sexual orientation is not considered a "risk factor" for sexual aggression, and is not associated with a proclivity to molest or rape. Far more sex offenders are heterosexual than homosexual. Even men who molest boys are not necessarily homosexual, as they may be married to women or have girlfriends. Sex offenders cannot be identified on thee basis gender, educational level, physical appearance, social class or sexual orientation. They are not typically "sex maniacs" who have no control over their sexual urges.

Sex offenders *are* people who have the ability to b aroused and gratified by sexual activities that are against the law, and which usually pose some type of harm to others. These acts include child molestation, rape, indecent exposure, voyeurism or "peeping," frotteurism (rubbing of the genitals against someone's private parts in a crowded place), incest, sexual contact with animals, obscene telephone calls, necrophilia (sexual contact with corpses), and stalking. It is a misnomer to call rape (or other acts of sexual aggression) an acto of violence, and not an act of sex. By their very nature, sex offenses are sexual acts. Rapists and other sex offenders commit their assault by abusing the sexual body parts of their victims, and it is often associated with sexual arousal and gratification for the offender. Many use the memories of the sexual offense as the basis of fantasies to which they masturbate and ejaculate afterward. This is not to minimize the violent nature of sexual abuse, or the roles of anger, violence and aggression. Emotions of anger, hatred, rage, and aggression often underlie sex offenses and contribute to the acting out of sexual abuse. In fact, physical aggression, poorly managed anger and impulsive expressions of anger can be risk factors for sexual offense. Anger management problems and misdirected rage are common traits among sex offenders. Many were sexually abused (at least 60%) prior to becoming perpetrators. Even more have histories of physical abuse and neglect. Their feelings about their own abuse are often unresolved and displaced onto others through sexual aggression. There are also issues of control, power and domination that contribute to sexual aggression. Many sex offenders derive a sense of ego strength and self-esteem by being able to control and dominate their victims. However, it is a fallacy that sex offenses are not sexual acts. To minimize the sexual aspects of these crimes is to ignore a crucial area that requires close attention in therapy, that is, the role of sexual fantasies and arousal response patterns. One of the characteristics shared by most sex offenders is that *they are sexually aroused and often gratified by their acts of sexual abuse.* If the acts were not sexually arousing and gratifying, they would not be as likely to be repeated. Another common trait shared by most sex offenders is that they are prone to repeat their crimes without special intervention and supervision. Most sex offenses are the products of cycles that involve a build-up of negative emotion and sexual arousal. There are also phases in the cycle called "cruising" (going out to locate a victim) and "grooming" (preparing the victim for assault, the so-called "buttering up phase" when the victim's trust is obtained and they are lured into situations conductive to abuse). Acting out the sexual assault is another phase of the cycle. And the final cycle, or the "post-assault" phase, consists of all the behaviors, fantasies and thoughts the offender has after the act of sexual abuse. Often, masturbation to fantasies of the assault takes place in the post-assault phase. These cycles are likely to repeat themselves, and in some cases, they become compulsive and habitual, unless intervention occurs.

The early part of this paper highlighted the commonly believed myths about sex offenders and who sex offenders *are not.* The following list highlights some facts about sex offenders, the common characteristics that many share, and who *they are:*

- Most sex offenders begin their cycles of assault during adolescence, sometimes even earlier.
- Most sex offenders have been physically, sexually or emotionally abused prior to becoming perpetrators.
- Some sex offenders are sexually aroused by the pain and suffering they cause to their victims, so called sadistic offenders. Others are aroused in spite of it.
- Most victims of sexual offense know the offender. Most offenses take place in the home of either the victim or the perpetrator.
- Adolescent sex offenders are most likely to commit acts of sexual abuse during babysitting situations.
- Fire-setting, animal cruelty, truancy, pre-mature use of pornography and physical aggression are common behavior problems among adolescent sex offenders.
- Sex offenders are more commonly diagnosed with character disorders or personality disorders, rather than with severe mental disorders.
- Many sex offenders aggressively deny their offenses when caught and are prone to blame their victims or other external sources for their problems.
- Fear, control and power are often used as weapons by scx offenders to manipulate or coerce their victims.

- Psychopathic sex offenders, exhibit impulsive, opportunistic habits. They take pride in tricking, conning and manipulating their victims to get what they want. They have a belief system of "entitlement." They show no signs of conscience. They are indifferent to the harm they cause. And they may use their interpersonal relationships, their jobs, or their status to gain access to potential victims.

Treatment

The treatment approaches most often endorsed in the research literature are cognitive-behavioral and social skills-based. Specific techniques include relapse prevention training, covert sensitization, victim empathy training and arousal re-conditioning. *Relapse prevention* teaches offenders self-control skills for managing sexual urges. It also teaches about the cycles of sexual assault and the triggers for re-offense. Offenders learn to avoid high-risk situations to reduce the chance for relapse. *Covert sensitization* is a treatment intervention that has three goals. It teaches offenders to recognize the antecedent factors that can lead to assault; it teaches offenders to pair natural negative consequences with the assault and with deviant sexual fantasies; and it teaches offenders appropriate outlets for the feelings that can lead to assault. *Victim empathy* training challenges the cognitive distortions, rape myths and defense mechanisms sex offenders use to justify their behavior and minimize the impact of the assault on their victims. It teaches them about the psychological and sexual harm that victims experience after assault. It teaches offenders to assume full responsibility for their actions, and fosters empathy for those they have harmed. It is considered one of the most important aspects of sex offender therapy. *Arousal re-conditioning* addresses the role of sexual fantasies and deviant sexual response patterns. Through the use of masturbation exercises, it teaches offenders to associate sexual pleasure with healthy sexual fantasies of age-appropriate consensual sex, and negative consequences with fantasies of deviant sex.

Sex education and social skills training are also part of treatment. Medication may be used when deviant sexual urges are compulsive and resistant to psychotherapy along. Certain anti-depressants, such as Prozac, have been used with some success in controlling deviant obsessive-compulsive sexual behaviors. Libido-reducing drugs, such as Depo-Provera, have been used with greater success, and work by reducing the level of testosterone (the sex drive hormone) in the blood.

Sex offender therapy is best provided in group settings. Group treatment is considered more effective than individual therapy. Confrontation by the peer group, and also the support of the peer group, is highly effective in resolving the denial that most offenders present with in the early stages of therapy. The intensive phase of treatment can be expected to last an average of 18 months, but sex offenders often require ongoing therapeutic maintenance after they complete treatment. There is no cure for sexual offending. A reasonable expectation is that sex offenders will learn the self-control skills necessary for relapse prevention, but they are not considered cured, even after completing treatment successfully. It is important that sex offenders have access to treatment, either in prison if they are incarcerated, or in the community if they are probationed or paroled. Those who are highly motivated to rehabilitate themselves, who are fully accountable for their offenses, and who have the support of families and treatment resources, will have the best prognosis for rehabilitation and successful adjustment in the community.

Complexities of Discussing the Erotic Lives of People with Disabilities

25

CHAPTER

Sandy O'Neill, Ph.D. (cand.)

Introduction

Many current textbooks on human sexuality include short sections discussing the matter of sexuality and people with disabilities. In preparing to write this article I reviewed several of them specifically from what I'll refer to as a disability rights perspective. Not surprisingly, I found some textbooks better than others. Yet, as a disabled person, I came away from this research troubled not so much by these specific visible sections discussing people with disabilities having sexual lives but by both our presences and our absences in many other places throughout these books.

For instance, few photographs or other illustrations include people with disabilities in any section except those specifically discussing this subject. One unfortunate exception is a text that in a section on problems encountered in pregnancy discusses chromosomal "abnormalities" as part of a list including toxemia, RH incompatibility, etc. A small photo of a boy with Down's Syndrome is included in a column of definitions of terms such as toxemia and eclampsia. The child's picture is unintentionally captioned in a manner that suggests he is a syndrome![1] Other introductory texts produce similar jarring juxtapositions in attempting to analyze this relationship of disability and sexuality.

The absence of a specific disability rights framework shows up particularly in accounts of the history of sexology. Disabled people are not generally mentioned. Yet, the fact of disability along with racist, ethnocentric views were central to the development of eugenics, which had an influential role in developing this and other social 'science' disciplines.

Reprinted by permission of Sandy O'Neill.
[1]Carroll, Janell L. and Wolpe, Paul Root, Sexuality and Gender in Society, Harper Collins College Publishers, 1996, p. 391–94.

This short article obviously cannot take up each issue in depth. Rather, I would invite the reader to think of some of the issues that arise in societal conceptions of disability/illness particularly as they pertain to the topic of sexuality. Posing the following questions from an anthropological standpoint conscious of cultural issues of power, oppression and liberation begins to get more clarity about the complex nature of intertwining sexology studies with a disability rights/disability studies perspective. Figuratively stepping back to situate larger questions of the role of disability in society in general places those specifically dealing with sexuality in a different, more differentiated conceptual framework.

These questions to be discussed include:

- What is a disability?
- How can we define people with disabilities?
- What is a disability studies/disability rights perspective?
- What types of societal conceptions and/or misconceptions about and expectations of people with disabilities might shape our ideas about them/us?
- Are people with disabilities culturally perceived as being asexual (non and/or under interested in sex) or in being over-sexed?
- Which stereotypes about disabled people affect views on their/our sexuality?
- What is it that mandates including discussions of disability issues in human sexuality texts and courses?
- How does including people with disabilities in thinking about sex change notions of sexuality and the erotic?
- A final section points the interested reader toward some literature mentioned throughout this article.

To avoid disappointments, I'll note here that readers who are seeking information on the how-tos of sex with people with a variety of disabilities will not find that information here. It can be gathered in a number of places in libraries, sex research programs, or from sexual therapists and most clearly from people with disabilities themselves. This article starts from a conception that people with disabilities are sexual beings despite societal prejudices and misgivings that have had the effect of making a specific discourse on disability and sex necessary.

Defining Disability

Defining disability moves into contested territory from several angles. Who defines who is disabled What does it mean to identify as such when some groups particularly from Deaf communities who are commonly thought of as disabled reject that definition of themselves? Those working for disability rights haven't always been and won't always be as clear as might be desired about these definitions either. Often terms such as able-bodyism are used not to define disability per se but to define the prejudices often expressed toward us. However, this terminology usually excludes those with mental or emotional disabilities from the group being considered. (This, of course, depends quite a bit on one's understanding of both the causation of these conditions and beliefs about defining the body and body/mind connections. See further reading for more material on this.)

I think it is most wise to see or define disability as a permeable category with self-definition as the major criterion, more so than in other social/political identity questions. Self-definition of disability can change depending on people's location in other cultural points as well. For example, a Japanese man who is a friend of mine is color blind and an artist. In Japan, he found his color-blindness to be a disability whereas here he doesn't. Another example is a Nicaraguan friend who is unable to have children; she considers this a disability.

In life people with some conditions may move in and out of being and/or identifying as disabled. Or people may become disabled for a lengthy time but return to "normal" status. There is a great deal of variation among this category ranging from people who are born with disabilities to those (the majority) who acquire them later. Differences also show up in distinctions between observable or noticeable disabilities and non-noticeable ones, between physical and emotional and/or developmental differences.

It's sometimes useful to break disability down to types such as physical disabilities, including mobility impairment,s hearing, sight, etc, and chronic diseases. Also, there are learning disabilities, developmental disabilities and emotional disabilities. Additionally, I include those with substance abuse addictions as members of the disabled population. Not everyone discussing disability does so. The government agencies involved in defining who is and isn't eligible for various benefits often define disability quite narrowly as many people with disabilities can attest to.

To make things even more complex, here in the United States we are immersed in a culture geared toward diagnosing and thereby medicalizing an increasing number of problems. For example, there has been a huge increase in diagnosing attention deficit disorders in children and all types of addiction in teenagers and young adults over the past 15 to 20 years. The wide penetration of a psychologized viewpoint of human behavior can be seen in the broad usage of terms like "road-rage" and the analysis of this and other phenomena as particularized forms of stress reactions. Guests on popular TV talk shows confidently attribute problems in their lives to a lack of self-esteem on their part.

This section in looking at ways to define disability and who is disabled is meant only to give an indication of some of the ways in which these classifications are made and, more important, to begin to get a grasp of the wide variety of people signified when discussing disability issues. Unfortunately, the complexities of defining disabilities are too often used as a rationale to dismiss questions of disability and ableism as a critical area of discourse.

Ableism and Disability Rights

The emergence of a disability rights movement and the concomitant creation of disability studies are important to understand in continuing to ask how we define the questions of disability identity. I think the clearest summation of the diverse viewpoints being put forward from these perspectives is that disability rights/studies rejects the medical definition of disability and posits that disability is not an individual medical or psychological problem. Rather disability is defined as a social problem, which is created and institutionalized by social attitudes and prejudices.

It is of some interest to note that the creation of disability studies curricula in some university departments is proceeding even while there is a popular conception that passage of laws, especially the Americans with Disabilities Act, have somehow already remedied any disparity in access to goods, services, education, housing, etc. also play into this. Unfortunately, the realities of life for many of us who identify as people with disabilities are still marked by the frustrations of encountering barriers, both physical and attitudinal, in our daily lives. Consider for example the social situation of many young people. Get-togethers of people in their early 20s often take place at bars or cafes. Even if one can get in the door, the percentage of accessible bathrooms is quite low.

On a larger social plane, few people seem to even know the history of genocide of people with disabilities. The murders, sterilizations and other forms of persecution directed at people with disabilities in Nazi Germany during the Third Reich are often omitted from history books. Yet, research shows that the idea of ridding the population of people with disabilities wasn't met with total shock anywhere in the world. In fact, eugenic ideology did not arise in Germany but was largely imported from the United States and England.

The two examples above obviously differ greatly in severity. Yet, this can be the nature of any specific social oppression. In defining and discussing the oppression of people with disabilities in diversity workshops and classes, I am often struck by how quickly comments about our own mortality come to the surface. This is probably a good part of the explanation of some of the fear and hatred expressed toward us. My fears are aroused more by the fact that people don't want to hear about the reality but are keenly interested in the disabilities themselves, which are simply different ways of being than that which is culturally dominant or normalized.

In defining ableism here as the systematic, pervasive, routinized, institutionalized mistreatment of people with disabilities, I am drawing on a model used in work aimed toward "unlearning" oppression that explores the subjective conditions of emancipation and domination and the ways in which social realities construct psychological realities. I've found the effective practice emanating from liberation theory to be a vital and necessary one for many reasons. Too often, in its concentration on the individual, the field of psychology ignores the manner in which societal relations of inequality affect people intrapsychically. Paradoxically, social movements can often dismiss the necessity of addressing subjective aspects of oppression thereby missing part of the problem.

This theory is rooted in a version of Critical Theory.[2] It contextualizes inter and intra psychological phenomenon. As in the disability rights/studies perspectives, power distribution and issues arising from this area seen as socially constructed products of society, while each particularized type of oppression is defined as the systematic, routinized, institutionalized, pervasive mistreatment of the targeted group based on their membership in that group. Oppressing others then is not viewed as innate in anyone. The differences in human beings are not responsible for oppression. Rather, everyone is conditioned to accept particular roles in society in relation to the power dynamics that are in operation at the particular sites or intersections of various cultural and subcultural groupings. This conditioning or socialization is understood as painful for everyone, no matter which side of the equation they are on in any particular grouping. (This is not in any way interpreted as excusing or ameliorating the horrors of oppression but a way to get at the source of prejudices.)

Conditioning to accept imbalances in power arrangements occurs in childhood. In a broader academic sense, it is part and parcel of the inescapable enculturation process of humanity. Everyone individually and in social groupings resists being oppressed and at least initially resists being oppressors. Yet, the circulation of misinformation about the targeted groups is ever present throughout society, both in dominant culture and in subcultures. The form that the oppression resulting from the misinformation takes is different for those targeted than from those in the dominant group. Internalized oppression is the form that this takes for those in target groups. This is a construct associated with the Frankfurt School and not a pathologizing form as presented in some humanist psychologies.

Delineating hierarchies of oppression is not seen as usually useful in any effort toward liberation. Nor is there a quantifying of pains or oppressions. I wouldn't say that since I'm oppressed as a woman and by being poor and disabled I am not only triply oppressed but am not capable of oppressing anyone else/any other group so I do not need to explore where and how I've not only been exposed to racism, but as a Euro- or white American, I have played a part, even passively and unwillingly in perpetuating racist thinking. Rather, although no one likes being regarded as an oppressor, I am called upon to investigate and oppose racism as an ally. No group can fully gain their liberation while others are oppressed.

There are differences between active right-wing oppression and subtle forms. The subtle forms though can and have led to a passive attitude toward the oppression of others, either by not seeing the oppression or acting to stop it. Individual or specific types of oppressions reinforce each other and are often intertwined.

---

[2]Often referred to as the Frankfurt School and/or Western Marxism. This work is located more precisely as an extension of the work that is known or identified as that of the first-generation Frankfurt school with an openness to both a postmodern variant and a multicultural emphasis.

Oppression that is learned can be unlearned. People can decide either altruistically or in recognition of their own interests to change their views/consciousness and act to stop oppression. The following exercise is one I've developed to get at the specific nature of ableism. In simplified form, it represents the breadth of the oppression. I think most people will find one or another portion of it resonates with some cultural message they have been exposed to.

Exercise Exploring Ableism

PEOPLE WITHOUT DISABILITIES

Think about whether you've ever thought that:

- you need to be tough on disabled people so they'll learn independence
- disabled are just too needy and dependent
- you'd rather be dead than blind or in a wheelchair
- (told) a disabled person how much you admire him/her because you couldn't deal with their life
- if people w/disabilities took better care of themselves they wouldn't be in this shape
- wished a friend or relative w/terminal or degenerative condition would hurry up and die
- ever chosen not to get close to person because he or she had disabilities
- ever felt really frightened about your body decaying
- been afraid of dying
- been afraid of becoming disabled
- felt confused about whether or not to help a person with disabilities
- felt confused about how to respond to advocates of civil rights for people with disabilities
- lived, worked, played, or prayed in inaccessible (segregated) places?

Think about the following: Where did you learn ableism? How did you resist? How have you been an ally? Think about how your own fears of becoming disabled may determine your relationship to the topic.

PEOPLE WITH DISABILITIES

Think about whether you've ever:

- heard people call you a cripple
- had teachers or bosses give you a hard time about needing time off or extra time on projects for medical reasons
- lost a job/place in a school/ because of your disabilities
- gotten a lot of unwanted advice about caring for yourself

- felt it was your own fault for getting sick
- felt you had to hide your disability even when it meant more pain or worsening of your condition.
- been refused housing
- felt that you were not really welcome if you make a fuss about having your needs met
- been upset when friends tolerated your being discriminated against
- felt you constantly had to prove how independent you are.

Many more things could have been chosen. There are entire areas of emerging literature focused on the specific nature of ableism and the emergence of disability cultures. A few titles of articles and books dealing with social theories of liberation and oppression, multi-cultural resources are included in the final section. We can now turn to some of the specific intersections of human sexuality and disability studies.

Nowhere or Everywhere? Too Little or Too Much?

I now will turn back to the questions posed in the introduction, utilizing the framework we are developing to problematize some notions of 'disabled sexuality.' Particularly, we'll briefly explore the question of whether people with disabilities are depicted only as asexual beings or whether there are more complex messages being expressed. By pulling examples both from current popular culture and the more arcane literature of sexual dysfunction, we can, in simple form, begin to pinpoint some of the specific stereotypes about disabled people's sexuality.

When thinking about how disability in general is represented in mainstream culture or even in some alternative or counter-cultural formats, I think the first "common sense" instinct is to conclude that people with disability are generally desexualized by society just as we are absent from the scene more often than we are included. This is true even in product advertisements. Disabled actors are rarely cast in movies or on TV unless the disability is the topic of the show.

One exception to this is the Carrie Weaver character on NBC's ER. Her disability is visible but not explained. Her character defies the sweetness stereotype and goes more in the direction of portraying the opposite stereotype of disabled people as bitter, frustrated individuals as she humorlessly pursues efficiency at the cost of relations with her coworkers. Yet, Carrie is shown at times as insecure, probably due to the fact that she was abandoned by her birth mother for not being "perfect."

Perhaps the most discussed character among disability rights groups over the past couple of years is not a TV character but a new friend of that popular sexual icon, Barbie. Barbie's new friend, Share-A-Smile Becky, fits more easily into the mold of an asexual character than the irascible Doctor Weaver. Becky, you unlike Barbie's numerous other friends, carries the introductory Share a Smile moniker appropriate for images of long-suffering but brave disabled girls, is the school photographer. While the "normal" girls prepare frantically for their big proms and parties, Becky loads another role of film. She won't need any of those revealing clothes the others wear. And, of course, Mattel's first version of Becky's wheelchair wouldn't fit in Barbie's house!

Many depictions of the desexualized disabled come to mind. Yet, people writing from a disability studies/rights perspective have pointed toward the other side of the equation.[3] Rather than only showing our absence, there are countless representations of disability in films. Unfortunately, disability is usually the symbol for tragedy, evil, or dependence with little attention to the disabled characters as full human beings.

Our initial efforts to survey the breadth of those falling into the category of people with disabilities comes back into play here. Many culturally held stereotypes involve people with disabilities as desexualized. Depending on the type of disability, we are discussing how other people with disabilities are viewed as oversexed and indeed dangerous sexual beings.

In the past few years alone, the very popular TV drama, *NYPD Blue* had two episodes focusing on how easily developmentally or emotionally disabled figures can be blamed for sexual assaults or murders of children. Of course, in these dramas, the cops are the ones who understand that it's not the homeless man who killed a child. Sipowitz and Simone again immediately sense that it is not the building supervisor's developmentally disabled son who hurt a young girl. Despite the lack of realism, these accusations of people with disabilities point toward an underlying prejudice about people with these types of disabilities.

Peter Knoepfler, in an article on sexuality and psychiatric disability, discusses the following three ways that psychiatric disabilities and sexuality can be linked:

SEXUAL BEHAVIOR IS THE DISABILITY

Mr. A. is a man in his twenties who functions well in most areas of his life. His predominant form of sexual expression is being an exhibitionist. Psychiatry considers this form of sexual expression a psychiatric disability.

SEXUAL BEHAVIOR IS UNRELATED TO THE DISABILITY

Ms. B. Suffers from a severe case of agoraphobia. Sexual behavior in a bedroom does not trigger Ms. B.'s phobia and it is therefore unimpaired.

---

[3]See for further reading, particularly Lennard Davis and Sander Gilman.

SEXUAL BEHAVIOR IS AN INTEGRAL PART OF THE DISABILITY

Mr. C. is suffering from a severe depression. While depressed, his sexual desire and interest are impaired. When the depression is treated and relieved, his sexual interest is likely to be awakened.[4]

Exploring sexuality literature on the specific topic of developmental disability, brain injuries, and emotional disabilities, reinforces the view that some disabled have dangerous libidinal urges. Therapists and others in helping professions in general pay much more attention to ways to instruct people about where to have sex than to explaining sex safe practices, etc.

The duality of sexual imagery concerning people with disabilities that is being pointed to in this section is quite similar to that discussed by other groups of people who are on the targeted side in various societal power dynamics. Women, for instance, are often sexually stereotyped as either Madonnas or whores. As people with disabilities, we are either long-suffering martyrs to be kept on a pedestal or lazy malingerers taking advantage of others. These dichotomized images put those in the marginalized groups into a classic dual bind situation. There is no way to win since one side or the other of someone's preconceived notions of who we are will come into the picture on some level.

The Strange Case of Abasiophilia

In an effort to further complicate the ideas one might have on disability and sexual practices, I thought surfing the Web might reveal an interesting facet of the developing discourse. While the following may seem a distraction from the major thrust of the article it serves the purpose of asking us to think even more deeply about the relationships of power in our society and how these are expressed and repressed culturally. This meditation will lead us into the concluding sections on the entangled and sometimes unpleasant history and relationships of those who study sex in its broadest sense and people with disabilities.

Abasiophilia is defined on a Web site devoted to "Legbrace (Caliper) Fascination" as a fascination with physical disability and the orthopedic appliances used in its management. Now, sexology and psychiatry have more exact and complicated definitions of this and characterize a few discrete paraphilias and fetishes. There have been established categories for what are seen as disorders in medical literature for over 100 years. There are indeed people who are sexually excited by leg braces, crutches and casts. Others are sexually attracted to amputees or others with a particular physical difference. Richard Bruno characterized those suffering from this collection of disorders "devotees, pretenders, and wannabes."[5]

---

[4]Knoepfler, Peter T., Sexuality and Psychiatric Disability in Marinelli, The Psychological and Social Impact of Disability, Third ed., Springer Publishing, 1991, p. 211.

[5]Bruno, Richard L. Ph.D., Devotees, Pretenders and Wannabes; Two cases of Fictitious Disability Disorder in Journal of Sexuality and Disability, 1997; 15:243–260.

Yes, like other oppressed groups, people with disabilities apparently have wannabes. I don't propose to offer a full analysis of this phenomenon except to note that the literature that exists on this topic points to people being envious about what they perceive to be the special treatment afforded those of us with disabilities. Case studies reflect that patients believe people with disabilities are admired for their courage and stand out from others in this respect.[6]

The problem I'm posing here is similar to the more widely reported fetishisms and paraphilias of infantilism. The adult babies as they prefer to be called appearing on his TV show even stumped TV host, Jerry Springer. Understanding them was much too difficult for even this ringmaster. I would not want to judge or stigmatize anyone's sexual practices particularly as what is known of fetishes and paraphilias indicates that this is not a conscious choice. The problem I wish to call attention to is twofold.

In the first case, of those attracted to people with particular disabilities and/or attracted to or aroused by disability paraphernalia, the underlying stereotypes about the experience of disability in this society are uninformed. In the second case, my objection after perusing their Web pages is that many of those active in various groups express a longing to not have bladder and bowel control. They express this by referring to those with incontinence problems as the "lucky ones" and even have sites devoted they say to helping young people who must wear protection feel better about themselves, raise their self-esteem and such. This attitude also reflects a real lack of information about the experience of living with a disability in an ableist society. It encourages a romanticized view of disability. (As for helping young people with disabilities feel better about themselves, I would posit that this is better done by having adults with disabilities as role models.)

The other question I want to pose about the phenomena discussed here is a more philosophical one to ponder. What does it say about our cultural values as a whole that (no matter how different they may seem to many of us) these specific attractions to items that symbolize disability or imitation of people with disabilities are classified as a type of mental aberration? Does this say anything about the social ranking accorded people with disabilities or is the classifying itself perhaps a move to protect us (people with disabilities) from people with a now defined type of mental problem?

Obviously many questions could be posed flowing from this particular intersection. While a bit out of the ordinary, this is also a reminder of just how medicalized and psychologized a society we live in. This brings us to the concluding section, which argues for a more thorough treatment of disability issues in social science disciplines, especially sexology. It also points to the potential advantages of a deeper inclusion.

---

[6]Ibid.

Moving Forward by Uncovering History

I began this piece by indicating some of the problems I see with omissions of people with disabilities from general introductory textbooks on human sexuality. The problem in reality is broader than this. Our absence is perhaps most noticeable in this field because there are so many intersecting points emanating from disability studies tied not to narrowly defined issues of sex but also those issues of reproduction, health, and medical research. For instance, how much medical research is given over to preventing the birth of disabled people rather than raising that intangible something called quality of life? It's not really so intangible.

And too often, when a disabled child is born, decisions are made to withhold medical treatment, as it is euphemistically termed. All treatment including food is sometimes withheld until the child dies. (I don't know how it's humane even if a baby can't be medically saved to allow her/ him to starve). Rarely if ever are parents facing this situation given a chance to talk to people with similar disabilities about what living with disabilities does and does not mean. It's impossible not to sympathize with the anguish of parents faced with these decisions. Yet people with disabilities are written off and parents are often told by experts that their child's future is bleaker than it could be.

These examples indicate only part of the problem. Another aspect, which was alluded to earlier and directly bears on teaching sexuality, concerns the history of sexology itself. When books refer to the work of Havelock Ellis, for instance, and his *Studies in the Psychology of Sex,* it is equally important to discuss his "The Task of Social Hygiene," which is written specifically in support of eugenics ideas. While he was a relatively mild "positive" eugenics advocate, this is a critical area of discourse in understanding the history not just of people with disability but many people of color and poor people in this country who were involuntarily sterilized under these doctrines. A better understanding of these issues can be obtained by including this type of historical analysis. Recent books on the history of eugenics along with many uncovering forgotten bits of disability history of eugenics along with many uncovering forgotten bits of disability history add a more complete picture. For example, the switch to defining norms rather than ideals in statistics is tied to the discourse around many of these questions as studies of demographics and populations took on a "scientized" tone.

In other words, just expanding sections on disability and sexuality, even if this material is more explicit about ableism, is not adequate. A more rounded inclusion of a disability perspective is needed. Invocations of the identity/diversity mantra remain superficial devices that aren't even prosthetic when only used to signify political awareness of oppression without regard for how these realities change the configurations discussed.

There is an emerging cultural creation or at least feelings of solidarity among some disabled cultural groupings that feel new. Better representations of our lives are already flowing from this, yet if these reflections remain isolated and only viewed by people with disability, we will not be the only losers.

The incorporation of disabled experience and history can add much to current discussions on sexuality as a whole. This is most obvious in the very definition of what is sensual and erotic. For example, an expansion of the meaning of sexual enjoyment sometimes including but sometimes bypassing the usual genital areas and discovering other erotic sensations is an obvious part of sexuality for some people with disabilities.

Conclusion

This paper has attempted to stimulate thinking around the complexities of the topic by touching on areas not always thought through adequately. Those interested in further reading may find some of the following books useful:

Adams, Mark B, 1996, *The Wellborn Science, Eugenics in Germany, France, Brazil and Russia,* Oxford University Press

Davis, Lennard J. 1995. *Enforcing Normalcy, Disability, Deafness, and the Body,* Verso New Left Books, London.

Fine, Michelle and Asch, Adrienne, Eds. 1988. *Women with Disabilities Essays in Psychology, Culture, and Politics.* Temple Univ. Press, Philadelphia

Kevles, Daniel J., 1985, *In the Name of Eugenics: Genetics and the Uses of Human Heredity,* Alfred Knopf Publishing.

Marinelli, Robert P. and Arthur E. Dell Orto, eds. 1997. *The Psychological and Social impact of Disability,* Third ed., Springer Publishing.

Morris, Jenny, 1991. *Pride Against Prejudice.* New Society Publishers.

Paul, Diane, 1998, *The Politics of HEREDITY, Essays on Eugenics, Bio-medicine, and the Nature-Nurture Debate,* SUNY Press.

Porter, Theodore M., 1986. *The Rise of Statistical Thinking, 1820–1900,* Princeton Paperbacks.

Proctor, Robert N. 1988. *Racial Hygiene, Medicine Under the Nazis.* Harvard Univ. Press, Cambridge.

Russell, Marta, 1998. *Beyond Ramps, Disability at the End of the Social Contract,* Common Courage Press, Monroe, Maine.

Shapiro, Joseph P. 1994. *No Pity, People with Disabilities Forging a New Civil Rights Movement.* Times Books.

Section 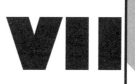 VII

Sexuality and Spirituality

Sexuality and Spirituality: The Relevance of Eastern Traditions

26

CHAPTER

Robert T. Francoeur, Ph.D. ACS

In recent years, the age-old association of sex with Adam and Eve's original sin in the Garden of Eden has lost its meaning as individuals increasingly accept sexual desire and pleasure as a natural good. Social turmoil, technological changes, increasing recognition of personal needs, and a sexual revolution have wreaked havoc with the meaning and relevance of the traditional Judeo-Christian sexual images, icons, and myths of the purpose of sex, monogamy and male primacy over female.

Because cultures draw their life blood from their myths and archetypes, human beings are searching for new myths and archetypes.[1] At the same time, Americans in particular are increasingly fascinated by the more sex-positive images of Eastern sexual philosophies. This article outlines two major Eastern sexual and spiritual traditions, Tantrism and Taoism, within the context of Hinduism and other religions and philosophies. After contrasting these Eastern views with Western values, some practical applications that complement Western sexology are discussed.

Eastern Sources

Even when the hidden roots of Eastern sexual traditions can be detected, they are found to be far more tangled than the origins of sexual values in Judaism, Christianity, and Islam. Archaeologists have found 8,000-year-old clay images of feminine power and fertility in the pre-Indus settlements on the northwest edge of India. Similar early expressions of a great Goddess who guarantees fertility have been found, with her subordinate male consort, in regions of ancient Egypt, the Aegean, the Danube, Asia Minor, and western Asia. Between 1800 and 1500 BC, waves of migrating Indo-Aryan people moved from eastern Europe, over the mountains, and into the Indus valley of western India. Their worship of a great Goddess intermingled with the fertility religions of pre-Aryan inhabitants they conquered in the Indus River valleys.[2,3,4] Historian Karl Jaspers calls this the pre-Axial period of human consciousness.[6] In this context, Jaspers is using the term Axial to mean turning point.

According to Jaspers and others, this striking transformation in human consciousness occurred in China, India, Persia, the Middle East, and Greece with the advent of Confucius, Lao Tzu, Buddha, Zoroaster, the Jewish prophets, and the pioneering philosophers of Greece. This opened the first Axial period. Everywhere male consciousness and power gained ascendancy over the female principle. In Christianity and Islam, phallic power virtually subdued the power of the female, except for the veneration of Mary, the Virgin Mother of God. After a male God gave man dominion over nature in Eden and ancient Greece gave priority to analysis and objectification, nature became Western man's toy to control and exploit. Although feminine images of sexual power persisted in the East, they were subordinated to the phallocentric male. But unlike the West, Eastern cultures maintained a respect for nature, emphasizing that health and spirituality are only achieved when humanity respects its place in the cosmos and places itself in harmony with nature.[5,6]

Hinduism

In India, the amalgam of pre-Aryan fertility religions with the emerging dominance of male consciousness produced Hinduism, a generic term for the traditional religion of India. Hinduism encompasses a wide range of seemingly contradictory beliefs, including reincarnation or transmigration of souls, atheism, and a pantheon of gods and goddesses who symbolize the many attributes of an indescribable supreme principle or being. Hinduism embraces both monistic and dualistic beliefs, and contains many popular local deities and cults. Thus it is not a religion in the same sense Westerners use that term to refer to a system of clear beliefs about a personal God and a spiritual world apart from this material world.[7]

The ideal life of a Hindu male embraces a wide spectrum of roles, from the student of religion to the householder who produces a son to carry on ancestral tradition, and from the hermit who tries to achieve indifference to everything in the world he previously found desirable to the homeless wanderer who renounces all earthly ties. Passing through these four stages is the *Way of Knowledge,* an expression that denotes the spiritual path, which leads to spiritual union with the Infinite. Along the Way of Knowledge, a Hindu male can pursue four goals: *kama* (sexual love), *artha* (power and material gain), *dharma* (spiritual duty), and *moksha* (liberation).[2] The first two goals deal with desire, the last two extol duty and renunciation. Typical of Axial thinking, Hindu sacred texts explain the paths of desire only from a male viewpoint, as if desire, pleasure, and power play no role in the lives of women whose primary activities are childrearing and household duties.

This mix of desire and duty in Hinduism allows a strong tradition of sexual abstinence by celibate monks to coexist with an equally strong religious celebration of sexual pleasure in all its forms as a path to the Divine. While sexual abstinence is favored at certain stages, Hindu sexual asceticism complements the celebration of sexual desire and pleasure, unlike Christian sexual asceticism, which is rooted in the need for redemption from original sin. Most Hindus, even the ascetics and monks, view sex as something natural, to be enjoyed in moderation without repression or overindulgence.

Hindu sacred writings, devotional poetry, and annual festivals celebrate married love, the fidelity of women, and the religious power of sexual union. Hindu myths of gods and goddesses are symbolic of spiritual powers and energies within and the daily challenges of life faced by all human beings. While monotheistic Western cultures tend to objectify and personalize their God, Eastern cultures view their mythologies as psychological and metaphysical metaphors that reveal the miraculous and natural wonders of human life and its desires.

Mythology provides a key to Hindu sexual views. *Brahma,* the Creator, *Vishnu,* the Preserver, and *Shiva,* the cosmic dancer of the cycle of destruction and rebirth form the basic triad of gods in the Hindu pantheon. Hindu sexual values are expressed in images and rituals associated with Shiva and his consort, the goddess *Shakti.* Shakti has several images, appearing as *Parvati,* the gracious embodiment of sensuality and sexual delights, as *Durga,* the unapproachable, and as *Kali,* the black wild one, the helpful, awesome goddess of sex's transcendent powers.[2,8] The *lingam,* a stone or wood phallus, represents Shiva and the concentration of sexual energy by asceticism. Triangular stone sculptures of the *yoni* represent Shakti and the vulva. Mystical geometric patterns called *yantras* combine the circular lingam with triangular yoni. Used in meditation, yantras reflect the belief that sexual practices can be a way of balancing the male and female energies of one's body and experiencing cosmic unity. The worship of lingam and yoni, of Shiva and Shakti, are a regular part of public and household rituals. *Kama,* the Hindu god of love, is also believed to be present during all acts of love. He represents love and pleasure, both sensual and aesthetic. His wife, *Rati,* is the embodiment of sensual love.

Hindu scriptures include hundreds of treatises on the art of eroticism, allegedly written by the gods and sages. Only three of these manuals, the *Kama Sutra, Kama Shastra,* and *Ananga Ranga,* have been translated into English. The *Kama Sutra* (second century BC) discusses the spiritual aspects of sexuality, with advice on positions and techniques for increasing the sensual enjoyment of sexual intercourse. The beautifully illustrated *Ananga Ranga* or *The Theater of God* (15th century AD) describes the sexual organs and erogenous areas of men and women, the cycles of erotic passion, and an encyclopedia of lovemaking positions. This spiritual tradition of erotic love appears in temple art depicting *mithuna,* loving couples in sexual embrace. Such sculptures reached their peak in the sensitive, emotionally warm, and intensely spiritual bas-reliefs celebrating all forms of sexual behavior (except adultery and violence) that cover the 1,000-year-old "love-temples" of Khajuraho and Konarak.[9,10]

Taoist Sexual Traditions

In their quest for spiritual and physical health, including longevity and immortality, the Chinese traditionally turned to Taoism, which originated from the teachings of the sixth century BC philosopher Lao-Tzu.[7] Taoism views nature and spirit as interdependent and mutually sustaining. Tao is "the Way," the "eternally nameless" path followed by the wise, the everchanging rhythmic source of life, and living in harmony with all things. Taoism advocates a life of simplicity, integration, cooperation, and selflessness, and has no formal dogma or church. It does not recommend asceticism or reject natural desires or cravings. It recommends self-cultivation, healthy living, and the fuller enjoyment of both earthly and heavenly joys.[2,11,12] Harmony in one's sexual desires, passions, and joys is a natural and important aspect of health. Sexuality is considered part of nature and is not associated with any kind of sin or moral guilt. In fact, lovers joined in ecstasy can experience a transcendent union with the cosmos.[13]

> ". . . Eastern cultures maintained a respect for nature, emphasizing that health and spirituality are only achieved when humanity respects its place in the cosmos and places itself in harmony with nature."

Some Taoists have sought the secret of longevity in an alchemical formula. Others have sought longevity by bringing the body and soul into a perfect, harmonious balance,[11,12] or by transforming the male or female essence into the "Elixir of Life."[14]

Taoist sexual traditions emphasize the importance of female satisfaction in all sexual relations. It talks of "a thousand loving thrusts," and the importance of nongenital touch for both the woman and the man.[11] In order to increase the enjoyment of sexual intercourse for both women and men, Taoist exercises help a man gain control over his ejaculation, with simple but sophisticated versions of the Sensate Focus, Stop and Go, and Squeeze Exercises popularized 2,000 years later by Masters and Johnson for treatment of premature ejaculation and inhibited female arousal and orgasm.[11] Taoism teaches that men cannot experience true sexual ecstasy unless they develop the ability to control their ejaculation.

This emphasis on male ejaculation is often misinterpreted. It is not the same as coitus reservatus (withdrawal followed by ejaculation) or the "male continence" practiced by the members of the Oneida Community in the 1800s to prevent unwanted pregnancies. It is not the same as the passive lovemaking of *karezza,* an ancient technique for prolonging sexual intercourse without ejaculation, popularized by Marie Stopes in her 1920s best seller *Married Love.*

Taoism also emphasizes the difference between male orgasm and ejaculation, a distinction rediscovered by modern sexologists. According to Taoism, men deplete their energy when they are driven to ejaculate too frequently. Specific Taoist exercises can enable a man to pleasure his partner and enjoy several "non-explosive" orgasms prior to ejaculation.[13]

The early Taoist traditions recognized the greater capacity of women for sexual pleasure and their vital role in introducing men to the treasures of sexual pleasure and ecstasy. But this mutual, harmonious concern for female and male pleasure did not last. In the Han Dynasty (206-219 BC), male interests began to dominate as Taoist exercises were converted into techniques that focused on men's pleasure, including intercourse with virgins and with numerous women in order to become immortal. Women became the footbound pleasure toys of men in the T'ang Dynasty (618-906 AD). During the Manchu Dynasty (1644-1912 AD), the egalitarian Taoist sexual philosophy practically disappeared in male obsessions.[12,13]

For guidance in the customs and proprieties of society and public life, the Chinese looked to the teachings of Confucius (551-479 BC). Early Confucian thought was quite sex-positive. Only in the last thousand years of imperial rule did Confucianism adopt a negative view of sexuality.

Both Taoism and Confucianism appear to have borrowed the basic idea of two vital energies, Yin and Yang, from earlier Chinese who lived centuries before Confucius and Lao-Tzu. Everything stems from the dynamic interaction of *Yin* and *Yang*.[15]

The polarity of Yin/Yang energies is very different from the body-soul opposition that underlies Western thought. Western thought maintains a very clear split between the body and spirit or soul. In Christian thought, salvation and redemption are achieved by subjugation of the body and its passions to reason and to the spiritual soul. In both Taoism and Confucianism, the vital energies of Yin (earth, dark, receptive, female) and Yang (heaven, light, penetrating, male) are complementary rather than opposing aspects of nature. The challenge of life is to achieve a healthy, dynamic balance between these two energies.[8,12,13]

Since both Yin and Yang coexist in every man and woman, in different proportions, everyone can cultivate, balance, and unite their psychosomatic energies. In sexual play Yin and Yang are aroused and can be channeled from the lower levels to the heart and head. According to some modern interpreters, this can be done in self-pleasuring, and in both heterosexual and homosexual relations.[11,13,16]

Some Taoist masters recommend that a male release his semen according to seasonal changes and infrequently, for example, only two or three times out of ten instances of intercourse, in order to direct and transform the vital life energies. Similarly, women are taught to use proper breathing exercises and meditation as ways of circulating and transforming their Yin energy. The mutual exchange of Yin and Yang essences in intercourse and orgasm is believed to produce perfect harmony, increase vigor, and bring long life.

Tantric Sexual Traditions

Some suggest that Tantric sexual traditions were derived from ancient Chinese Taoism, or that Taoist sexuality was derived from Tantra.[13,14,17,18] Others believe that the earliest

Tantric traditions predate Hinduism, Buddhism, and Taoism and that they were derived from the pre-Aryan religion of Indus Valley natives and religious symbols brought from paleolithic Europe by the Indo-Aryan invaders about 1800 BC.[19] Whatever their origins, Tantric ideas are found in Hindu, Buddhist, Jain, and Taoist writings in Nepal, Tibet, China, Japan, Thailand, and Indonesia.[2,19]

Over the centuries, the ecstatic, and at times orgiastic, cults inspired by Tantric visions of cosmic sexuality were attacked by ascetic Hindus and buddhists, denounced by the invading Muslims, opposed by the British colonial government in India, and outlawed by the Chinese communists.

Tantra is a Sanskrit word meaning thread" or "continuity." Tantra involves active ways of transforming one's perceptions and energies that plunge one back into the roots of personal identity to nakedly experience the truth and reality of oneself and the world. Tantric rituals are kept highly secret, and require severe discipline and every kind of physical, sexual, mental, and moral effort. Instead of recommending abstinence from the pleasures of life as celibate asceticism in other religious traditions do, Tantra cultivates the realization of an ultimate bliss in order to experience awareness of the true nature of reality, beyond all dualistic conceptions. In Philip Rawson's modern wording, Tantra urges its practitioners to "Raise your enjoyment to its highest power and then use it as a spiritual rocket-fuel."[4] The original Tantras use a cryptic "twilight" language difficult to understand. Some modern books on Tantra such as *Sexual Secrets* by Nik Douglas and Penny Slinger are filled with such symbolic terms, while other writers such as Mantak Chia mix traditional with Western terms to more clearly elucidate the meaning of esoteric terminology.[11,17,20]

Hindu Tantric Doctrine (Shaktism)

In Hinduism, Tantric rituals became associated with the worship of Shakti, Shiva's consort. Hindu Tantra reached its most profound external expression in the "love temples" of northeastern India (700-1100 AD).[7,9,10] Right-handed Shaktism is a refined philosophy that focuses on the benign side of Shakti as the energy of nature and mother-goddess. Left-handed Shaktism focuses on Durga and Kali, the violent side of Shakti, and sweeps one into conventionally forbidden expressions of natural impulses to achieve transcendence. Ritual violation of social taboos against adultery and incest, and coitus for otherwise celibate monks, are an important part of these left-handed Tantric rites.[2,19] In Victor Turner's social dialectics of structure-antistructure, Tantric taboo-breaking (anti-structure) rituals may play a vital role in maintaining the flexibility, dynamism, and creativity of a social structure or culture.[21]

Participants in the *Rite of the Five Essences,* a Tantric love ritual, for instance, use the five forbidden *Ms: madya* (wine), *mansa* (meat), *matsya* (fish), *mudra* (parched grain), and *maithuna* (sexual union) in a kind of holy communion.[2] It includes enhancement of the environment with flowers, incense, music, and candlelight, a period of meditation designed to hasten the ascent of the vital energies of the kundalini (see below), the chanting of a mantra, and the couple's visualization of themselves as an embodiment of Shiva and Shakti, the supreme couple.

Buddhist Tantric Doctrine

In Buddhism, Tantra refers to a series of teachings delivered to humans by the Buddha. According to Buddhist Tantra, the most effective means of awakening to the true nature of reality is not by intellectual pursuits, but by experiencing the state of voidness and bliss through one's own body and mind. The Buddhist Tantrik controls his/her body and its psychic powers to attain Buddhahood by coming face to face with the elemental forces of the world and transcending the desires aroused by them.

In Tibetan Buddhism, devotion to male and female deities stresses the interaction of external and internal energies.[4] *Yabyum* is the Tibetan term for the mystical experience of oneness and wholeness men and women can achieve through sexual intercourse.[22] In mystical sexual union, the male and female principles are combined in an experience that resolves all dualities and reflects the union of wisdom and compassion. Because all natural forces and the deity are a union of male and female elements, the highest and most harmonious energies are experienced in such unions as the realization of the inherent luminosity and emptiness of all phenomena.[22]

Tantra and Yoga

The system known as yoga was first mentioned in the Hindu *Upanishads* (eighth-fifth? century BC). Yoga, literally translated from the Sanskrit as "union," means being aware without thinking. It is the silence of the mind that is broken by trying to tell another person what one experienced in a yoga meditation/exercise.

Yoga is a highly evolved technique of meditation and concentration for disciplining mind and body and purifying the senses from their bondage to limiting concepts. Yoga combines physiological and psychological methods, which involve postures, breathing, and in some cases the rhythmical repetition of proper sound-syllables or *mantras* that suppress the conscious movement of the mind in body.[23] When the whole body is disciplined to aid the gradual suspension of consciousness, one can experience a state of pure ecstasy that is without thought or sensation. In this ecstasy, the yoga practitioner may use ritual, devotion, meditation, the intellect, or physical pleasure to find a complete freeing of the true self from the external world and natural causation.[24]

Both early Tantra and Taoism adopted yogic exercises to gain access to the spiritual through physical pleasure and discipline. The central concept in sexual yoga is a physiology that conceives of the body as interconnected by many channels, or *nadis,* that are conduits for energy. Two main channels run along either side of the spinal column, connecting power centers known as *chakras,* which correspond to the Taoist *tan tien,* located between the loins and throat. The third conduit, the *susumna,* runs from its base in the perineal region to the crown chakra. The *kundalini,* named for the goddess Kali, is the powerful but latent energy source that lies coiled like a serpent at the lowest chakra. The kundalini is also believed to represent Shakti, the feminine aspect of the creative force, the serpent power or mystical fire in the subtle body. The aim of sexual yoga is to arouse the kundalini or serpent power and channel it upward.[25] Once aroused, the kundalini can be channeled upward through the seven chakras of the subtle body until it merges with the eternal Shiva to confer freedom and immortality. By redirecting the body's most basic and vital generative energies of semen and ovum to the brain, the yoga practitioner hopes to gain spiritual energy, cosmic consciousness, and salvation, the experience of real self completely freed from earthly bonds and joined with all reality.[24]

In developing the idea of kundalini energy, the Tantriks and Taoists may have adopted earlier Persian ideas, using meditation, breathing control, postures, and finger pressure to prolong sexual intercourse without ejaculation. In the process, they added the goal of transforming and circulating the sexual energy upward in the body and in exchanges with a partner, thereby extending the enjoyment of many orgasms without ejaculation.

Orgasm and ejaculation are two distinct processes and can occur apart or together. William Hartman and Marily Fithian, for instance, report that men are capable of experiencing multiple orgasms as long as they do not ejaculate.[26] While most Tantric teachers urge males to avoid ejaculation at all times, Taoist teachers place more emphasis on gaining control of ejaculation rather than eliminating it altogether.[11,13]

The !Kung of Africa, Sufi mystics, and ancient and contemporary practitioners of yoga, Tantra, and Taoism, have cultivated the awakening of kundalini energy. Descriptions of these experiences bear intriguing similarities to reports of spontaneous experiences of Christian mystics and secular contemporaries. Strange as these reports sound in terms of Western physiology, their consistency and persistence over thousands of years deserve serious attention from Western scientists. There are hints in the preliminary research of neurophysicist and author Itzhak Bentov and psychiatrist Lee Sannella that a serious clinical and experimental investigation of the kundalini experience may reveal important new insights, much as modern medicine has benefited from clinical investigations of acupuncture and Ayurvedic herbal medicine.[27,28]

Blending East and West

To understand the Tantric and Taoist sexual systems and appreciate their rich messages, one has to go beyond the surface of sexual acts, rituals, and roles to get in touch with the cosmology, philosophy and world view that frame these exercises. One also has to deal with Eastern erotics, the way the Taoists and Tantriks interpret sexual feelings, ideas, fantasies, excitements, and aesthetics—what is beautiful or ugly, luscious or nauseating, dull or titillating.[29] Unfortunately, too many manuals, especially those presenting Tantric sex, are exotic recipe books or tourist brochures for a sexual Shangri-la. Fang-fu Ruan rightly notes that many books on Oriental sexology, while useful, ". . . are limited by either concentrating on a specialized topic or presenting a popular treatment of their subject. Some, by treating sexuality as a domain of pleasure independent of the changing contexts of medicine, religion, family life, reproductive strategies, or social control, effectively reinforce stereotypes of exotic Oriental cultures."[12]

Complicating any effort to evaluate the extent to which Westerners, raised with very different, even opposing world views and erotics, can understand, practice, and incorporate these sexual systems into their daily lives, is the fact that, while some proponents rhapsodize about the potential for ecstatic and cosmic experiences in Tantra and Taoism, very little can be actually known about the subjective experiences of men and women who practice these systems.[11,20]

These ancient traditions celebrate the naturalness of sexual pleasure and the spiritual potential of sexual relations, a view that may fit well with many people's sensitivities and yearnings. They also accept female sexuality and women's unlimited sexual potential, a view that is congenial with contemporary feminist awareness. Contemporary sexuality can be enriched and broadened by a reawakening of the experience of sexuality as integral to whole-person connectedness. It can also benefit from seeing sexual satisfaction as a fluctuating, non-goal-oriented, continuum of responses that includes pleasuring, orgasm, and ecstasy.[30] Can these ancient and yet very modern views be translated into the Western consciousness without being trapped by faddism? Advocates of yoga and acupuncture have succeeded in similar challenges.

In Western religions, spirituality refers to a loving, personal union of a human being with the Creator who has no gender or sex, although we are said to be created in "His image and likeness." In the Bible, sexual pleasure is commonly associated with an original sin—a fall from grace. Sexuality tends to be viewed as antagonistic to spiritual liberation.[31,32] In the words of Joseph Campbell, in the West, "eternity withdraws, and nature is corrupt, nature has fallen . . . we live in exile."[1] Neither Hinduism nor Buddhism have a concept of an original sin or primeval fall. Tantric and Taoist sexual union is viewed as a way to spiritual liberation, a consciousness of and identification with the Divine, and a way of becoming enlightened through one's embodiment and interaction with another. Can Western religious thought incorporate these sex-affirming Eastern views without scrapping much of our religious myths and beliefs? Can the spiritual and cosmic sense of sexuality be expressed in a Western world view without sanitizing or weakening sexual passion, or reducing its playful element?

> "These ancient traditions celebrate the naturalness of sexual pleasure and the spiritual potential of sexual relations . . ."

Despite these questions and challenges, we need to remember that nuclear physicist Werner Heisenberg acknowledged that Indian philosophy helped him make sense of some of the seemingly "crazy" principles of quantum physics. And Western science and medicine increasingly acknowledges the value of ancient traditions, such as Ayurveda, the Hindu system of medicine, and techniques of acupuncture originating from China.

The life cycles of past civilizations clearly suggest that as they degenerate, their cultures tend to exaggerate the great primordial insights that led to their greatness. Western cultures have overvalued individualism at the expense of the environment, separated human nature from nurturing nature, and turned everything, including the human psyche, into objects to be manipulated, controlled, and exploited. The resultant technological superiority has given humankind dominance in our global village. It has given Western culture the leisure and affluence that has allowed women to regain some of the gender equality they experienced in the pre-Axial era. However, the violent, exploitive extremes of Western intellectual and moral assumptions contain the seeds of self-destruction. History suggests that Western culture may avoid self-destruction and achieve a transformation into a new global consciousness if it can integrate values that will bring forth a more balanced culture, respectful of the unit and harmony of all reality. Jaspers and others see in this renaissance the possible advent of a second Axial Period.[5,6,33]

Many critics have deplored the objectification of sex and the Western obsession with sexual performance. Christianity, for the most part, has not been able to integrate sexuality into a holistic philosophy or see sexual relations, pleasure, and passion as avenues for spiritual meaning and growth. There have been a few prophetic efforts in this direction, but many Christian churches are having difficulties dealing with sexual pleasure, apart from reproduction, and along with the spiritual dimension. For individuals or couples, the Eastern views may have rich meaning, but they will not help with the problem Western religions face in accepting and affirming alternates to heterosexual, exclusive monogamy in today's world.

Eastern sexual and spiritual traditions can help Westerners break out of the prevailing reduction of sexuality to genital activity. Taoist and Tantric sexual practices highlight all the senses and involve the whole energies of both partners in slow, sensual dances that are rich variations of what Western sexologists label the "outercourse" of the Sensate Focus Exercises. In addition, Eastern thought may help refocus our understanding and appreciation of male orgasm. The obsession in sexually explicit films and videos with ejaculation as the affirmation of masculinity leaves the male with an inevitable flaccid vulnerability that requires denial in a vicious cycle of repeated "conquests" followed by inevitable detumescence. Taoist practices can help a male achieve some parity with the multiorgasmic woman by controlling his ejaculation, much to the benefit of both sexes.

Conclusion

Over the centuries, Tantriks and Taoists adopted philosophies and practices involving yoga from others and Yin and Yang from earlier Chinese, and borrowed aspects of the cultures of the pre-Aryans and (possibly) the paleolithic Europeans. Some Americans have already borrowed from the riches of Eastern sexual views. In the future this cross-fertilization may increase and become more sophisticated. The outcome could lead to new icons, archetypes, and meanings for sexual relations as expressions of love, passion, commitment, procreation, playful fun, and friendship as well as mystical transcendence and spiritual oneness.

The Western technological imperative needs a strong antidote to regain its health in the 21st century. Western culture may find a corrective to its highly successful but dangerously exaggerated technological imperative (Yang) in the ancient Eastern tradition of the nurturing potential of a panerotic sensuality (Yin). The health of Western culture can be improved by learning from key elements of the Taoist and Tantric traditions. At the same time, Eastern cultures are also caught up in the current revolution of human consciousness that some see as the advent of a second Axial Period, which is based on gender equality and a global and cosmic consciousness, sensitivity, and shared responsibility. This requires mutual collaboration and cross-fertilization on all sides.

References

1. Campbell, J. The power of myth. New York: Doubleday, 1988.
2. Bullough, VL. Sexual variance in society and history. Chicago: University of Chicago Press, 1976.
3. Gimbutas, M. The language of the Goddess. New York: Harper and Row, 1989.
4. Rawson, P. Tantra: The Indian cult of ecstasy. New York: Avon Books, 1973.
5. Jaspers, K. The Origin and goal of history. New Haven, CT: Yale University Press, 1953.
6. Cousins, EH. Male-female aspects of the Trinity in Christian mysticism. In B Gupta, ed. Sexual archetypes: East & West. New York: Paragon House, 1986.
7. Noss, DC. A History of the world's religions. New York: Macmillan, 8th edition, 1990.
8. Sivaraman, K. The mysticism of male-female relationships: Some philosophical and lyrical motifs of Hinduism. In B Gupta, ed. Sexual archetypes: East & West. New York: Paragon House, 1986.
9. Watts, A. Erotic spirituality: The vision of Konorak. New York: Collier Macmillan, 1971.
10. Deva, SK. Khajuraho. New Delhi: Brijbasi Printers, 1987.
11. Chia, M & Winn, M. Taoist secrets of love: Cultivating male sexual energy. Sante Fe: Aurora Press, 1984.
12. Ruan, FF. Sex in China: Studies in sexology in Chinese culture. New York: Plenum Press, 1991.
13. Chang, J. The Tao of love and sex: The ancient Chinese way to ecstasy. New York: Viking Penguin Arkana, 1977.
14. Van Gulik, RH. Sexual life in ancient China. Leiden, Netherlands: EJ. Brill, 1961.
15. Srinivasan, TM. Polar principles in yoga and Tantra. in B Gupta, ed. Sexual archetypes: East & West. New York: Paragon House, 1986.
16. Anand, M. The Art of sexual ecstasy: The path of sacred sexuality for Western lovers. Los Angeles: Jeremy Tarcher, 1989.

17. Douglas, N, & Slinger, P. Sexual secrets: The alchemy of ecstasy. New York: Destiny Books, 1979.
18. Needham, J. Science and civilization in China. Cambridge, England: University Press, 1956.
19. Rawson, P. The art of Tantra. Greenwich, CT: New York Graphic Society, 1973.
20. Chia, M & Chia, M. Healing love through the Tao: Cultivating female sexual energy. Huntington, NY: Healing Tao Books, 1986.
21. Turner, V. The ritual process: Structure and anti-structure. Ithaca, NY: Cornell University Press, 1969.
22. Blofeld, J. The Tantric mysticism of Tibet. Boston: Shambhala, 1970.
23. Sharma, PS, & Sharma, Yoga and sex. New York: Cornerstone Library, 1975.
24. Campbell, J. Transformations of myth through time. New York: Harper and Row, 1990.
25. Radha, S. Kundalini yoga for the West. Boston: Shambhala, 1985.
26. Hartman, W, & Fithian, M. Any man can. New York: St. Martin's Press, 1984.
27. Bentov, I. Stalking the wild pendulum. New York: E.P. Dutton, 1977.
28. Sannella, L. The Kundalini experience: Psychosis or transcendence. Lower Lake, CA: Integral Publishing, revised edition, 1987.
29. Herdt, G. Representations of homosexuality: An essay on cultural ontology and historical comparison, Part 1. *Journal of the History of Sexuality*, 1991, 1(3), 481–504.
30. Ogden, G., Women and sexual ecstasy: How can therapists help? *Women and Therapy*, 1988, 7(2,3), 43–56.
31. Lawrence, Jr, RJ. The poisoning of Eros: Sexual values in conflict. New York: Augustin Moore Press, 1989.
32. Rainke-Heinemenn, U. Eunuchs for the kingdom of heaven: Women, sexuality, and the Catholic Church. New York: Doubleday, 1990.
33. Paglia, C. Sexual personae: Art and decadence from Nefertiti to Emily Dickinson. New York: Random House, 1990.

Section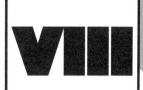

The Sex Industry and Sex Technology

Sex Work: A Contemporary Introduction to the World's Oldest Trade

27

CHAPTER

Carol Queen, Ed.D.

Introduction

"Sex work" is a term that serves a dual purpose. First, it allows us to consider the provision of sexual services or entertainment in terms of economic exchange, not in terms of sexual or legal deviance. "Sex work" is now a preferred term for referring to prostitution, for example, because it emphasizes that prostitution is in fact a form of work, a prostitute one category of laborer.

Second, providing erotic goods or entertainment or sexual service is work not done only by prostitutes, and so the term "sex worker" also lets us consider a wider range of types of work within what is often called the "sex industry" or "sex trade." Besides prostitutes, the sex industry employs people as peep show workers and strippers; porn models and performers; professional dominants and other S/M practitioners; phone and computer sex "operators"; writers, editors, and publishers of pornography; adult industry distributors and retail sales workers; and in diverse other capacities. In fact, I will argue that a case can be made for using the term "sex worker" to describe anyone who works primarily with sex, including in a research or educational capacity, although this use of the term is not very common.

It should be noted that reference to the "sex industry" does not mean that all elements of it are connected. They are not. Nor are all sex workers employed by someone else. Many are self-employed or small-business owners. There exists no overseeing corporation that ties the disparate elements of the sex industry together, although some businesses that run sex shops, publishing ventures, video production and distribution, etc., are sizeable, and the industry as a whole is big business.

Prostitution is often termed "the oldest profession." There is no doubt that discussing it (and related professions) is of interest in virtually all eras. Even where they are socially stigmatized, prostitutes elicit fascination because they supposedly have access to great sexual knowledge and hidden information. Most early written pornography used prostitutes as main characters, because whores were seen as the only real female representatives of explicit, active sexuality. But looking at sex work today sheds light on more than a culture's sexual secrets. It also provides a window on the sexual attitudes of a society and on its gender issues.

This discussion of sex work is intended to serve as a wide-ranging overview, including some history, a look at the diversity within contemporary sex work, and more. It is focused especially on the US, but does not exclude information from other parts of the world. Topics covered will include feminism and gender politics, criminalization, research, and the sex workers' rights movement. However, it *is* an overview, and interested readers are urged to explore the topic more thoroughly than is possible here.

My approach owes a great deal to the contemporary sex workers' movements, especially the academic/research arm of these movements. They are attempting to describe and analyze working conditions and other related issues from an insider's point of view, something that has rarely been done in the past.

Research

Some of the earliest modern social science research focused on prostitutes (and the possibility that they might spread sexually transmitted diseases). Since then, research about sex workers has fallen into many categories. It can be done from various points of view: historical, anthropological, psychological, sociological, criminological, epidemiological, and more. Archaeology has even gotten into the act, excavating ancient brothels in Pompeii and elsewhere.

Particularly as "hands-on" research goes—participant observation and survey research, in particular—academics who wish to study sex workers can face an extreme version of the problems confronting all researchers who wish to gain knowledge about taboo or little-understood topics from human subjects. As with the subjects of any research on sex or illegal behavior, many sex workers will not easily trust a researcher. They may answer questions incompletely or incorrectly, tell the researcher what they think s/he wants to hear, or refuse to participate in the research at all. Finding study subjects in the first place can be challenging. It is next to impossible to do a random sample on a secretive subgroup, so most survey research on sex workers uses convenience or snowball samples, less generalizable than other forms of research. Sample size may also be too small to be really useful.

This problem is worse when the research is being done on prostitutes and others whose work is criminalized. Still, other sex workers share some of the stigma attached to prostitutes and may be equally hesitant to stand up and be counted, much less questioned in depth.

Additionally, much general sex research does not even ask sex workers to stand up and be counted, so any opportunity such research may offer to query a general population about sex work experience goes unexploited. Research that asks about frequency and variety of sex practices usually includes nothing that would allow the researcher to identify and analyze the responses of sex workers.

Bias can enter into a research project from many directions. Convenience sampling, as I have noted, is not considered highly generalizable to large populations, although if done well it can usefully describe a particular subgroup. Substantial bias and misinformation enter such a sample when the researcher makes the mistake of assuming the sample s/he got adequately describes the population as a whole. For example, many studies on prostitution conducted by sociologists rely on populations that are incarcerated. Similarly, much research is done simply by applying the federal government's own crime statistics; this, too, counts only those who have been arrested. Prostitutes who work the streets are much more likely to be arrested and convicted than those who work indoors as escorts or "on call," so prison studies disproportionately include streetwalkers. Furthermore, however street workers are more likely than other prostitutes to be poor, of color, less educated, and drug-using—so prison and crime statistics-based studies disproportionately describe the "average" prostitute (a creature no researcher has adequately described) as drug-addicted and downtrodden.

Researcher often includes built-in biases. Some researchers approach sex workers with fascination others with distaste. Pre-existing, unexamined attitudes about prostitution, pornography, and sexual entertainment can taint a study and make its conclusions open to debate, but for too long such debate was rare in academics. That tendency is changing today partly because more current and former sex workers have spoken up to debunk the bias inherent in much so-called research.

An interesting source of bias in most contemporary research on sex work is a form of gender bias: We are much more likely to think of sex workers (especially prostitutes) as female than male, even though men work in the sex industry in virtually every capacity women do. Potentially interesting comparisons between female and male sex workers are made. Sex workers are often described generically, as it were, as female, since the culture tends to see provision of sexual service as part of the "normal" female role, not the male's. The experiences of male sex workers are hence more hidden and less examined, and it is harder to differentiate male and female experiences.

There is also substantial class bias in research, as noted in the discussion of prison studies, above. Researchers may expect to find sex workers who come from the underclass and fail to look very hard for exceptions to the "rule"—or when they find such exceptions they may assume they are anomalies and not listen to the alternative information they may offer. Conversely, researchers may find educated and articulate sex workers and look no further. Either bias misrepresents the real diversity among sex workers.

In short, although there is a lot of research that looks at sex workers, much of it is not very useful outside the context of the specific group profiled in each particular study. Beware of researchers who generalize their findings to all prostitutes, all porn performers, etc.

History

"The oldest profession" has been practiced in one form or another in a great many epochs and cultures. There is even recent evidence that sexual favors traded for valuable exchange (food, nesting materials, etc.) may be practiced in the animal kingdom. Considering historical sources or sites (such as archaeological digs) for information about the sex trade in other times and cultures is made difficult by several things. Historical sources may be just as tainted by bias as contemporary researchers' work. Information about a vanished culture can be simply incomplete or speculative. A real gender bias exists in most historical information—much more has been written about female than male prostitutes. Some cultures are relatively open about sex, while others maintain a high level of privacy in sex and gender relations.

Perhaps most interestingly (not to mention confusingly), since female prostitutes get the most scrutiny, historians' interpretation of the role of sex workers in any given culture is affected by the role of women within that culture—particularly as relates to sexuality. In cultures in which women have a high degree of sexual freedom and autonomy, prostitution may take very different form than it does in societies that seek to control women's sexual expression and outlets. When the larger question of gender roles is not addressed, the picture painted of prostitution can be rather misleading.

Prostitution is intimately related to the history of pornography, at least in the West. The word pornography translates as "writings of or about whores," and as we have seen, prostitutes became fixtures in pornographic writings because they were openly sexual when other women of the times were not supposed to be.

History gives us glimpses of times and cultures in which prostitution was not as marginalized and demonized as it is today. Sacred prostitution may have been practiced in some pre-Christian Middle Eastern cultures: in these goddess-worshipping societies, priestesses made themselves available for sex with the men of the community, who paid them for the privilege of having this encounter with the divine. Funds raised this way went into temple coffers. It is thought that this practice is the reason the Bible rails against the "Whore of Babylon." Some prostitutes today feel that they are re-creating this form of prostitution and may term themselves Quadesha or sacred whores. In some cases they may attract clients who appreciate their spiritual approach, but in most cases the spiritual importance of this identity helps support the sex worker herself, allowing her a stronger self-image in a society that does not value her or her work.

More historical material is available on prostitutes who worked with the wealthy and titled than on those who provided sexual service to the lower classes, just as there is more documentation of every kind about the lives of the powerful. Hetaerae in ancient Greece, courtesans in Middle Ages Europe, and geisha in imperial Japan led very different lives from other women, often being among the most well-educated and cultured women of their societies. Prostitutes were sometimes the only independent women in cultures that restricted women's freedom and required male oversight of their lives.

There is an exception to the historical blackout of common prostitutes. It is generally recognized that at times of social change, especially wars and migrations, prostitutes emerge to provide sexual service to men who are single and separated from their wives. This occurred in Europe's great period of urbanization, in America's Western migrations, and it is commonly associated with military encampments and troop movements. We typically do not know much about the individual prostitutes who made their living under these conditions, but we often know something about how they lived, how their businesses worked, and who their customers were. Much historical documentation is available about certain red-light districts, such as Storyville in New Orleans, which were a recognized part of their communities for many decades.

Developments in technology have historically impacted the sex industry, in two main ways. The first has to do with the way new technologies can change an entire society's economic circumstances, as implied above: Europe's great migrations were set in motion by the Industrial Revolution, and urbanization changed traditional communities and provided the opportunity for the growth of red-light districts and an expanded economic niche for prostitutes. The second involves the way certain new technologies can be used by the sex industry itself: this list of specific technologies is long and involves contraceptive methods, prophylactics, photography, film, video, telecommunications, and computers. Totally new inventions can be exploited for sexual purposes and may involve the development of entirely new branches of the sex industry; pornographic movies would not exist without motion picture and/or vide technology, for example.

Different Jobs Within the Sex Industry

As noted above, sex workers come in many diverse subtypes. Though "sex worker" is often used as a synonym for "prostitute," many other types of erotic or sexualized labor can also be described as sex work, and most of the workers doing other jobs in the sex industry do not understand themselves as prostitutes of any kind. Of course, it often happens that an individual does several jobs in the sex industry; a porn star may pose for photos as well as doing videos and may also do live shows and strip or even turn tricks. But there are definite lines between different kinds of work, and they are not always crossed. This section will briefly explore the various types of work sex workers do.

PROSTITUTION

Prostitutes may be male, female, or transgendered. They may work the streets of an urban red-light district, linger at truck stops, gather in massage parlors or brothels, or work discreetly in their own or their clients' homes. The fee they receive for the sexual service they provide may range from just a few dollars to several hundred dollars or more. Because their work is illegal in most parts of the US (and in many other parts of the world), prostitutes do not often speak for themselves, and so many stereotypes abound about their work, lives, habits, and histories. Some of these stereotypes are essentially true for some prostitutes. But no stereotype adequately describes the "average" prostitute, because there is such great diversity among these sex workers that no one type could be called average.

Common stereotypes include: Prostitutes are drug-addicted; they are repulsed by sex with strangers but are forced to it by economic necessity or inescapable pimps; they can't do any other sort of work; they are young; they are female; they are more likely to have sexually transmitted diseases than non-prostitutes; they have been sexually abused.

Many of these elements are more commonly seen in the lives and experiences of street workers than among prostitutes in general. Street workers' experience can definitely be harsh, and many are well served by leaving prostitution, when and if they can find other economic alternatives. But the majority of prostitutes probably do not work the street. In fact, researcher Priscilla Alexander has estimated that only about 10% of prostitutes in America are street-based. Far more are employed in brothels and massage parlors or by escort services, while still others work independently. The latter, often called "call girls" (men will often be called "escorts" or "models"), advertise in the classifieds or work with a madam or other individual who helps procure clients.

Because independents work in a less-organized and obvious fashion, they are less likely to risk arrest, and so they are harder for researchers to locate and study. In between well-publicized busts of madams whose rings of call girls service wealthy or famous men (think Heidi Fleiss or "the Mayflower madam," Sydney Biddle Barrows), the general public does not see call girls in their midst, because they don't hang out on street corners wearing skimpy outfits. Rather, they blend in, and one of the many qualities they offer their clients is discretion.

Class background and education level help determine the future of a prostitute, and this distinction underlies the great diversity among prostitutes. As we have seen, this has been as true historically as it is today. While it would be incorrect to say that poor, undereducated women and men always end up on the streets while individuals with a more privileged class and educational background end up working solo or with an escort service or a madam, this split exists more often than not. Some street prostitutes say they prefer the flexibility and freedom of such work, but most are probably there because their life choices are circumscribed. Conversely, many escorts are better-educated and often do have more choices; often people gravitate to this level of the sex industry because they like the money, the freedom, and the fact that, at rates of $200 per hour or more, they have to work relatively little to make ends meet. Many prostitutes save to buy businesses, go to school, or devote time to art, activism, or other interests. These people are more likely to think of themselves as professionals and to view customers not as johns but "clients;" they may start prostitution when they are older, and they often rely on regular clients (contradicting another common stereotype, that prostitutes have sex with "strangers").

Prostitutes are sometimes termed "sexual slaves" who "sell their bodies" for money. But in fact they are not "selling" anything except their time and their skills, just as anyone does who labors for a wage, and they typically are not enslaved by their clients, even for an hour at a time. It is commonly supposed that a prostitute will do, or has to do, anything a client wants her or him to do, but this is not the case. Most prostitutes have clear limits about what they will and will not do for money, and they negotiate with clients about issues like safe sex, specific or intimate practices like anal sex or kissing, time availability, and more.

It is true that some prostitutes are forced (by dire circumstances, or by another person) to turn tricks. It's difficult to say what number do not practice prostitution of their own free will, but it is clear that not all prostitutes with pimps are forced into sex work. (And not all prostitutes work with pimps; probably a minority does.) Pimps are, if anything, more subject to stereotype (often race-based) than prostitutes. In the US, the stereotypical pimp is a black man who has "stable" of female prostitutes who work for him, turning tricks and bringing him all or most of their money. He may control them through sweet talk, violence, drugs, or all three, but (still stereotypically speaking) he calls all the shots.

In fact, the legal definition of pimping has to do with receiving money from a prostitute, meaning that anyone who is supported by, or even simply residing with, a prostitute could be charged with pimping, as long as the prostitute was covering household expenses. Prostitutes' spouses or lovers are often charged with pimping; it can happen whether or not they are involved with the prostitutes' business. In many places it is a more serious charge than committing an act of prostitution, because it is assumed—sometimes correctly, other times not—that the pimp is the person in charge. (Many prostitutes argue that this is an inherently sexist assumption—someone else, probably a man, *must* be in control.)

Street prostitutes may work with a pimp for safety: someone to keep an eye on possibly violent clients, watch out for vice officers, and hold the day's take to guard against theft. Often, though not always, the pimp is the prostitute's spouse or lover. However, many street workers do not work with a pimp. Instead they work solo or develop a network of other prostitutes so they can watch each other's back.

A related role is that of "madam." A madam works, depending on the context, as an employer or manager (as in a brothel), or as a referring agent, putting prostitutes in touch with clients. Often the madam is a former prostitute who has moved into this management or agenting role. For the work s/he does, the madam or agent is paid a cut of the prostitute's fee. This legally makes her or him a pimp, and other laws may be used against a madam too, including pandering and keeping a bawdy or disorderly houses.

The issue of international trafficking will be addressed below.

PEEP SHOW WORK AND STRIPPING

From the exotic dancers of the nineteenth century whose work evolved into tease-oriented burlesque to present-day strippers who "show pink" and leave nothing to the imagination, the sex industry has made a place for artistes whose work is too bawdy for the prevailing standard of the times. Live shows range from stripping, with at least some focus on dance and movement, to shows featuring masturbation and live sex acts. These are now mostly centered in adult theaters and strip clubs in or near urban areas, although strip clubs (also known as "titty bars," "gentlemen's clubs," or by other names) are on the rise in the US and can sometimes be found outside of cities. While most such places feature female performers only, there are clubs featuring only male performers too, either oriented toward female audiences—like the famous Chippendales dance troupe—or toward male ones.

Depending on the location of the club and the laws and zoning of the area in which it operates, full nudity and even explicit sex may be the norm; in other places erotic dancing is available, but dancers must cover genitals and sometimes breasts, and explicit behavior is illegal. Strip clubs usually feature a stage with a surrounding audience, and in many of these venues an attraction beyond the stage show is called lap dancing, in which a scantily clad performer sits on an audience member's lap and wiggles to stimulate him (or, more rarely, her). Table dancing, wall dancing, and couch dancing are all variants.

In some countries live heterosexual sex shows can be viewed. These are not common in the US, whose clubs feature male and female masturbation as well as lesbian (or "girl-girl") sex shows when live sex is featured at all. Nevada brothels may feature heterosexual shows as well as girl-girl acts. Peep shows often feature porn video booths as well as booths allowing a view of dancers or performers on a stage. Sometimes one-on-one talk and masturbation shows are available.

PORN MODELS AND PERFORMERS

Pornography is available in various forms: written, photographic, film, or video. It is published in magazines and books as well as online. In most cases visual porn involves models and performers, some of whom are well known to their fans and appear in dozens of photo layouts and movies; others are amateurs who may appear just a few times or only once. Successful porn performers tend to be sexually exhibitionistic, and many see themselves as actors. Some viewers might disagree—porn is almost never very highbrow—but many performers prefer working on more elaborate productions because it reinforces their sense of themselves *as* performers.

All the personnel involved in a nude photo shoot or a porn movie can also be described as sex workers, at least when such work is their primary way of making a living.

PROFESSIONAL DOMINANTS

Professional dominants (a.k.a. "pro doms") are usually self-employed or work in a loose affiliation of other dominants; occasionally they work for a "house," which is owned by someone else, and they pay part of their fee to the house in much the same way that a prostitute who works in a brothel contributes a percentage of her fee to the madam. Pro doms are not prostitutes, however; they work with clients who want sadomasochistic or dominant/submissive scenes. They do not have sex with their clients (at least, not the way most of us think of sex). In session they may do widely varying activities, depending on their interest and expertise and the desires of the client. Some of these include: bondage; whipping; cross-dressing; psychodramatic erotic roleplay; piercing; and "slave training," in which the paying submissive is trained to serve the dominant as s/he specifies.

Males as well as females work as pro doms, with either male or (more rarely) female customers. The women tend to be more high profile, with publications such as *Dominants' Directory International* devoted to showcasing them in their fetish garb. Female doms may also be known as mistresses, dommes, or dominas, while males are usually known as masters. In some cases pro doms may employ or work with professional submissives, so that they can accommodate a client who wants to be the dominant partner in a session.

Professional dominance is a highly specialized type of sex work, requiring substantial specialized knowledge. In spite of this, it usually pays a little less than escort work, probably because it is not as illegal as prostitution. Few, if any, locales specify S/M and D/S practices in laws and ordinance. However, pro doms are sometimes charged with operating a disorderly house, and even with prostitution, especially when authorities do not clearly know the difference between professional domination and prostitution.

PHONE AND COMPUTER SEX

In both phone sex and live computer sex a person makes her/himself available to customers for erotic talk. In the case of computer sex, a camera often allows the customer to see the sex worker live. In this case the computer becomes a virtual peep show. In the case of phone sex, though, the worker's only salient qualities are voice and imagination. Customers often call with specific fantasies they want to talk through, though others let the phone fantasy worker take the lead; customers often also request a phone partner of a particular body type, hair color, or ethnicity, and phone sex workers are adept at portraying themselves as blonde or African American, brunette or lesbian, depending on the desire of the customer. Both phone sex and computer sex workers may work either from home or from a group "office" where several people can take calls at once. Both types of erotic entertainment may cost the customer a fair amount of money; but often the worker gets only a fraction of it.

PORN WRITERS

A sex industry job that requires no fancy clothing and little human contact, writing may cover the range from porn movie scripts to *Penthouse* letters, literary short stories to smutty paperbacks. It usually does not pay a great deal, so successful porn writers are the ones who can produce fast, especially if they can write a variety of scenarios and from various erotic points of view. It is not unusual to find erotic writers working for heterosexual and gay porn magazines simultaneously. A really professional writer may be prepared to tailor her or his work to the venue at hand.

ADULT INDUSTRY DISTRIBUTION AND RETAIL

The sex industry obviously includes people who directly provide sexual services and entertainment, but it also encompasses people whose job it is to get sexual products into the hands of those who want to use them. From video and sex toy importers and distributors to sales staff in retail sex emporia, sex workers in distribution and retail are hidden behind a veil of commerce. These may be mom and pop businesses or sizeable corporations. Many cities now have erotica shops that cater to and/or are owned by women. The largest of these have catalogs and ship to all parts of the globe. Many of these businesses operate on the Web, too; whether a retail staffer sees her/his customers or simply downloads their e-mail, they remain sex workers.

These businesses, large and small, differ from other retail businesses, which are not at risk for obscenity prosecutions, as some retail sex businesses are. Moreover, the legal definition of obscenity is vague and undefined enough that many distributors and retail staff have a hard time protecting themselves. Many sex workers in the retail and distribution side of the industry have been charged with crimes.

SURROGATE PARTNERS

Surrogate partners, also known as sec surrogates, may do all the things that prostitutes typically do, but they do not do them for the erotic entertainment of the client, but rather to teach him or her sexual skills and assist in the client's therapy. Surrogates almost always work in conjunction with, and by the referral of, sex therapists, which helps protect them against prostitution charges. Surrogate therapy was pioneered by sex researchers and therapists William Masters and Virginia Johnson, who felt people would benefit better from sex therapy if they had a partner with whom to go through a series of experiential exercises, many of which are explicit. A client will work with a surrogate partner for a prearranged number of sessions, and the client's therapist may recommend further work after the basic program is done.

Sex Educators and Therapists

Many people's idea of sex work stops with surrogate partners. But a case can be made that anyone who works primarily with sex is a sex worker, and that definition would clearly include therapists, educators, and other academics, whose professional focus is about sexuality and sexual health. Surrogates often describe the difference between their work and a prostitute's by saying, "Going to a prostitute is like going to a restaurant. Seeing a surrogate is like going to cooking school." Therapists and sex educators are also instructors in that school.

Porn Crusaders and Vice Officers

People who earn their living by focusing on sex may be neither restaurateurs nor cooking school instructors; they may be trying to shut the restaurant down. Seeing vice cops and prosecutors as sex workers may be stretching the definition to the breaking point, but it bears noting that these people, too, make a living from society's focus on, and contradictory feelings about, sex—and some of them are as closely focused as any copy editor on a porn magazine.

Using this definition, while not one all sex workers (and certainly not all vice officers) will concur with, allows us to look at sex work from a neutral distance, one unclouded by the moral assumptions that underlie so much discussion about the sex industry.

Clients and Customers

Sex workers' clients and customers have little in common with one another—except the majority of them are male, whether they prefer their sexual entertainment from women or from other men. They tend to be able to compartmentalize the sexual entertainment or services they purchase, since many are married or partnered and tend to keep their dealings with the sex industry private as far as their spouses or partners are concerned. In many cases, these customers say they have sexual interests they can't share with their primary partners. This is particularly true of the clients of pro doms, clients who want to explore variant sex practices with prostitutes, and male, heterosexually partnered clients of male prostitutes.

In other cases, clients want very ordinary sexual experiences, but they want these experiences with a variety of partners, without emotional entanglements, or according to a specific schedule their partner does not wish to accommodate. A stereotyped view of clients presents them as unable to find partners because they are unattractive or otherwise unsuitable, but in fact, while certainly some men who patronize the sex industry are not likely to find partners elsewhere, most *are* partnered, and they use the sex industry as an outlet or entertainment source separate from the life they share with their partner or spouse.

Clients are stigmatized just as prostitutes are, and many tend to keep their involvement with the sex industry to themselves. Hence it is difficult to say what percentage of men patronize prostitutes, strip clubs, and other sex industry venues, or take advantage of the more private entertainments of adult video rental, phone sex, and sex on the Internet. However, it is clear that the sex industry is established and in many places thriving, that it exists on a global scale, and that in most cultures today there is either a tolerance for the sex industry or at least a "boys will be boys" attitude about men who patronize it.

Countering this, though, is a newer trend that attempts to further criminalize men who patronize prostitutes. Many jurisdictions in the US have adopted tougher laws in recent years, and the trend may be going global. Sweden passed such a law recently in the name of protecting prostitutes, many of whom say they would prefer not to be protected from engaging in their livelihood.

Though the majority of clients and customers are men, some change is occurring today; women are increasingly becoming consumers of pornography, which has changed somewhat in an effort to attract more women and couples. (This change is not seen across the board, but many videographers and publishers have seen the writing on the wall and are purposely making porn for women to enjoy.) Other sex industry venues are seeing more women customers, too: sex toys stores that cater to women, like San Francisco's Good Vibrations and Boston's Grand Opening!, can be found in several cities; many traditionally male-oriented places have cleaned up and tried to make themselves more women-friendly; more women are venturing into strip clubs as patrons. Although the industry as a whole has not embraced this change (nor, for that matter, have the majority of women), there are signs that it may continue and transform at least some corners of the business into welcoming female patrons.

Women who do *not* patronize the sex industry today sometimes say they would if they had more money, and indeed, there still is a pay differential between women and men that may allow men more disposable income to spend on erotic entertainment. Many women also view sex industry venues as dangerous places and avoid them for safety reasons. This complex (and sometimes real) association between sex and sex-related venues and danger is clearly a stumbling block for women who might otherwise explore sexual interests outside of relationships. Also a factor is the lack of visible female sex industry patronage. Men can explore the sex industry and justify it by saying that other men are doing the same; far fewer women are blazing the trial for other women. (When they do venture in, however, the erotic entertainers at strip clubs and peep shows are often very happy to see them.)

Laws Affecting Sex Workers

Prostitution is illegal everywhere in the US except in certain counties in Nevada. Prostitution-related offenses range from actual acts of prostitution—exchanging sex for money—to soliciting for prostitution, frequenting or maintaining a house of prostitution (also called "bawdy house" or "disorderly house" laws, giving a clue as to their archaic origins), and pimping or pandering. Prostitution is regulated, if not illegal, in most places in the world. In many places, including the Nevada brothels, a prostitute must obtain a license to legally practice the trade. In these locations certain areas are usually set aside as red-light districts, and the state attempts to confine prostitution to these areas. In some British Commonwealth countries, the act of prostitution is not illegal, but many of the surrounding activities are: "communicating for the purposes of prostitution" is a crime, for example.

In the US prostitution-related offenses may vary by state and municipality. Offenses may be misdemeanors or felonies, depending on the offense and the place in which it is committed. Prostitutes who work when they have HIV are sometimes guilty of a more serious offense, even if they limit their sexual contact with customers to a hand job. And as we have seen, in many venues there are also laws against customers: johns may be ticketed, have their cars impounded, or be arrested.

Laws meant to control prostitution can also affect pro doms (especially disorderly house laws, which are usually written so broadly that anything from a brothel to a swing club to a crack house to a loud after-hours party might fall under them). They could theoretically be applied to sex surrogates, as well, although such prosecutions rarely happen.

Laws and ordinances may control or criminalize what goes on in a peep show or strip club, especially as regards full nudity, contact with customers, and live sex acts. Zoning laws are also routinely used to keep such businesses in certain parts of town. Any sort of adult industry venue may be subject to these zoning regulations, including erotica shops.

Obscenity law is the other sort of law that is most relevant to sex industry workers. Laws against obscene behavior can affect erotic performers (as, we should note, can local laws regulating *any* sexual behavior: in a state with a sodomy law that includes lesbian sex in the definition of sodomy, a live lesbian act would invoke that statutes as well as any public indecency, lewd and lascivious, or obscene behavior laws on the books).

Obscenity statutes are most often used in the US today to regulate certain kinds of pornography, although in the past they were regularly used to regulate sexually explicit literature as well, or even literature that is not especially explicit but is considered socially harmful for its era, as in the prosecution of Radclyffe Hall's lesbian novel *The Well of Loneliness* in the late 1920s. In fact, much of the "smut" hunted down by morals crusader Anthony Comstock (after whom the Comstock Act, regulating sending obscene material through the US mail, was named) would be considered sex education or literature today.

Statutes may be interpreted to cover pornography performance, as in a movie or video; but most at risk are the distributors and sellers of the material. Since obscenity law typically cites "community standards," conservative areas host obscenity trials far more frequently than liberal urban areas. After the Meese Commission on Pornography was held in the 1980s, more federal prosecutions of pornography were done, always held in areas with conservative populations.

International Issues

The sex industry is global, but it takes different forms depending on the cultural context of each region, country, and locale. For instance, in Senegal there is no local word for "prostitute"—instead, the women who exchange sex for money in that culture are known as "women who go out." (Women there are typically overseen by husbands, fathers, or brothers, so women who go by themselves to conduct their own business apparently need no further definition.) Certain cultures place much more judgment on prostitution and other types of sex work than others do.

Partly because of the opprobrium sex workers, especially prostitutes, may face at home, many go elsewhere to work. Border crossings like this happen all over the world. Some travel to another country within their region, others emigrate to the other side of the globe, and some merely go to the next town, but the phenomenon is often made more complex by xenophobia in the host country. Still, it is in many places more acceptable to spend time doing sex work elsewhere than to do it at home.

An extreme form of this phenomenon is known as trafficking. This is most often seen when people from an impoverished area or Third World country come to an urban, usually First World area to do prostitution, exotic dancing, or other form of sex work. Since this form of immigration is extremely costly, a broker will often help the person make the trip—paying for travel expenses, living expenses in the arrival country, and often papers and visas—and the immigrant must pay the broker back, sometimes at extremely inflated rates. This is known as "debt bondage," and it is not done only in the context of sex industry jobs. Resident aliens in many kinds of jobs (mostly menial) have been relocated by these brokers.

Trafficking is often represented as a nonconsensual situation in which women are kidnapped or duped into going to another country to work, only to find themselves in the power of the broker or the broker's associates. In fact, while this does happen, it is frequently the case that the trafficked individual wants to immigrate, knows s/he will be doing sex work, and has even done it before. Still, a life that amounts to indentured slavery in the arrival country, often to pay back tens of thousands of dollars, is abusive no matter what. Trafficking is a big business, and it is being organized against around the world. To the trafficked individual, however, it may not seem entirely positive to be released from a brothel only to face deportation. This is usually the fate of these illegal residents, since the visas provided by the trafficker are often faked.

Prostitutes are not deported only because their papers are not in order. Globally, the HIV/AIDS epidemic has been hard on prostitutes. Many sex workers, especially in the West, have been scapegoated as AIDS carriers even though a prostitute is more likely to practice safe sex than a non-sex worker. In poorer cultures, though, information and prophylactics are not so readily available, and it is the most disadvantaged sex workers who have thus borne the brunt of the epidemic—and of blame for it. However, even in enclaves of disadvantaged prostitutes, education and organizing has helped empower sex workers and save lives. Grant money has become available through governments and NGOs, and it has been used in literacy campaigns, economic development projects that aim to make prostitutes self-sufficient in other trades, safe sex education projects, and more. Such organizing has occurred in Thailand, India, Brazil, Mexico, and many other Third World countries, as well as in Australia, the US and Canada, and several European countries.

The strategies and needs of sex workers in developed countries may be very different from those in developing nations. Several global organizations work with prostitutes and other sex workers, but the best approach seems to involve regional focus and local autonomy.

Sex Workers as Abuse Victims/Survivors

Among the most prominent recent stereotypes about sex workers is that a very high percentage have been sexually abused. The underlying suggestion seems to be that non-abused adults would not choose to provide erotic entertainment or services unless something had predisposed them to do so, and those who advance the abuse theory clearly cannot imagine someone doing sex work of his or her own accord. In fact, some sex workers *do* recognize such a connection in their own personal histories, but many more do not. Studies that suggest an extremely high percentage of sex workers were abused mostly fall prey to the research problems described above. Until good research is available, this will likely remain an open question, but sex worker advocates remind us to think of all the people with histories of abuse who do *not* become sex workers—clearly a cause-and-effect relationship is not present, at least in most cases.

Feminism and Sex Work

Modern feminism has had an extremely mixed and often difficult relationship with sex work. The contemporary sex workers' rights movement (about which more below) derived great inspiration from the women's movement of the 60s and 70s. Many sex workers are staunch feminists, and many more *would* identify as feminists if mainstream feminism were not so openly hostile to the sex industry. Virtually any sex worker could give a critique of the sex trade; nobody thinks it is perfect and without worker abuses; but sex workers and sex worker advocates often get rather defensive about mainstream feminism's seemingly total discomfort with (and their harsh judgments about) the facts of sex workers' lives.

Feminists have been among the most vociferous anti-pornography and prostitution crusaders since the 1970s. By the end of that decade "the sex wars" were in full swing. Feminists developed strong (if not rigid) positions against porn, prostitution, S/M, and other sexual activities with which most mainstream feminists were uncomfortable. These positions seemed to be grounded in ideas about sexuality, female autonomy, and gender that seemed anything but feminist to women who disagreed with their moralistic tone, and a substantial split within feminism resulted. The tendency that made theorist Gayle Rubin call feminism as "system of sexual judgment" left some women feeling judged, and many felt this judgment was unfair and unduly conservative. "Sex-positive feminism" emerged to allow women (and others) to continue to identify with feminism's larger goals of equal treatment and an end to misogyny, while allowing more room for feminists to lead the kind of sexual lives they preferred. Sex-positive feminists argue that if feminism means that a woman owns her own body, the things she can choose to do with it should not be unduly restricted.

In fact, mainstream feminism is not monolithic, and feminists' attitudes about the sex industry are gradually being affected by the increasing numbers of sex workers (especially feminist ones) who are speaking up and telling their own stories. Sex workers have made many trips to national NOW (National Organization for Women) conferences to lobby and communicate with that organization, and the result is that the discourse among feminists now leaves more space (and support) for sex workers and their advocates. It remains an uneasy relationship, because both feminism and sex work are diverse, opinions multifaceted and strongly held. But progress is slowly being made.

SEX WORKER RIGHTS ORGANIZING

This progress would probably not be happening without the unified voices of the sex work advocacy movement. This movement is global, though in many countries talking to feminists takes a far back seat to priorities like human rights abuse issues, standard of living issues, and health education and support. Still, international whores' congresses are held a couple of times a decade, and organizers are united in a loose network of affiliation that spans the world.

COYOTE (Call Off Your Old Tired Ethics) was started in the early 70s in San Francisco by Margo St. James. It created a standard for US (and other western) organizations: a strong emphasis on advocacy and support for sex workers, plus a high public profile designed to raise consciousness and dispel stereotypes. Organizations inspired by COYOTE include COYOTE Los Angeles, Prostitutes of New York (PONY), Hooking Is Real Employment (HIRE, in Atlanta), and Willing Women Workers (WWW, in Minneapolis/St. Paul). In the San Francisco area other spin-offs included CalPEP (the California Prostitutes' Education Project), which focuses on AIDS and safe sex education and was founded by Gloria Lockett; BASWAN, the Bay Area Sex Worker's Action Network, helmed by Carol Leigh (a.k.a. performer Scarlot Harlot, who coined the term "sex work"); the Exotic Dancer's Alliance, which formed to organize strippers to fight workplace abuses in strip clubs; and the Cyprian Guild, which organizes for support, advocacy, and to promote professionalism among prostitutes.

Another wing of the prostitutes' rights movement originated in England with the socialist-feminist Wages for Housework movement. A radical anti-poverty organizing effort, it soon added prostitutes' rights to its list of issues. It supported sex workers' strikes in France and Britain in the 1970s and 1980s, and inspired organizers in the US as well. It is known as the English Collective of Prostitutes in Britain and US-Pros, or the US Prostitutes' Collective, in the US.

A big issue in the US sex workers' rights movement is the legalization of prostitution. Really the question is whether to support some form of legalization, as Nevada has, vs. decriminalization. At issue is whether prostitutes should be licensed by the state or whether laws against consensual prostitution and related offenses should simply be removed from the books. At this writing one state in Australia has completely decriminalized prostitution, and while decriminalization is generally preferred by sex worker activists, it is recognized that in the often-moralistic US, that goal might be difficult to achieve. Certainly legalization is supported by many who feel the state needs to monitor prostitution for health reasons; those who disagree feel prostitutes' attitude of "My body's my business" will be sufficient to ensure safe sex. An issue in some other parts of the globe (notably Europe) is probably far in the future for the US prostitutes' movement, namely state pensions, health care, and other worker benefits.

However, a step in that direction may be occurring in the US with a recent emphasis on occupational health and safety issues among sex workers. This emphasis goes fa beyond safe sex and AIDS education and includes all kinds of health issues relevant to sex workers: how to find a physician one can trust, stress management, substance abuse issues, OSHA violations in workplaces, and much more. The first health clinic for sex workers, the St. James Infirmary, has just opened in San Francisco as of this writing. This health focus is the brainchild of Priscilla Alexander, a sex worker advocate who spent several years working with the World Health Organization.

In the strip club industry a wave of organizing has occurred to protest policies that allow the clubs to hire dancers as independent contractors. They are paid no wages or benefits, and often have to pay the house for the privilege of being booked. Arguing that this practice is illegal, the EDA, individual dancers, and other organizations have brought lawsuits and instituted organizing efforts in various clubs. Union organizing has even been attempted in some clubs, successfully at San Francisco's Lusty Lady Theatre. The union-busting firm hired by the club's management was completely unprepared to deal with articulate, college-educated, union-savvy workers, rather than the unclothed bimbos they had been expecting. The Lusty Lady victory was not only a union victory, but also a blow against perhaps the commonest sex worker stereotype, that of the bimbo: the dumb female without other life choices.

In addition to the occasional Whores' Congresses, mentioned above (which are now commonly held in conjunction with International AIDS Conferences), and International Conference on Prostitution was held in 1997 in conjunction with University of California at Northridge (followed by a similar conference on pornography in 1998) and attended by sex workers, sex work advocates, and academics. This gathering could not have come together without Whorenet, an Internet news group that connects activist sex workers all over the world.

Finally, an interesting new organization has emerged that puts a new spin on sex work organizing. Helmed by Norma Jean Almodovar (head of COYOTE L.A. and author of *Cop to Call Girl*), the International Sex Work Foundation for Art, Culture, and Education (IWSFACE, pronounced ice-face) is working to buy the historic Dumas brothel in Butte, Montana to use as a museum, cultural center, and research institute.

Conclusion

As noted above, the topic of sex work is enormous, and this discussion has really only provided an introduction to a series of issues that deserve much more attention. A list of selected readings is included below for readers who would like more information and a more nuanced discussion of issues briefly addressed here.

The sex work movement is not monolithic by any means, and many sex workers claim no affiliation with it. A prostitute in Calcutta and an adult video distribution clerk in Los Angeles don't have much in common—except that they are both, in separate ways and cultural contexts, laboring to provide for someone else's erotic entertainment, and in certain ways both are at risk because of it. Since the desire for such entertainment seems to persist over time and across many cultures, the trade that has developed to cater to it (or control it) brings these and other disparate people somehow together.

Because sex and the economy are both basic facts of human existence, though developed very differently in different cultures and epochs, sex work and the many issues that devolve from it are to some degree universal. Because sex is rarely a neutral fact of cultural life, but is embedded in a nexus of kinship and relationship structures, taboo, religious prohibition, and state control, examining the particulars of any culture's sex industry opens multiple windows of enquiry into that culture's core issues. It is hoped that this abbreviated tour of sex work-related issues opens such windows of enquiry for the reader.

Recommended Readings

There are many books on prostitution, in particular, not listed here because they are out of print and/or are based in not particularly useful, often stereotypical, views of the sex industry. Of these, the ones dealing with history are probably most worthwhile for contemporary scholars and those interested in sex work-related issues.

The list below should not be viewed as a comprehensive bibliography on the subject, but a place for the interested reader to start developing a deeper grasp of the issues.

Alexander, Priscilla and Frederique Delacoste, ed. *Sex Work: Writings By Women in the Sex Industry.* San Francisco: Cleis Press, (1987) 1998.

Bell, Laurie, ed. *Good Girls/Bad Girls: Feminists and Sex Trade Workers Face to Face.* Seattle: Seal Press, 1987.

Bell, Shannon. *Reading, Writing, and Re-Writing the Prostitute Body.* Bloomington: Indiana University Press, 1994.

Chapkis, Wendy. *Live Sex Acts: Women Performing Erotic Labor.* New York: Routledge, 1997.

Doezema, Jo and Kamala Kempadoo, eds. *Global Sex Work.* New York: Routledge, 1998.

French, Dolores and Linda Lee. *Working: My Life as a Prostitute.* New York: E.P. Dutton, 1988.

Keefe, Tim. *Some of My Best Friends Are Naked.* San Francisco: Barbary Coast Press, 1993.

Nagle, Jill, ed. *Whores and Other Feminists.* New York: Routledge, 1997. Pheterson, Gail. A Vindication of the Rights of Whores. Seattle: Seal Press, 1989.

_____ *The Prostitution Prism.* Amsterdam: Amsterdam University Press, 1996.

Queen, Carol. *Real Live Nude Girl: Chronicles of Sex-Positive Culture.* Can Francisco: Cleis Press, 1997.

Roberts, Nickie. *Whores In History: Prostitution in Western Society.* London: Grafton (HarperCollins), 1992.

Stubbs, Kenneth Ray, ed. *Women of the Light: The New Sexual Healers.* Larkspur, CA: Secret Garden, 1997.

Sycamore, Matt Bernstein, ed. *Tricks and Treats: Sex Workers Write About Their Clients.* Binghamton, NY: The Haworth Press, 1999.

Vance, Carole, ed. *Pleasure and Danger: Exploring Female Sexuality.* Boston: Routledge and Kegan Paul, 1984.

Sex Sells, Especially to Web Surfers: Internet Porn a Booming, Billion-Dollar Industry

28

CHAPTER

Jeordan Legon

Gone are the furtive visits to seedy theaters and the fear of being outed as some perverted purchaser of porn. Now, all you need to indulge anonymously in the "XXX" world is your trusty personal computer and a good connection to the Internet.

It's difficult to derive reliable figures from an industry that, despite flirtations with the mainstream, is made up of many small shops that prefer to keep a low profile. But the figures that exist paint a picture of a booming online field, fueled by the relatively low costs of setting up shop, fickle consumers in constant search of new thrills and the promise of quick profits.

The flood of sites competing for attention is fueling a torrent of X-rated spam, resulting in minors being exposed to adult content and annoying marketing ploys that spurred the recent approval in Congress of the first national effort to stem the flood of unwanted e-mail.

Attorney General John Ashcroft's office has launched dozens of investigations of adult content businesses and filed an obscenity case against Extreme Associates, a California porn firm that sold violent sex videos by mail and over the Internet.

"It's an enormous business . . . There's a lot of money to be made," said Sean Kaldor, an analyst with Nielsen/NetRatings, which estimated that 34 million visited porn sites in August—about one in four Internet users in the United States.

The average user is "looking at 121 pages, going back six times and spending an hour and seven minutes every month looking at adult-related material," Kaldor said.

All that browsing has caused the number of pornography Web pages to soar during the past six years, with over 1.3 million sites serving up about 260 million pages of erotic content, according to a study released in September by the Seattle, Washington-based Web-filtering company N2H2.

N2H2's database of porn sites, a company spokesman said, includes man low-budget, fly-by-night and sometimes unscrupulous operators hoping to rake in their share of a market that the National Research Council estimates to be in the $1 billion range annually.

The council, which advises Congress on technology, issued a report in 2002 that predicts the online porn industry will grow to a $5-$7 billion business within five years.

People should be concerned, said N2H2's David Burt, "because of the ease with which children can stumble on porn sites accidentally and the ease with which people can stumble upon this in the workplace, creating liability issues."

Kathee Brewer, technology editor of porn industry news site AVN Online, said the increase in adult Internet pages has spurred opposition from conservative groups and heightened government scrutiny. She said critics of porn sites are attempting to blur the lines between law-abiding adult content and banned obscene material.

"People can be easily led, and the mere twist of a phrase—like substituting 'obscenity' for 'pornography'—can have a profound effect on basically good folk who want to do the right thing but don't know exactly how to go about it," Brewer wrote recently in an essay about conservative groups that support porn-filtering software.

Instead of government intervention, Brewer urged the industry to police itself by keeping minors away from explicit content and cutting down on spam e-mail. At the same time, she said, it should be acknowledged that porn has been one of the few profitable Internet businesses from the start, employing thousands of people and generating millions in revenues for site owners, Web hosting companies and computer-hardware firms.

Experts say the industry has been on the forefront of many innovations that have been adopted by mainstream sites, such as new payment systems, ad revenue models, chat and broadband.

"One of the most interesting things is to watch how these sites pioneer new technologies," said Kaldor, the Nielsen/NetRatings analyst.

Online Porn Grows Up

Kaldor said the industry is showing signs of maturity.

Password services have sprung up, often charging an annual fee to deliver access to hundreds of small sites, which share the subscription revenues.

Large firms also have consolidated power by providing free content to smaller "affiliate" sites. The affiliates post the free content and then try to channel visitors to the large sites, which give the smaller sites a percentage of the fees paid by those who sign up.

Another way some adult Webmasters make money is by forwarding traffic to another porn site in return for a small per-consumer fee. In many cases, the consumer is sent to the other sites involuntarily, which is known in the industry as "mousetrapping." Surfers who try to close out a window after visiting an adult site are sent to another Web page automatically. This can repeat dozens of times, causing users to panic and restart their computers in order to escape, the National Research Council found.

A fourth trend is for adult sites to cater to niche audiences.

"There's a Web site for just about every kink," said Scott Fayner, who writes for Luke-Ford. com, a site that posts porn industry news and gossip.

Experts say tech advances and the growing use of broadband will fuel even more growth in the industry.

Porn and the Future

All of which is prompting concerns about what impact the onslaught of porn might have on future generations raised on a steady stream of adult images. Some believe porn is creating unrealistic expectations among couples.

A recent article in New York magazine contained interviews with men who said they were hooked on Internet porn.

"Dude, all of my friends are so obsessed with Internet porn that they can't sleep with their girlfriends unless they act like porn stars," a 26-year-old businessman told the article's author.

"Just imagine the adolescents who, you know, their sexual coming of age has totally coincided with the Internet and high-speed connections," reporter David Amsden said. "As opposed to the 13-year-old-boy [before the Internet existed] who is lucky to find one Playboy magazine."

Like it or hate it, Internet porn is here to stay, Amsden said. And the key, said sex therapist Laura Berman, is to keep it in check.

"There's always a role for pornography and for fantasies, if it's used to the benefit of the couple," Berman said.